WHY SO TIRED?

A 101-Day Guide to
Clearer Thinking,
Lasting Energy,
and Better Sleep

Athan Smyrlis, MD

Copyright © 2025 Athan Smyrlis, MD
All rights reserved.

Cover Design by The Publishing Pad
www.thepublishingpad.com

No part of this book may be reproduced, stored in a retrieval system, or transmitted in any form or by any means — electronic, mechanical, photocopying, recording, or otherwise — without the prior written permission of the author, except for:
• brief quotations used in reviews, articles, or educational materials with appropriate citation, and
• short excerpts shared privately with friends or family for personal, non-commercial use (for example, a line, a short paragraph, or a photo of a single page).

This book is provided in print and eBook formats with the understanding that the author is not engaged in rendering individual medical, psychological, nutritional, or other professional services to any specific person through these pages. The information contained here is offered for general educational and wellness purposes only and is not a substitute for personalized medical care, diagnosis, or treatment. Readers should consult their own licensed healthcare professionals regarding any questions or concerns about their health, medications, or treatment plans. The author and publisher (True Health Compass LLC) expressly disclaim responsibility for any adverse effects, loss, or damage resulting, directly or indirectly, from the use or application of any information contained in this book.

All characters and patient stories are based on composites, with identifying details changed to protect privacy.

True Health Compass™ (and associated logos) are trademarks or service marks of the author and may not be used without written permission.

Published by True Health Compass LLC.
ISBN: 979-8-9942521-0-9 (paperback)
ISBN: 979-8-9942521-1-6 (hardcover)

Dedication

To my mother,
who inspired this work.

And to you, the reader —
who has long felt tired or unlike yourself, trying to make sense of it…
who left doctor visits with more questions than answers…

May this book help you feel clear, steady, and well again.

Inspiration

"The best doctor gives the least medicine."
— attributed to Benjamin Franklin

"It is health that is real wealth and not pieces of gold and silver."
— attributed to Mahatma Gandhi

"The doctor of the future will give no medicine, but will interest his patients in the care of the human frame, in diet, and in the cause and prevention of disease."
— attributed to Thomas Edison

Table Of Contents

Legal Disclaimer & Safety Notice 9
A Note to the Reader..11
How to Use This Book 14
Three simple ways to move through the book 16

PART I: THE MINI COMPASS 17
    Chapter 1 — My Story: The Gap Between Better and Well.....................19
    Chapter 2 — Early Drift Signs...22
    Chapter 3 — In Need of a Compass, Not a Map 23
    Chapter 4 — First, Let's Define Health...24
    Chapter 5 — The Foundations of True Health..26
    Chapter 6 — The 7 Roots of Health 27
    Chapter 7 — My Conviction 30
    Chapter 8 — Why You're So Tired
        The Fog Loop That Makes Life Harder Than It Should Be..................32
    Chapter 9 — It's Not You — It's Your Clock
        Why "Normal" Labs Miss the Real Problem 34
    Chapter 10 — How Your Life Fell Out of Rhythm
        The Hidden Forces That Pulled You Off Course 37
    Chapter 11 — Your Roots
        The Real Reasons Energy, Mood, and Sleep Fall Apart 40

TOOLS..45
    Tool 1 — Head-to-Toe Health Self-Check 45
    Tool 2 — The Score Game — Simple Rules...49
    Tool 3 — Begin Tonight (two minutes) 51

PART II: THE GUIDED JOURNEY 53
    A 101-Day Guided Journey to Clearer Thinking, Lasting Energy, and
        Restful Sleep 55
    101-Day Guided Journey..57

PART III: THE COMPASS EXPLAINED 385
    Chapter 12 — Your Energy Grid
        How Your Body Makes Power (and How Life Quietly Steals It).........386

Chapter 13 — The Domino Game
　How to Start Without Overhauling Your Life 389
Chapter 14 — Sleep
　The First Domino 392
Chapter 15 — Movement
　Your Daily Dose 397
Chapter 16 — Food
　Instructions for Your Brain, Energy, and Sleep 403
Chapter 17 — Gut Health
　Soil Before Seeds 413
Chapter 18 — From Redline to Rhythm
　Stress, Screens, and How to Stop Running on Empty 420
Chapter 19 — Hidden Saboteurs
　The Things You Can't See But Your Body Can 425

PART IV: LIVING WITH THE COMPASS 435
　BONUS: "THE COMPASS" 439

NOTES & SOURCES 441

MEET THE AUTHOR 461

Legal Disclaimer & Safety Notice

Educational Purpose Only. The information in this book (including text, charts, protocols, and examples) is for educational purposes and general wellness guidance. It is not medical advice, not a diagnosis, and not a treatment plan. Do not disregard professional medical advice or delay seeking it because of something you read here.

No Doctor–Patient Relationship. Reading this book, using any worksheets, or following any suggestions does not create a doctor–patient relationship with the author or publisher.

Consult Your Clinician. Always consult your licensed healthcare professional before starting, stopping, or changing:

Medications (e.g., anticoagulants, diabetes drugs, blood-pressure medicines, psychiatric medications, thyroid or hormone therapy).

Supplements, fasting regimens, or detox protocols.

Exercise programs or significant diet changes — especially if you have chronic illness, are pregnant or breastfeeding, are immunocompromised, or have a history of eating disorders or heart, lung, kidney, or liver disease.

Do Not Ignore Urgent Care. If you have symptoms that could signal an emergency — such as chest pain, severe shortness of breath, one-sided weakness, confusion, high fever, or thoughts of self-harm — call emergency services (911 in the U.S.) or seek immediate medical care.

Supplement & Product Disclosures. Any discussion of nutraceuticals, devices, labs, or brands is informational, not an endorsement. Dietary supplements are not evaluated by the FDA for safety or efficacy and are not intended to diagnose, treat, cure, or prevent any disease. Quality varies; consider third-party testing and discuss risks with your clinician.

Individual Results Vary. Outcomes depend on many factors, including genetics, environment, medical conditions, adherence, and timing. There are no guarantees of specific results.

Assumption of Risk & Limitation of Liability. You agree to take full responsibility for your choices and actions. The author and publisher disclaim liability for any harm, injury, loss, or adverse outcome resulting from the use or misuse of the information herein, to the fullest extent permitted by law.

Evolving Knowledge. Science evolves. Recommendations may become outdated as new evidence emerges. The content reflects the author's understanding at the time of writing and may be updated in future editions.

Institutional Independence. The views expressed are solely those of the author and do not represent the views of any employer, hospital, or institution.

This book is a guide, not a substitute for your own clinician.

A Note to the Reader

If you're holding this book, something inside you is tired.

Not the kind of tired a nap can fix.

The kind that makes you wonder if you're slowly becoming someone you don't recognize.

The kind where your body feels heavier than it should.

Where your mind, at times, can't hold a thought steady.

Where small tasks cost more than they used to.

Where your whole system feels unpredictable — quietly alarming, even if you don't show it.

Maybe your body is doing things you can't explain — and you don't quite have words for it.

Your concentration slips.

Names vanish right when you need them.

Ordinary things take more effort — and more time — than they should.

Some days it's headaches, dizziness, or a sudden wave of weakness.

Some days you're wired-but-tired: your mind won't quiet, and sleep feels strangely far away.

And sometimes your heart flutters or races and you wonder, What is happening to me?

Most people won't recognize every line here.

If you recognize even a few, you're in the right place.

I want you to know something clearly:

You are not alone.

I wrote this for my patients — and for anyone who has been trying to function while their body no longer feels like home.

I've sat with thousands of bright, responsible, hardworking people who look "fine" on paper and feel anything but in real life.

And I've had seasons when my own body didn't match my responsibilities.

I've felt the 3 a.m. dread.

The brain fog that makes you doubt your own mind.

The tight chest. The racing thoughts. The sense that you're running out of runway.

And then comes the part almost no one names:

The quiet panic.

How long can I keep going like this?

What if this is something serious?

What if it gets worse — and I can't be who my family needs?
Stay with me.
There is a pattern to this.
And patterns can be understood.
You don't say these fears out loud because they sound vague or "not concrete enough."
You've probably already heard some version of, "You're just stressed," or "Your labs look fine."
Meanwhile, you're trying to live a normal life while your symptoms quietly make everything harder than it needs to be.
So you soldier on.
You patch the cracks with caffeine, late-night scrolling, supplements, podcasts — and good intentions.
The wellness world tells you the answer is one more product.
A powder. A pill. A protocol. A hack.
But deep down, you know this isn't the whole story.
The deeper truth is simpler than you think:
Most of us have been trained — consciously or not — to override our body's signals.
Do that long enough, and the body doesn't betray you.
It pulls the alarm.
That alarm is what you're feeling.
There's an unfairness here.
Most people were never given an owner's manual for their body.
This book is my attempt to hand it to you.
And here is the part I want you to hold onto:
You are not crazy.
You are not weak.
You are not broken.
More often, you are misaligned — your timing is off, and your system is overloaded.
The good news is simple:
Alignment can be restored.
Not through extreme measures.
Not through magic pills.
Not through punishing yourself.
But by working with the basic laws of human physiology — in plain language — and by learning to send your body the signals it was built to recognize.
Sleep depth matters.
Light matters.

Food timing matters.
Nervous-system load matters.
Small, consistent inputs change the whole trajectory.
This book is not a lecture.
It's a map and a compass.
It won't replace good medical care.

It will help you understand your body more clearly so you can use medical care wisely — and reduce how often you need it.

It's structured as a 101-day journey — one small step a day — to bring your rhythm back online.

Not overnight.
Not perfectly.
But genuinely.
When I finally found my way out of the fog, I made myself a promise:
If I ever understood this clearly enough to explain it,
I would turn around and light the path for the next person.
That person is you.
As you read, I want you to feel two things:
Relief — that there is a reason you feel the way you feel.

And direction — that doesn't require perfection, only small honest steps repeated with compassion.

I can't promise a life without stress, aging, or hardship.
Here's what I can offer:
A clear explanation.
A workable plan.

And a path that many people find leads to steadier energy, clearer thinking, deeper sleep, and a calmer nervous system.

You are not at the end of your story.
You're at the end of a chapter that has lasted too long.
This book is the start of the next one.
Walk with me.
Let's reset your rhythm — one small step at a time.

— A. Smyrlis, MD

How to Use This Book

Most health books quietly assume you can sit, focus, and power through long chapters.

This one assumes the opposite.

Chances are you picked up this book because you're tired, foggy, overwhelmed — or all three. Your days already demand more than you feel you have. The last thing you need is another 500 pages of "shoulds" that you can't realistically use.

A lot of excellent books fail for one simple reason: the science may be right, but the structure assumes more time, energy, and concentration than the reader actually has.

I'm fully aware of those limits. I see them in clinic every week.

So I built this book differently on purpose.

The book has four parts.

Part I — The Mini Compass:

A quick orientation so you don't feel lost.

In a few short chapters, you'll understand:

- **why you feel this way (the Fog Loop),**
- **why "normal" labs can miss the real problem,**
- **how life falls out of rhythm (and how to climb back),**
- **your likely roots (the patterns driving your symptoms),**
- and what matters most for sleep, movement, food, gut health, stress, and your environment.

You do not have to memorize this to start getting better.

If you want to start immediately, jump to Part II. If you want the "why" first, read Part I straight through.

Part II — The Guided Journey:

This is a 101-day journey made of small, daily steps. You'll see why it's 101 days right at the start of Part II. Each day gives you:

- a short reflection,
- one simple action,

- **and (when helpful) a pointer to a deeper chapter in Part III if you want more "why."**

These entries are designed for real life:

- one idea at a time,
- one doable step,
- no need to "catch up" if you miss a day.

If all you can do right now is open to today's entry, read one page, and do one small thing — you're using the book exactly as intended.

Part III — The Compass Explained:

These are the full-length chapters that unpack the deeper "why," including:

- what's happening in your energy grid and mitochondria,
- how sleep, movement, food, gut health, stress, and environment work at a deeper level,
- and what the research actually says.

Think of this section as your "why" library. Dip in when your energy and curiosity allow.

Many people find that understanding the "why" first makes the daily steps feel easier and more motivating — so if your energy allows, consider reading a chapter here before you begin the guided journey, or anytime you feel stuck.

Each part of this book can stand on its own, but each new part adds another layer of depth to the same core ideas.

Part IV — Closing Reflections:

This is where you zoom out, take stock, and decide how you want to carry the work forward.

It's not heavy. It's meant to feel like a calm landing.

Three simple ways to move through the book

There's no "right way." There's only what feels doable for you right now.
Choose one path, then ignore the others for now.

Path A — You're in deep fog

If you're bone-tired and long explanations feel impossible, go straight to Part II (The Guided Journey). Start at Day 1. Read one entry per day — just today's page. Then stop.

Let the journey carry you.

As you feel clearer, circle back and read Part I (only about 12 pages — easy to read), then visit Part III slowly when you want the deeper "why." When your brain is underwater, start with oxygen — not textbooks.

Path B — You're tired, but you can focus in bursts

If you can read a small chapter at a time, start with Part I for quick clarity. Then move into Part II for daily practice. Use Part III when a topic grabs you—no need to read it in order.

Path C — You're here for optimization and performance

If you're not in crisis but you want to sharpen your edge, start with Part I for a quick, big-picture overview. Then go straight to Part III for a deep dive into the core concepts that drive your energy, focus, and sleep. Use Part II as your daily practice (5–10 minutes a day). Revisit Part I anytime you want the map again.

One rule that matters most

Never "catch up." Just come back. One small step today beats ten perfect steps you never start.

PART I
THE MINI COMPASS

CHAPTER 1
My Story: The Gap Between Better and Well

I was in a hurry to be born. My mother used to joke that I arrived a few weeks early — on Doctors' Day. I don't read it as fate. If anything, it was an early hint of a habit that can feel productive — until it starts stealing from your body: urgency.

For the past twenty-five years, medicine has been my life's calling. I poured myself into it with everything I had — eighty-hour weeks, nights that dissolved into mornings, weekends swallowed by the fluorescent glow of the hospital. And yet it never felt like a sacrifice. Not once. It felt like purpose. I wanted to be the best I could possibly be for my patients, and I believed I knew what that would take.

But I need to admit something honestly — something many physicians feel but rarely say out loud.

In my effort to be the best doctor I could be, I became overzealous. I pushed too hard, too long. I lost my balance. And my own health paid the price.

I carried the pager like a badge of honor, but I ignored the quiet truths my body was whispering. I could teach physiology all day, but I wasn't always living it. And I learned something no textbook ever taught me: it's hard to guide someone back to health if you've abandoned your own.

That realization opened my eyes.

Because I began to see a hard truth: even with evidence-based, state-of-the-art care, many people weren't becoming truly healthy. Their labs improved, their numbers stabilized — but their lives didn't. They functioned, but they didn't flourish. They survived, but they weren't well.

That gap — the space between better and well — is why I wrote this book.

As you'll see clearly in Chapter 8, these symptoms aren't random — they follow a pattern.

What struck me most was how predictable the complaints became over time. Different ages, different jobs, different stories — yet the same quiet refrain: "My labs are normal, but I don't feel like myself." People came into my office with:

- brain fog
- low morning energy
- restless, non-restorative sleep
- afternoon crashes
- cravings and reactive eating
- stress they couldn't shake, and a sense that something inside was slipping

These symptoms were often brushed aside as "aging," "anxiety," "your labs look fine," or "just life." But they aren't small. They are early alarm bells — subtle, but specific — telling us the body's rhythm is off, the foundation is weakening, and the system is running under strain. Ignore them long enough, and health doesn't usually collapse in one dramatic moment. It unravels quietly.

That realization forced me into questions my training had not fully prepared me to ask. Do medications truly restore health — or do they mostly stabilize disease? What is the real root cause beneath the diagnosis? And what actually maximizes health, not just treats illness?

So I began a second education — not through another residency or fellowship, but through deep reflection after each patient visit, with curiosity and humility. I learned from pioneers like Sidney Baker, Jeffrey Bland, Matthew Walker, and others who dared to look "under the hood" of modern chronic disease. Their ideas rang true. Slowly, a picture emerged: many diseases share the same roots. Heart disease, diabetes, dementia, cancer — different branches, often the same tree.

Sleep deprivation, nutritional mismatch, chronic stress, environmental overload, disrupted circadian rhythms — these are the forces bending the branch long before it breaks.

Picture health as a chain. Every person has a weakest link. For one, it's the brain. For another, the heart. For another, the immune system. When enough stress accumulates, the chain breaks where it's already thin. But before it breaks, the body usually sends warning lights: foggier thinking, lighter sleep, lower morning energy, irritability, congestion, afternoon crashes — more days that just feel "off." These aren't random annoyances. They are early chapters in a disease story you don't want to finish.

One reason these symptoms are so widespread is what I call the Time-Lag Trap. Most modern habits don't make you sick right away — unlike a bad oyster that drops you in hours. They act like a drip, not a flood. Small daily insults accumulate quietly: sugary breakfasts, ultra-processed "health" snacks, late screens, poor light exposure, repetitive stress, and disrupted sleep. The cause happens here. The effect shows up months or years later. We miss the connection — but the body never does.

And we all carry blind spots — habits we don't question because they feel "normal" in our families or culture:

- bread or cereal as the default start
- sugary drinks "just to keep going"
- ultra-processed foods — and frequent fried or packaged foods — as everyday fuel

- late nights followed by early mornings
- bright screens flooding the brain at 11 p.m.

We wonder why our labs inch up. Why our minds feel slower. Why inflammation markers creep. Why sleep stops restoring us. But the roots often live in daily life — in plain sight.

I've also come to believe something essential: we do not inherit a fixed fate from our genes. We inherit habits. And habits change gene expression. In my own family, "diabetes" seemed hereditary — until I realized the real inheritance was bread at breakfast, bread at lunch, bread at dinner, and dessert as the evening ritual. Genes respond to the environment you place them in. And when you change that environment, the body often remembers how to heal.

Finally, I've learned that God — or nature, if you prefer — built us on rhythm. Every healthy system oscillates: wake and sleep, feast and fast, effort and rest, cortisol (your wake-up signal) and melatonin (your sleep signal), light and dark. When we honor these cycles, the body tends to stabilize. When we violate them — slowly, quietly, daily — symptoms start to speak.

At first, this may sound abstract. Keep reading; it will become concrete. Once you see the pattern, you cannot unsee it. And once you begin living in rhythm, a lot of things that felt "stuck" start to soften — energy returns, sleep deepens, mood steadies, cravings quiet, and health stops feeling like a fight. Life begins to feel light again.

This book is my invitation — and my promise — that the path back is real. And you're closer to it than you think.

CHAPTER 2
Early Drift Signs

These drift signs show up quietly, long before a diagnosis:

Fatigue: She wakes up tired no matter how long she stayed in bed. By 10 a.m., her third coffee stares back at her like a dare. She crawls into bed drained, but her mind flips on like a bright light. At 2 a.m., thoughts race, to-do lists multiply, and she feels wired and tired — and she knows the alarm will still ring on time.

Brain Fog: He opens his laptop and watches focus slip through his fingers. Even a short email feels heavy.

Weight Gain: Same meals, same routine, yet the waistband pinches. A half-pound at a time, the scale creeps upward.

Forgetfulness: Keys vanish, names hover just out of reach, sentences trail off mid-thought.

Sugar Cravings: At 3 p.m., the vending machine starts calling. One bite becomes a slide — cookies, chips, promises to "start Monday."

They are not "sick enough" for a diagnosis — just heavy enough to make every day harder. These are the water stains on the ceiling that hint at a deeper leak. Not a flood, so they're ignored — until the studs are rotten and the foundation weakens.

You bring them to your doctor. The paper on the exam table crackles as he says, "Your labs are fine. Eat well and exercise. Come back in six months." You nod, gather your things, and carry the same tiredness back to the parking lot.

Beneath the frustration is a quiet fear: maybe this is how life will always be.

I wrote this book for you. I've lived through these same "manageable" issues myself — until I hit my own breaking point. I've watched my patients wait until a heart attack, a biopsy, or a diagnosis forced their hand. But you don't have to wait for crisis.

CHAPTER 3
In Need of a Compass, Not a Map

Most health advice is like a map: step-by-step directions, assuming everyone starts in the same place and follows the same road. Maps fail when the terrain shifts — new jobs, new stresses, new seasons of life. What you need is a compass — something that orients you no matter where you are, no matter how the landscape changes.

That's what this book offers. Here you'll find:

A clear vision of what true health feels like, so you'll recognize it when you arrive.

A practical, adaptable framework that fits your unique life, so you can always find your way back when you drift.

My goal is not to hand you a rigid program. My goal is to make sure that wherever you are, whatever changes, the arrow on your compass always points toward health.

We'll begin with first principles: circadian rhythm (your body's internal clock), the timing and type of food, sleep habits, movement and stillness, feasts and fasts, clean air and water, and the mindset that makes change last. You won't need perfect discipline — just the right levers, pulled in the right order.

Some of these ideas may feel new. That's by design. If what you've tried hasn't worked, doing more of the same won't help.

But you can test this. These steps are practical, humane, and trackable. Many people notice steadier energy, clearer thinking, deeper sleep, fewer cravings, and a body that feels easier to live in. Your relationships will benefit, too — because when you feel better, you bring more patience, presence, and generosity into every corner of your life.

If your shell has cracked — if you feel the turning point — start now. You'll find answers, hope, and real solutions here. If your shell is still intact, that's okay. Place this book nearby. Let the idea of a Compass sit with you. When the moment comes, you won't need willpower — you'll need orientation. And you'll have it.

CHAPTER 4
First, Let's Define Health

The alarm buzzes on a Tuesday. You open your eyes feeling rested and clear-headed. You smile with gratitude for a night of deep, uninterrupted sleep. You get out of bed without pain or stiffness. Your chest feels light. Your mind is calm.

You look forward to working on the things that really matter to you. You have the focus to stay with them and the energy to finish. When problems show up — and they always do — you feel confident you can tackle what comes your way.

That picture is a better compass for health than any lab number.

The Physical Dimension: A Body in Harmony

Physical health is a body free of chains: no heartburn after meals, no dull headache settling in the temples, no joints stiff and swollen before their time.

Instead, it is the fresh feeling of waking up renewed. It is stretching without pain and feeling the muscles respond with supple readiness.

It is the delight of climbing stairs without breathlessness. It is walking in nature and feeling the legs strong beneath you. It is carrying your child or grandchild without strain. It is hiking up a hill and feeling your heartbeat as a rhythm of vitality — not distress.

A healthy body is not fragile; it carries you like a trusted vessel across the journey of life.

It is abundant energy — not just for survival, but for pursuit. For goals. For dreams. For work that matters. It is the delight of a body that feels like a trustworthy companion.

The Mental Dimension: A Mind at Peace

Mental health is the quiet confidence that you can find your way through life.

It's focus that doesn't scatter. Patience that bends instead of snapping. Clarity that holds steady when life gets loud.

When your mind is well, you wake to calm rather than chaos. You look at the day with readiness, not dread. You're creative and resilient, able to solve problems without being paralyzed by them. You can laugh, remember, plan, and forgive. You know when to pause, how to listen, and when to wait.

Mental health gives you patience in difficulty, perspective in conflict, and creativity when challenges arise.

When the mind is well, it's like a clear, still lake. It reflects what is true without distortion. Thoughts and feelings still come and go, but they don't churn the surface or pull you under.

A healthy mind isn't one that never struggles; it's one that returns, again and again, to balance.

The Spiritual Dimension: Connection and Integrity

Beyond body and mind lies the domain of spirit — the dimension of meaning and belonging.

Spiritual health is not confined to religion, though it may blossom there. It is the felt connection to something larger than the self.

It is standing before a sunrise and feeling renewed, or watching a sunset and sensing that endings are not the end. It is the quiet power of integrity — choosing honesty when deceit is easier, choosing compassion when judgment tempts.

It is alignment with life's values, the sense that your steps follow a compass not drawn by whim, but by principle.

A spiritually healthy person is not flawless, but they are oriented. They walk with direction, anchored in something greater than themselves. To tend the spirit is to tend the body as well.

More Than a "Clean Bill of Health"

You can walk out of your doctor's office with a "clean bill of health" and still feel unwell. Numbers can look fine while your days do not. Health isn't a printout.

Think of it like a symphony — body, mind, and spirit playing together. When the body is strong, the mind clear, and the spirit steady, life has a richness no blood pressure reading or lab test can measure.

You know you are healthy not only because pain is absent, but because joy is present. You feel connected — to your work, your family, the natural world, and the divine mystery that whispers through all creation.

This vision of health matters because without it we aim too low. You cannot hit a target your eyes are not fixed upon. If health is defined only as "not sick," then we stop short of the fullness of life. But if health is seen as this radiant wholeness, then every choice — what we eat, how we rest, how we think, how we love — becomes a step toward true health.

Now that you can picture what true health feels like, we'll turn to the foundations that can build it from the roots up.

CHAPTER 5
The Foundations of True Health

Doctors, medicines, and emergency rooms are vital in a crisis — but they are not where everyday vitality begins.

True health grows only one way: from the roots up, from the inside out.

Outside-in fixes can make the surface look better. Pain pills lower pain scores. Procedures and patches can quiet numbers. But if the soil underneath stays the same, the problem returns.

It's like painting over a moldy wall without fixing the leak behind it. The room looks cleaner — but the damage continues.

This book takes the opposite path. Roots first. Inside out. Not to reject medicine when it's needed, but to give your body what it has been missing for years: sleep that repairs, food that truly nourishes, movement that restores, and rhythms that let every system work the way it was designed.

We will rebuild, not just patch.

We will grow new — from the roots up.

CHAPTER 6
The 7 Roots of Health

Here are the seven roots we'll return to throughout the book. Each one gets its own chapter later. For now, I want you to see the whole map.

1. Sleep — the night shift that restocks and cleans

Think of your body as a store.

Sleep is the night crew.

When the store closes, the crew restocks the shelves — energy, hormones, neurotransmitters — and takes out the trash — cell and brain waste, stress signals, and inflammation. If the store never really closes, shelves run bare and garbage piles up in the aisles.

Skimp on sleep and you feel it: low energy, more cravings, foggier mood, shorter fuse, "tired but wired" at night. Over time, blood pressure creeps, weight drifts, and even motivation shrinks.

Sleep isn't laziness. It's logistics. Let the night crew in most nights — long enough to do the job — and everything you try in this book works better.

2. Nutrition — food as building blocks and instructions

Think of your body as a house under construction.

Food is both the blueprint and the bricks.

Each bite sends orders: build muscle or store fat, calm or inflame, steady or spike.

Donut + coffee → fast sugar surge → order: store, spike, fog.

Eggs + greens + olive oil → steady fuel → order: repair, build, stabilize.

Most people think of food as calories. Your body reads it as information and materials. Ultra-processed foods are cheap, brittle bricks with confusing instructions. Whole foods are solid bricks with clear plans.

Every bite is a vote for the body you're building. This book will show you how to choose better bricks — without perfection or fancy rules.

3. Movement — repair in motion

Think of your body as a city.

Blood and lymph circulation are the traffic; movement turns the lights green.

When you move, deliveries arrive — oxygen, nutrients, immune cells — and garbage trucks roll out — waste, extra fluid, and stiffness. If traffic stops (couch, long sitting, bed rest), supplies stall, potholes deepen, and trash quietly collects on the streets.

Start walking and you feel it: warmth in your hands and feet, smoother joints, lighter mood, better sleep that night. You don't need brutal workouts; you need regular green lights.

This book will help you find small, realistic ways to keep the lights green — most days, in a body and schedule like yours.

4. Stress & Safety — your RPMs and brakes

Think of your body as an engine.

Stress is your RPMs.

RPMs are meant to rise for short bursts when needed, then settle back to idle. That surge-and-settle pattern is normal and healthy. The trouble comes when you stay red-lined — always on, always braced.

Running hot like that cooks parts, wears down bearings, and eventually blows gaskets. In a human body, that looks like anxiety, poor sleep, blood pressure issues, gut flare-ups, headaches, and a brain that never really feels "off duty."

Your brakes are simple: deep breathing and long exhales, a 10-minute walk, a few minutes in nature, a brief call with someone who cares. Use them consistently and you feel it: heart rate eases, jaw unclenches, shoulders drop, sleep comes easier.

Stress isn't the enemy. Getting stuck in the red without working brakes is. This book will help you rebuild both: the ability to accelerate when life calls for it, and the safety systems that let you truly slow down again.

5. Purpose (Ikigai) — your fixed point

Think of learning to balance.

Stand on one leg and stare at one spot — you're steady. Look around the room and you wobble.

Health is the same. When you have a clear "why" — "I want energy to play with my kids," "I want a clear mind to do my best work," "I want to be present for my partner" — daily choices get simpler. You're no longer just saying "be good" or "try harder"; you're aligning with something that matters.

Without a fixed point, every stress, craving, or late-night show pulls you off center. With it, you can say, "Does this choice move me toward or away from that picture?" That's a very different kind of motivation than fear or guilt.

This book will help you name a purpose you can feel in your chest, and then use it as the quiet anchor for all the small changes ahead.

6. Light & Timing (Circadian Rhythm) — the conductor of your day

Think of your body as an orchestra.

Light is the conductor.

Morning light gives the downbeat: "It's daytime — wake up, burn energy, think clearly."

Evening darkness lowers the tempo: "It's night — repair, clean, and store."

Hormones, digestion, temperature, and even immune function all listen for that baton.

Bright nights + no morning light → off-beat hormones, late melatonin, restless sleep, groggy mornings, and cravings.

Catch morning light + dim evenings → earlier natural sleepiness, deeper sleep, steadier daytime energy.

You can't control everything in your schedule, but you can send clearer signals. This book will show you how to follow the conductor — day by day — so your internal orchestra plays in rhythm again.

7. Environment — keep your fishbowl clean

Think of a fish and its bowl.

You are the fish; your air, water, food, and surfaces are the water.

If the environment is dusty, smoky, moldy, chemically scented, or full of junk, the fish struggles — even if the fish is "doing everything right." Clear the water — ventilate when cooking, filter bedroom air if you can, dry damp spaces, avoid heavy fragrances and sprays, choose safer pans and containers — and the fish comes back to life.

You feel it as a clearer head, calmer airways, fewer headaches, and steadier sleep. The body has less background "noise" to fight and more room to repair.

You don't need a perfect, toxin-free life that's almost impossible. You need fewer daily drips into the bowl and better cleanups. This book will help you clean your fishbowl one small step at a time.

CHAPTER 7
My Conviction

True health is a birthright in a simple sense: whether you call it God or nature, the same quiet instruction is written into your DNA:

Your body and mind are designed to drift toward balance when they are given a fair chance.

This birthright is not for the fortunate few — it is for everyone.

Our job is to learn how to work with nature, not against it — to stop blocking what the body is trying to do every day: repair, reset, and restore.

Health can be cultivated, restored, and pursued when you know how.

Let me say this plainly: wherever you stand now — burned out, broken-hearted, or even bed-bound — meaningful improvement is possible for everyone. Over the past twenty-five years, I have watched with my own eyes as bodies rebuilt, minds grew calm, and spirits quietly rekindled. I don't just hope this; I know it.

The human body carries a remarkable capacity to heal. Our task is to assist it, and most of all, to stop getting in its way with daily habits. Much of healing is surprisingly simple: support what your body is already trying to do, and gently remove what keeps interrupting it. This is one of the most common patterns I see — and also one of the most hopeful, because it's changeable.

Three Non-Negotiables

To return to true health, three things are non-negotiable.

- **A clear picture**
  See your true-health image in detail—how you move, think, love, work, pray, and play.
  Name it. Feel it.
  Let it be your last thought at night and your first thought in the morning.
  Hold it in mind until it becomes your guiding image.

- **An unshakable belief**
  No pain, setback, or scary result gets to decide your direction.
  Walk it step by step.

Let your actions lead—one small step at a time—until your nervous system learns to trust again.

- **Courage over fear**
  Fear and worry are headwinds. They don't mean you're off course.
  Courage is choosing the next right step while fear is still present.
  Support is your engine.
  And your inner compass—the steady part of you that still wants to live—can be invited back, gently, day by day.

Practice Is the Bridge

Conviction without practice is just noise.

In the pages ahead, you'll learn to harness nature's best healers — sleep, food, movement, light, and connection — to rebuild your capacity. You'll learn how to protect yourself from the quiet drips in daily life — plastics, fragrances, PFAS "forever chemicals," common pesticides, and heavy metals such as mercury — using clear, evidence-informed shields and simple recovery plans.

You'll also learn how to move more safely through a health system that can sometimes over-rely on pills and tests, so you can choose wisely and protect yourself — not instead of medical care, but alongside it.

My vow to you is this: I will share what I've seen help real people, in real lives, over real time. Your vow — if you choose it — is to practice, one small step at a time, until your body and life begin to prove these truths to you.

CHAPTER 8
Why You're So Tired

The Fog Loop That Makes Life Harder Than It Should Be

In the introduction, we described a kind of tiredness that doesn't go away with a weekend off.

It sinks into your mornings, stretches across your days, and curls around your nights.

This chapter is about the pattern hiding underneath that feeling — what I call **The Fog Loop**.

The Fog Loop is a cycle many people fall into quietly over months or years, without realizing what's happening. Foggy morning. Drained afternoon. Wired night. Shallow, broken sleep. You wake up tired, push through the day, finally collapse into bed… and then your mind hits the gas. Thoughts race. Problems replay. To-do lists march through your head. Morning comes, and the same day begins again.

If this sounds familiar, hear this: you're not imagining it, and you're not weak.

You're misaligned — and that can be repaired.

People often blame themselves. They say things like, "I should be stronger," or, "I used to handle more," or, "Maybe I'm just getting older." But the truth is much simpler: your body's rhythm — the internal clock that coordinates your energy, focus, sleep, and metabolism — has drifted out of sync with your life. Once that rhythm slips, everything feels harder.

This isn't something you caused on purpose. It's something that happened slowly, almost invisibly. A few late nights. A few early mornings. One stressful month. Too much screen light after sunset. Too little sunlight in the morning. Skipped meals. Late dinners. Too much doing and not enough recovering. One small shift at a time, until your inner timing fell out of alignment with the world around you.

I think of people like Maria, a 42-year-old teacher who sat across from me and said, "Mornings feel like walking through glue." She used to be sharp, patient, and lively. Now she wakes up groggy, forgets names and simple words mid-sentence, and watches her temper shorten for reasons she doesn't understand. At night, her thoughts spin, and she wakes up every few hours without knowing why. Her routine labs were normal. But she didn't feel perfect. She didn't even feel functional. What she needed wasn't a new diagnosis. She needed someone to explain the pattern.

That's what I wish for you — to understand your pattern.

When your rhythm is off, life feels one notch too hard. Patience is thinner. Focus slips faster. Small tasks feel heavier than they should. You feel like you're living behind a pane of fogged glass. Because this fog isn't dramatic or visible, you may start to wonder if you're imagining it. You're not. Your life is showing you real data.

People often tell me, "I feel like I'm disappearing," or, "I don't feel like myself," or, "I'm not depressed but something is wrong," or, "I'm trying so hard and still falling behind." And I tell them what I want to tell you now:

You're not disappearing. You're misaligned.

And misalignment is reversible.

Once your rhythm slips, it touches almost every system connected to it — your sleep, your hormones, your appetite, your focus, your mood, your energy, your resilience, your libido. That's why everything feels connected. Because it is.

Relief begins when you stop blaming yourself. Healing begins when you understand that your body is not broken — it's confused and out of sync. Transformation begins when you start sending your body the right syncing signals again.

This book will teach you how.

Before we move on, I invite you to take a moment and name the three symptoms that impact your life the most. Not with judgment, but with honesty. Circle the one that hurts your days the most. You're not circling a flaw — you're choosing a starting point.

Name the symptoms:

_____

_____

_____

Circle the one that affects your day the most.

As you keep reading, remember this: you are not stuck like this. Your body can find its rhythm again. And when it does, you will feel like yourself again — clearer, calmer, lighter, stronger.

This is where your return begins.

CHAPTER 9
It's Not You — It's Your Clock

Why "Normal" Labs Miss the Real Problem

There is a particular kind of frustration that settles in when your doctor looks you in the eye and says, "Everything looks normal." You nod, because you want that to be true. You smile politely, because you don't want to be difficult. And you go home thinking, **"Then why does my life feel so hard?"**

I want to tell you something gently but truthfully: your tests were not wrong — they were just answering the wrong question.

Most medical lab panels are designed for one main purpose: to detect disease at the point where it clearly crosses a line. Is your blood sugar high enough to call it diabetes? Is your cholesterol high enough to put you at clear risk? Is your thyroid low enough to be officially "hypothyroid"? These are important questions. Lives are saved every day because we can measure those thresholds.

But they are not the same questions your body has been asking.

Your body has been asking things like: "Why am I wiped out all day?" "Why do I get my second wind at 10 p.m.?" "Why do I feel wired when I should be sleepy, and sleepy when I should be awake?" Those questions live in a space bloodwork doesn't measure well — the space between disease and health.

That space is the space of dysfunction and misalignment. The space of timing problems and stress-load problems. The space where most people's suffering actually begins.

Let me give you a real example.

James is a 38-year-old bank manager. He came to me after years of dragging himself through his days. He was always "on" at work, answering emails late into the night. By morning, his alarm felt like an assault. By afternoon, he needed coffee just to feel halfway human. By evening, he was too tired to play with his kids, but somehow still too wired to fall asleep.

He had done "all the right things." He went to his primary doctor. Then a neurologist. Then an endocrinologist. He had multiple rounds of bloodwork, a brain MRI, and more. The conclusion was always the same: "Good news — everything looks fine."

One day, sitting across from me, he said quietly, "I don't understand how I can feel so terrible and be so 'normal' on paper."

I told him, "Your labs tell me you don't have a clear-cut disease. They don't tell me anything about your rhythm."

You see, your body runs on a 24-hour cycle — a deep, ancient timing system wired into your cells. It coordinates when you feel sleepy and when you feel alert. It helps decide when you digest best, when your brain can focus, when your body repairs.

James wasn't "mysteriously sick." He was misaligned.

And misalignment doesn't show up on a standard lab panel.

His life looked like this: late-night business dinners pushed his metabolism too late. Bright screens in bed pushed his melatonin (your sleep signal) too late. Early alarms pushed his cortisol (your wake-up signal) too early. Weekend "catch-up" sleep pushed his internal clock off-center again and again.

If you could see his inner wiring, it would look like a clock whose hands had been nudged a little more out of place every week. Nothing was "broken enough" to flag as a disease. But nothing was lined up enough to let him feel well.

Here's one of the biggest gaps in modern medicine:

You can feel truly unwell long before anything looks abnormal on a standard lab test.

And that gap creates suffering — not because your doctor doesn't care, but because the tools we use are not designed to see what you're feeling.

The truth is, most people in James's situation don't need a new label. They need orientation — someone to explain what their body has been trying to say.

You can be "normal" on paper and still be unwell in real life — because timing, stress load, and rhythm aren't captured well by standard labs.

There is almost always a cause — or a pattern — even if it isn't visible on a standard lab panel. It just often lives outside the narrow window we use for disease detection. And it almost always lives inside your rhythm — inside the way your days and nights are arranged.

When your internal timing drifts, sleep gets lighter and more fragile. Energy sinks in the morning and spikes late at night. Mood swings more easily. Digestion becomes unpredictable. Hormones start to whisper, then shout. It's as if the conductor of your internal orchestra has lost his place in the score. The instruments are still there. The players are still talented. But they're no longer playing together.

I need you to hear this clearly: you are not a mystery. You are not weak, lazy, or imagining things. You are a human being living in a world that constantly pulls your biology out of sync.

Once you understand that, the story of your symptoms changes. You stop feeling like a broken machine. You start to see yourself as a mistimed orchestra that can be retuned.

Fear softens. Hope returns. The path ahead becomes clearer.

In the next chapter, we'll look at how modern life — light at the wrong times, food at the wrong times, demands at the wrong times — slowly pulled your clock off its center.

Your return doesn't begin with a new pill or a new label. It begins with timing.

Your healing begins with rhythm. And your best days come back once your clock does.

CHAPTER 10
How Your Life Fell Out of Rhythm

The Hidden Forces That Pulled You Off Course

Most people don't fall apart overnight.

You didn't simply wake up one morning suddenly exhausted, foggy, emotional, or unable to sleep.

It happened gradually — so gradually that when you look back, it's hard to find the moment it began. The truth is, it didn't start in one moment. It began in dozens of small ones.

A slow drift, not a collapse.

Your body is built to follow a rhythm older than civilization — a 24-hour cycle (your circadian rhythm) shaped by sunrise, movement, meals, sunset, darkness, and rest. For thousands of years, that rhythm was reliable. Then modern life changed the environment faster than biology could adapt. You're living in a world your body was never programmed for, and that mismatch quietly pulls you out of alignment.

Think about how your days actually unfold.

You stay up a little later to finish work. You answer one more message. You scroll for a few minutes to "unwind," and those few minutes turn into thirty. Screens cast daylight into your brain long after the sun has gone down, telling your internal clock that night hasn't really begun. Melatonin — your navigation signal for sleep — gets delayed.

You go to bed tired but not sleepy, or sleepy but unable to let go. You tell yourself, "I'll catch up this weekend," not realizing that "catching up," as we will see, pushes your rhythm even further off-center.

Then mornings begin rushing you. Instead of sunlight, calm, and a little movement, your day starts with alarms, stress, and artificial light. You skip the slow morning your biology expects. Maybe you skip food too — or you grab something quick, sweet, and convenient, fuel that lifts you fast and drops you faster.

Your body tries to rise, but the timing is off. It's like slamming the gas in a cold car that never had a chance to warm up: it moves, but every part is straining.

And then there's the afternoon.

You feel heavier than you should. Not sick, not faint — just unable to access the energy you used to count on. You push through with caffeine because that's what responsible adults do: they push. But caffeine in the afternoon raises adrenaline and nudges melatonin further into the night, and the drift widens: later energy, later hunger, later sleepiness, later wakefulness.

Stress adds its own layer. Not emergency stress — the quiet, constant kind. Emotional tension. Overcommitment. Pressure without relief. A nervous system with no true off-switch. You're alert when you should be unwinding. You're holding your breath without noticing. You're carrying responsibilities into bed with you, long after your body is begging for rest. Stress hormones rise when they should fall, and your inner clock loses clarity about when to be "on" and when to be "done."

Even the structure of your week works against you. On weekends, you stay up later because it's your only window to breathe. You sleep in because you're exhausted. But shifting your wake time by even one hour can confuse your brain's timekeeping system for days. Monday morning becomes a form of jet lag, even though you never left home. We call it "Monday brain," but it's misalignment — the same mismatch frequent travelers feel when they cross time zones.

And then come the pressures you barely even notice. Screens sit a few inches from your eyes all day, pouring bright light and tiny alerts into your nervous system. You sit for hours at a desk or in a car, hips locked, blood flow slow, brain humming but body still. Dinner slides later because the day ran long, so takeout lands heavy at a time your biology expected to be winding down. Alcohol takes the edge off; sugar tries to make up for energy you don't actually have. You lose contact with nature and real sunlight — signals your body needs almost as much as oxygen to function. Life becomes something lived indoors, glowing, stimulated, and rushing, even though your biology was designed for light and dark, movement and pause, effort and recovery, predictable rhythms instead of constant noise.

Given the way modern days are built, your drift makes sense.

Broken sleep, foggy mornings, and thin patience aren't moral failures — they're predictable signals of a system pushed off tempo.

This did not happen because you're undisciplined, or neglectful, or "getting old." It happened because the structure of modern life is fundamentally out of sync with the way human biology actually works.

You didn't break your rhythm.

Life pulled it away from you.

But here is the part I need you to hold onto with both hands:

If your rhythm drifted gently, it can return gently.

If your timing slipped in small steps, it can return in small steps.

Your body is not stubborn — it is listening, responding, adapting, trying. It has been trying to rebalance this whole time.

What you'll learn next is how to speak to your body in the language it recognizes: light and dark, food rhythm, movement, calm, and consistency. These aren't punishments or restrictions. They're signals — the signals your body has been missing, the ones that will guide it home.

Before you turn the page, please take a breath and release any guilt you've been carrying. You didn't cause this on purpose. You lived your life the best way you could in a world that demands too much from the body and gives too little back.

Now we begin the part where your body comes back into rhythm — not through force, but through understanding. Not through pressure, but through alignment. Not through perfection, but through gentle correction.

This is where the drift starts to reverse.

One cue at a time.

One day at a time.

One rhythm slowly coming back into place.

CHAPTER 11
Your Roots

The Real Reasons Energy, Mood, and Sleep Fall Apart

If you put ten tired people in a room, you'll hear the same sentences over and over:

"I'm exhausted."
"I can't think straight."
"I don't feel like myself."

From the outside, their stories sound almost identical.
On the inside, the reasons can be completely different.
That's what this chapter is about: Same canopy leaves. Different roots.

Three tired people, three different stories

Aisha: blood sugar and chaos

Aisha is forty-four. She teaches fourth grade and crashes after lunch every single day. Not because she's lazy, but because her blood sugar is on a roller coaster. She snacks all day to keep going, drinks coffee at 3 p.m. because she feels she has no other choice, and scrolls in bed at night to "unwind."
Her body isn't broken.
Her main roots are **sugar swings, late caffeine, and chaotic meals**.

Mark: time zones and light

Mark is twenty-nine, a consultant whose passport looks more worn-out than his running shoes. He crosses time zones constantly. He eats dinner when his body thinks it's midnight. He has drinks at hours that trick his internal clock into thinking it's still evening when it should be slowing down. On weekends, he "recovers" by sleeping in, not realizing that waking later in the morning will push his sleep cycle even further.
His main roots are **travel, late light, and constant schedule changes**.

Nora: depletion and duty

Nora is fifty-two, a nurse with a heart that has carried too many heavy shifts. Her legs feel heavy by afternoon, her thoughts feel slower than they used to, and her sleep has become unpredictable. She blames aging. But years of heavy periods left her iron low. Years of shift work pulled at her clock. Years of always being "on duty" kept her nervous system braced.

Her main roots are **nutrient depletion, shift work, and long-term stress**.
Same fog. Same fatigue. Same restless nights.
Completely different root mixes.

Stop staring at the leaves

Most people only see their "leaves": the fog, the fatigue, the irritability that wasn't always there, the strange heaviness that settles over the afternoons. Leaves tell you that the system above the ground is struggling.

Roots tell you why.

When you zoom out, the roots of your fatigue and fog are not random. They're made of rhythms and routines — the things you repeat without even thinking.

That's the good news: if patterns are the roots, then changing even a few patterns begins to change the roots. And here's the comforting part: your roots are not mysterious or unreachable. If you know how to look, you can usually trace which ones belong to you. Once you see them clearly, you can begin to correct them — and only then can the canopy above (your energy, mood, and sleep) truly recover.

A quick "root check" for you

You don't have to know everything today. But it helps to notice a few likely culprits.

Check any statements that describe your habits or patterns most weeks.
Be honest — no one will see this but you.

Fuel & sugar patterns

- ☐ I often start the day with coffee and carbs but very little protein.
- ☐ I grab food on the run or eat while working instead of sitting down for real meals.
- ☐ I snack or "graze" most of the day instead of having clear meal times.
- ☐ I regularly reach for sweets or refined carbs (bread, crackers, energy bars, pastries) to push through dips.

Clock & light patterns

- ☐ My bedtime and wake time jump around by more than 1–2 hours across the week.
- ☐ I'm on a bright screen (phone, tablet, TV, laptop) in the last hour before trying to sleep.
- ☐ I rarely get outside into real daylight within the first two hours after waking.
- ☐ I "catch up" on sleep on weekends by sleeping in much later than usual.

Gut & inflammation patterns

- ☐ I rely on packaged or ultra-processed foods (bars, chips, fast food, frozen meals) on most weekdays.
- ☐ I often eat my largest meal late in the evening or within two hours of going to bed.
- ☐ I use over-the-counter pain relievers (like ibuprofen, Motrin, Aleve) several times a week.
- ☐ I drink alcohol on several nights per week to relax or fall asleep.

Nervous system & stress patterns

- ☐ I check my phone, email, or messages within the first 5–10 minutes of waking.
- ☐ I leave notifications on all day and respond to them immediately by default.
- ☐ I rarely have a protected block of time (45–60 minutes) to focus on one thing without interruptions.
- ☐ Most nights, I go to bed still thinking about work, problems, or my to-do list.

Movement patterns

- ☐ I sit for more than six hours on a typical day (desk, car, couch) with few movement breaks.
- ☐ I rarely walk for ten minutes or more at a stretch on an average day.
- ☐ When I do exercise, it's usually a hard workout after many days of doing almost nothing.
- ☐ I don't have any planned "easy days" of gentler movement or active recovery.

Environment patterns

- ☐ I spend most of my day indoors under artificial light.
- ☐ I rarely open windows or air out my home or workspace.
- ☐ I wear perfume or use plug-in air fresheners, scented candles, or strong fragranced cleaners most days.
- ☐ I've lived or worked in a place with past leaks, dampness, or a "musty" smell — and I'm not sure it was fully fixed.

Take a moment and look at what you've checked.

Your fatigue and fog are not random.
They follow a pattern.
And patterns can be changed.

Why this matters before we move on

In the guided journey, we will learn how to use the big levers — sleep, movement, food, gut health, stress — that help almost everyone. But how you use those levers should depend on your roots.

- If your roots are mostly fuel and sugar, the right breakfast and walking after meals will do the heavy lifting.
- If your roots are mostly clock and light, morning light and a steady wake time will matter most.
- If your roots are mostly depletion and stress, gentle repair and nutrients will need to come first.

Two people can follow the same general plan and get very different results if they're aiming at the wrong roots.

That's why this chapter exists: to help you stop asking, "What's wrong with me?" and start asking, "Which roots are driving my leaves?"

For now, hold onto one gentle thought:

The way you feel is not the whole story. It's a clue. When you follow that clue down to the roots, the whole picture becomes solvable.

Your roots are discoverable.

Your roots can be worked with.

And once we tend them, the canopy above — your energy, your mood, your sleep — can be restored to health, piece by piece.

TOOLS

Tool 1 — Head-to-Toe Health Self-Check

Before we go any further, let's pause and listen to your body.
This simple checklist is a way to put on paper what you already feel.
Self-reflection is the foundation of change.
When you can see your patterns, they stop feeling random and overwhelming.
Foggy mornings, restless nights, crashes after meals, heavy moods — all of that becomes visible, not just vague.
Over time, this list becomes a quiet record of your progress.
You'll be able to look back and see how your score shifts — week by week, season by season — as your body remembers how to heal.
Take a few minutes.
Be honest and gentle with yourself.
There are no "good" or "bad" scores here — only information.

How to use this page

- Look back over the past 2–3 months of your life.
- Put a checkmark next to each statement that fits you.
- Each checked box = 1 point.
- When you're done, add up your points and write down your total.

You'll use this same checklist again later in the book.
Each time you revisit it, you'll see just how far you've come.

Head & Mind

- ☐ I lose my train of thought or misplace things more than I should
- ☐ I feel "foggy" or mentally slow during the day
- ☐ I often feel down, worried, or on edge
- ☐ Falling asleep or staying asleep is hard for me
- ☐ Mornings feel heavy; I'm slow to get going
- ☐ I get headaches without a clear reason

Eyes
☐ I have frequent blurry vision
☐ My eyes feel tired, dry, or burn by afternoon

Ears / Nose / Sinuses
☐ My nose often feels stuffy
☐ I have constant ringing in my ears
☐ I get sinus infections or colds more than most people

Mouth, Teeth & Gums
☐ My gums bleed when I brush
☐ I've had dental infections or frequent mouth issues
☐ I notice bad breath or a white tongue

Throat, Neck & Thyroid Signals
☐ I get frequent neck/shoulder tightness or spasms
☐ My energy is low in the morning and better late at night
☐ I notice thinning hair, dry skin, or constipation along with low energy

Lungs & Breathing
☐ I'm short of breath climbing a single flight of stairs
☐ I get bronchitis or chest infections frequently

Heart & Circulation
☐ I've been told my blood pressure is high
☐ I get heart racing spells
☐ My hands/feet are cold a lot of the time

Blood Sugar & Metabolism
☐ I feel very sleepy after meals
☐ I carry most of my weight around my belly
☐ I've been told I have high cholesterol, triglycerides, or blood sugar

- [ ] My weight changed more than ~15 pounds in the past 5 years (not on purpose)
- [ ] I've noticed significant muscle loss over the past 5 years

Stomach & Upper Digestion

- [ ] I often get heartburn, indigestion, or reflux
- [ ] I get stomach pain or discomfort after eating
- [ ] High-protein meals sometimes upset my digestion

Intestines & Bowel

- [ ] I swing between constipation and diarrhea
- [ ] My stools sometimes look oily, float, or seem unusual
- [ ] I feel bloated or gassy after meals

Liver & Gallbladder Hints

- [ ] Rich or fatty foods sit heavily in me
- [ ] I feel nauseated or queasy after certain meals

Kidneys & Urinary

- [ ] I've had a kidney stone
- [ ] I've been told I have kidney problems or protein in my urine
- [ ] I wake to urinate more than once most nights

Reproductive & Hormone Balance

- [ ] My sex drive is lower than I'd expect for my age
- [ ] I have hot flashes or night sweats
- [ ] I have frequent mood swings or feel "wired and tired"

Skin, Hair & Nails

- [ ] I get rashes, itching, or sun sensitivity
- [ ] I've had recurring fungal issues (athlete's foot, yeast, etc.)

Muscles, Joints & Bones

☐ I have ongoing back or neck trouble
☐ My joints feel sore, stiff, or swollen
☐ I've been told I have low bone density or "weak bones"
☐ I have posture or flexibility problems
☐ I've had frequent sprains or joint pains (hips, knees, etc.)

Nerves

☐ I feel tingling or "pins and needles" in my hands or feet
☐ I get unexplained muscle aches or shooting pains

Energy & Recovery

☐ I feel exhausted even after a full night in bed
☐ Light activity leaves me unusually tired or sore
☐ A simple cold knocks me out for a long time
☐ I seem to catch every cold or flu going around

Environment & Sensitivities

☐ Strong smells (perfume, cleaners, smoke) bother me
☐ Alcohol, caffeine, or certain medicines make me feel unwell
☐ Processed foods, fast food, or MSG make me feel "off"
☐ I sometimes wake groggy, like I've been drugged

Your Totals

- Today's total: _____
- Date: _____

This checklist is an educational self-reflection tool, not a diagnosis or medical advice. If any of these symptoms worry you, please discuss them with your clinician.

Tool 2 — The Score Game — Simple Rules

Use this to watch your health change over time.
It's a game, not a diagnosis.

1. Start today
   - Count your checked boxes on the Self-Check. That number is your score.
   - Write it down with today's date somewhere you'll find again — a notebook, your phone, or the inside cover of this book.
   - Think of it as your "before" picture, taken in numbers instead of photos.

2. During your 101-day journey
   In Part II of this book, you'll walk through a 101-day journey — one small step at a time.
   You do not need to repeat the checklist every day.
   Just keep your original score handy as your starting point.

3. After your 101 days
   - When you finish the 101-day journey, repeat the Self-Check.
   - Add up your new total and write it next to your first score.
   - Even a drop of 3–5 points is worth celebrating.
   - What matters most is the trend: over time, you want your score gently drifting downward.

4. Long-term check-ins
   After the 101 days:
   - Use the checklist once a month (or every few months) as a quick early-warning system.
   - If your score starts climbing again, it's a friendly nudge that your rhythms are slipping and it's time to reset a few basics.

5. What your number means
   - A higher score usually means more symptoms and more strain on your system.

- A lower score usually means your daily life is feeling easier — more energy, clearer thinking, better sleep.

Your score is not a verdict on your worth as a person.

It's simply one way to listen to your body.

Again, the purpose of this tool is not to diagnose you. It's to help you notice what your body may be trying to communicate. If anything you're experiencing feels worrisome, new, or worsening, please discuss it with your clinician.

Tool 3 — Begin Tonight (two minutes)

Write one sentence that captures your picture of true health — in your own words:

_____

_____

Then read this to yourself (or say it out loud if it helps):

**"Change is possible for me.
Today I'll take one small step."**

PART II
THE GUIDED JOURNEY

A 101-Day Guided Journey to Clearer Thinking, Lasting Energy, and Restful Sleep

The pages you've just read were written to give you something most people never get: a clearer sense of what may be happening in your body — and why.

Now comes the part that changes your days.

Information can calm your mind.

Practice changes your life.

This section isn't meant to be skimmed or binged. It's meant to be taken one day at a time — and turned into action, even if the action is small. Think of these 101 days as compass checks and course corrections. One small adjustment won't move you across an ocean overnight. But hold the new angle, and over time you arrive on a different shore.

I first imagined this as a year-long guide, because health is a lifelong practice. But as I wrote, two things became clear: a full year can start to repeat itself, and most people need momentum sooner. So I shaped this into 101 days — a focused three-month season — because it's long enough to build traction without getting lost. Many habits start to feel easier after a couple of months, but they hold better when you practice them long enough to survive busy weeks and imperfect days.

A note on the science: many findings referenced in these entries come from large studies. They often show patterns, not guarantees. Your goal here isn't perfection — it's steady course correction.

Timelines vary, and that's okay. If you've been running on empty for a long time — or working around medical conditions, medications, or real-life constraints — your body may need more time. The good news is that small steps still work. They just work at your pace.

How to Use the Guided Journey

There's no wrong way to move through this part of the book, but there is a way that works best: slowly, intentionally, and consistently.

Each day, do two things.

First, read one entry slowly and choose one small action you can actually do today.

Second, write one line by hand. It turns intention into something physical — and helps the idea stick.

If you miss a day, don't catch up. Just return.

Over 101 days, these small practices compound. Some will feel easy. Some will challenge you. Some you'll skip and come back to later. That's okay. This isn't a test. It's a relationship — between you and your body, and between you and your future self.

I recommend starting at Day 1 and letting the structure carry you. The early days reinforce foundations. Later days add depth. Each day ends with a small checkbox — when you finish, mark it and move on.

Remember: you're not trying to become a different person in 101 days.

You're learning how to live as yourself with less fog, less strain, and more alignment.

So take a breath.

Pick up your pen.

Turn the page.

Today, you don't have to fix your whole life.

You just have to live one idea from one page as best you can.

The rest will come.

One last important note before we start the journey

Some ideas in this 101-day experience will show up more than once — and that's intentional. Healing isn't just collecting new information. It's rewiring old patterns. And the brain learns best through gentle repetition. Core ideas are revisited from different angles. That's also why this part of the book isn't meant to be read in one sitting. These entries are designed to be taken in daily, then practiced, so the ideas can move from "I get it" to "I do it." If a prompt feels familiar, don't skim it as more of the same. Treat it as a reminder meant to land deeper this time. Each pass is a small recalibration — and over weeks, those small shifts compound into real change.

When you see one reference number at the end of the Quick science section, it applies to all three bullets above and points to the matching source in the Notes & Sources section at the back of the book.

101-Day
Guided Journey

DAY 1

> "You can't stop aging, but you can slow the clock inside your cells."
> — A. Smyrlis, MD

Two people can share the same birthday and live in two different bodies. You can't slow the calendar — but you can slow the wear it writes into your body. What you do today is a quiet vote for how old you'll feel tomorrow.

Reflection

Most people think age is just a number on a birthday cake. In reality, you carry two ages: the one on your driver's license (chronological age) and the one written into your cells (biological age).

Chronological age moves at the same speed for everyone. Biological age does not. It speeds up with stress, poor sleep, processed food, toxins and loneliness. It slows down with aligned living: quality sleep, real food, movement, connection, and meaning.

This is why two 55-year-olds can look and feel completely different. One moves like they're 40 — clear-headed, mobile, curious. The other moves like they're 70 — stiff, foggy, and always recovering from something. The years on the calendar are the same. The pace of aging has been different for decades.

Inside your body, clocks are always running. Some are written into your DNA; most are influenced by how you live. Chronic stress and sleep loss accelerate wear on your brain, blood vessels, and immune system. Highly processed foods, smoking, inactivity, and heavy drinking push your biology into fast-forward. By contrast, real food, daily movement, good sleep, sunlight, and strong relationships are like pressing slow-motion on the aging process: less damage, better repair, more reserve. Your face, skin, and posture eventually show what your cells have known for years.

Cosmetic treatments can change what you see in the mirror — and there's nothing wrong with that. But they don't always change how old you feel inside. The deepest "youth work" is inside-out. It's healthier arteries, steadier nerves, clearer thinking, more flexible joints, deeper sleep — a body that recovers well and feels lighter to live in. That's biological age slowing down even as the calendar keeps moving.

The point is not to fear aging; it's to realize you have influence over the speed dial. *"You can't stop aging, but your daily choices can 'game the clock' a little in your favor."* Every night of decent sleep is a small nudge toward younger biology. Every real-food meal is quieter inflammation and steadier hormones. Every walk is a signal to your cells to stay resilient. You can't control everything, but you can stop pouring gasoline on the fire and start giving your body the inputs that help it age more gracefully — and sometimes even reverse some of the acceleration.

So when you blow out the candles and think, "I'm getting older," ask a deeper question:

"How old am I on the inside? Am I aging faster or slower than I need to? And what am I doing today to change that trajectory?"

That single question can become one of the most powerful motivators in your life.

Real-life snapshot

Lena and Laura are identical twin sisters. Same genes, same birthday. But after college, their lives unfolded very differently.

Lena chased a high-pressure career — late nights at the office, fast food at her desk, red-eye flights every month. She smoked "just socially" and joked that coffee was her blood type and sleep was a premium feature she hadn't unlocked yet. Her calendar had a recurring event called "Start Gym Monday" — always rescheduled by Monday.

Laura became a teacher. Her job wasn't stress-free, but her days had rhythm. She packed simple home-cooked lunches, walked most evenings in the park with her family, and guarded her sleep like a meeting she couldn't miss. Weekends were for cooking, friends, and laughter more than catching up on email.

On their shared 55th birthday, the family gathered for a party. Same age, same cake, same candles. But everyone could see the difference.

Laura moved easily — posture open, eyes bright. Her skin carried a few honest lines, but also that rested, healthy glow. Lena's joints hurt. Her blood pressure was up. Her skin looked dull and tired, with deeper lines that made her seem older than her years.

"It's not fair," Lena said quietly. Their father — a doctor who knew them both — gently replied, "Your birthdays are the same. But the way your days have treated your bodies hasn't been."

Same genes. Same dates on the calendar. Daily choices — not luck — had written two very different stories of aging.

Quick science

- Biological age is an estimate of how much "wear and tear" your body has accumulated, and scientists can approximate it using tests like DNA methylation ("epigenetic clocks") and other biomarkers.
- Lifestyle factors such as physical activity, diet quality, sleep, smoking, alcohol, stress, and social connection are consistently linked to faster or slower biological aging in large studies.
- Regular movement and healthier habits are associated with "younger" biological ages — sometimes several years younger than peers of the same chronological age — while ultra-processed diets, chronic stress, and inactivity are linked to accelerated aging and higher disease risk.[1]

Inspiration note

You can't rewind the calendar, but you can stop living on fast-forward — and your body will feel the difference.

Today's Invitation

One thing I will do for myself today:

- ☐ Sleep first: Set a lights-down time 20–30 minutes earlier tonight.
- ☐ Strength signal: Do 10 minutes of simple strength (sit-to-stand/squats + wall push-ups + plank).
- ☐ Real meal: Eat one balanced plate today (protein + vegetables + healthy fat).

Action Step:
Choose the easiest one today. Do it now or set one reminder and do it when it best fits your schedule.

Reflection:
After I took the step today, I felt: ☐ calmer ☐ clearer ☐ steadier ☐ proud ☐ no change yet (effort still counts)

Bottom line

You can't change how old you are today, but you can absolutely change how fast you age from here.

Your lines

(write one thought, one insight, or rewrite one sentence that rang true)

_____

_____

_____

☐ Done for today

Why this matters
Writing just a few lines by hand locks the concept into memory and gently primes your subconscious mind to adopt and act on it, leading to better recall and follow-through.

DAY 2

"Your cellphone is your kryptonite."
— A. Smyrlis, MD

It's not just a tool in your hand.
It's a drain on your time, focus, and peace.
If you don't cage it in small, reasonable ways, it quietly cages you.

Reflection

A smartphone looks harmless. Small, shiny, "helpful." But every time you pick it up, it makes a tiny withdrawal: a little attention, a little energy, a little presence. One or two withdrawals don't hurt you. Hundreds a day do.

Your phone quietly taxes your health — later nights, blue light, stress spikes. It taxes your relationships — half-listening to the people you love while your thumb scrolls. It taxes your productivity — fractured work, forgotten intentions, tasks that take twice as long. It even taxes your money — subscriptions and impulse buys you never planned.

Over time, the cost is huge, but the damage feels "normal," so we don't question it.

Knowing this is not enough.

The people who stay healthy aren't the ones who know more facts.

They're the ones who treat their phone like kryptonite: create distance, use a container, and choose when they'll touch it.

Your phone is not neutral. It is built to win.

If you don't have a plan for it, it has a plan for you.

Real-life snapshot

This quote was born on an ordinary morning. I teach my patients about time, focus, dopamine, and circadian rhythms. I know the science. I know the tricks. I also have a structured morning routine — reading, thinking, writing — the kind of routine that keeps me steady.

And yet one morning, I picked up my phone "just for a second" to check my sleep on a health app. One tap became another.

Sleep score → shopping app → scrolling a long shopping list.

When I looked up, thirty minutes were gone.

No decision was made. There was no clear moment of, "Yes, I choose to spend half an hour scrolling." The brain simply slid down the slope the app was built to create.

That was the moment of clarity: the phone is not neutral. If I can be caught that easily — with everything I know and practice — what chance does the average person have without safeguards in place?

Quick science

- Smartphones and blue-light screens at night suppress melatonin and disturb circadian rhythms, leading to poorer sleep quality and higher long-term health risks.
- Excessive smartphone use is consistently linked with more anxiety, more depression, and more perceived stress, especially in younger people and heavy users.
- High daily screen time is associated with lower physical activity, more weight gain, and poorer overall well-being over time.[2]

Compass link: If you want the deeper "why," see Part III — The Compass Explained — Chapter 18: From Redline to Rhythm — Stress, Screens, and How to Stop Running on Empty. *(Optional. Not required today.)*

Inspiration note

Every superhero has a weak point. Kryptonite didn't make Superman a bad person; it just made him weaker and less himself. When you step away from your phone — especially during deep work and family time — you're not being extreme. You're simply making room for your best self to show up.

Today's Invitation

One thing I will do for myself today:

- ☐ Quiet the pings: Turn off non-essential notifications (or use Do Not Disturb for one block).
- ☐ Bedroom boundary: Keep the phone out of the bedroom tonight.
- ☐ Check windows: Pick two times to check messages/social today (instead of all day).

Action Step:
Choose the easiest one today. Do it now or set one reminder and do it when it best fits your schedule.

Reflection:
After I took the step today, I felt: ☐ calmer ☐ clearer ☐ steadier ☐ proud ☐ no change yet (effort still counts)

Bottom line

Every time you pick up your phone, you are either serving your real life — or handling kryptonite that drains it away.

Your lines

(write one thought, one insight, or rewrite one sentence that rang true)

_____

_____

_____

☐ Done for today

Why this matters

Writing just a few lines by hand locks the concept into memory and gently primes your subconscious mind to adopt and act on it, leading to better recall and follow-through.

DAY 3

"Move the body; clear the mind — ten minutes is a real reset."
— A. Smyrlis, MD

Stuck mind? Move the body.
Ten minutes can change the weather inside.
Motion first; clarity often follows.

Reflection

When your mind jams, your first instinct is often to push harder — stare at the screen, re-read the same line, drink more coffee, try to "force" focus. But your nervous system doesn't respond well to force. It responds to signals. One of the fastest, most reliable signals you can send it is simple movement.

Even ten minutes can shift your internal climate. A short walk outside, a loop around the block, a hallway lap, or two flights of stairs sends fresh blood to the brain, wakes up attention networks, increases oxygen flow, and shakes loose the static that builds up during long sitting or heavy thinking. You don't need a "workout." You need movement, rhythm, and a message to the brain that the body is awake and safe.

Think of movement as a reset button you carry everywhere. When you move the body, the mind often unknots. Stress hormones ease. Blood sugar smooths out, especially after meals, which can prevent the classic afternoon crash. Sleep later that night often improves because your system got to spend some energy. Creativity and solutions show up not because you thought harder, but because you walked.

Ten minutes is small enough to repeat. One reset helps; two — one around midday and one in the mid-afternoon — can change the whole feel of your day. These tiny bouts add up: better sleep, steadier energy, fewer headaches, clearer thinking, and a calmer evening. When in doubt: move. Your mind will thank you.

Real-life snapshot

By 3 p.m., a working parent hit a wall every day. Her attention slid, fog rolled in, and cravings kicked up. She responded the usual way: more caffeine, more staring at the screen, more frustration with herself. The last few hours of the afternoon felt like wading through mud.

At her clinician's suggestion, she tried a small experiment: schedule a 10-minute "reset" on her calendar. Just ten minutes, labeled like any other meeting.

On clear days, she stepped outside for one loop around the building and two flights of stairs. On tighter days, she walked her hallway and climbed one stairwell. She ended each reset with a glass of water and two slow breaths.

Within a few weeks, she noticed fewer headaches, softer emails, and a surprising surge of focus in the hour after each reset.

"I didn't change my job," she said. "I just walked out of the fog instead of trying to think my way out of it."

Quick science
- Brief walking bouts (5–10 minutes) can improve alertness and mood within minutes and help stabilize blood sugar when done after meals.
- Walking activates motor and associative brain networks, which is one reason it tends to boost creative thinking and problem-solving.
- Accumulated movement (two or three short sessions) supports better sleep and next-day energy without requiring long, formal workouts.[3]

Inspiration note
A short walk can do what hours of trying cannot — it frees the mind.

Today's Invitation
One thing I will do for myself today:

☐ Reset walk: Take a 10-minute walk when you feel stuck or tense.
☐ After-meal dose: Walk 5–10 minutes after one meal today.
☐ Beat the slump: Set one reminder for your low point and do a quick reset then.

Action Step:
Choose the easiest one today. Do it now or set one reminder and do it when it best fits your schedule.

Reflection:
After I took the step today, I felt: ☐ calmer ☐ clearer ☐ steadier ☐ proud ☐ no change yet (effort still counts)

Bottom line

A short walk now is better than a perfect workout later.

Your lines

(write one thought, one insight, or rewrite one sentence that rang true)

_____

_____

_____

☐ Done for today

Why this matters
Writing just a few lines by hand locks the concept into memory and gently primes your subconscious mind to adopt and act on it, leading to better recall and follow-through.

DAY 4

> "Sleep is that golden chain that binds
> health and our bodies together."
> — Thomas Dekker

Sleep is the foundation under every healthy choice you make.
When sleep improves, everything else becomes easier.
Rest is not the reward — it is the requirement.

Reflection

Sleep powers everything. Creativity, clarity, even courage rise from sleep. Yet in our age, sleep is treated as optional — a luxury instead of the foundation. We stay up to get "one more thing done," believing we've gained time. But biology doesn't bend.

Your brain is like a busy city that has to close roads at night so crews can clean, repair, and reroute. If the roads never close, trash piles up, potholes deepen, and traffic jams spread everywhere. In the brain, that "trash" is the day's wear and tear — loose ends that need sorting, clearing, and filing. When deep sleep is cut short, memory frays, mood fades, and the night shift doesn't get to finish its work. You can still push through tomorrow, but it costs you: foggier thinking, a faster heartbeat, a heavier body, and a shorter fuse with the people you love.

Skimping on sleep is like running your phone on low battery mode all day while opening more apps — you stay "on" longer, but everything lags, freezes, and eventually crashes. You can't out-hustle a drained battery. You recharge it.

The path back isn't complicated, but it does require respect. Try to protect bedtime like an appointment with someone you love. And if your season is hard — a new baby, night shifts, caregiving, anxiety, pain — this isn't about perfection. It's about protecting what you can. You may not control every night, but you can still build anchors: a consistent wake time when possible, morning light, a wind-down cue, and a bedroom that supports sleep instead of fighting it.

When you give your body the sleep it was designed to receive, life stops feeling like an uphill battle. Health stops being a grind and starts to feel like your body is quietly working with you, not against you.

Real-life snapshot

Henry prided himself on working harder than everyone else. Late nights at the office, emails in bed, alarms before dawn — he called it "putting in the extra work for the promotion." Then the cracks appeared. He started making small mistakes, forgetting names and details, rereading the same paragraph three times. His performance reviews slipped. Instead of a promotion, he was warned he might be on thin ice.

Convinced he had an "attention problem," Henry went to his doctor asking for a stimulant, the pill his colleagues swore by. After a long conversation and a careful sleep history, the doctor said, "Your brain isn't broken. It's exhausted. A stimulant is like slamming the gas pedal on an empty tank. It can give you a short burst, but it can also raise your heart rate and steal even more deep sleep. You need the opposite: a calmer nervous system and deeper rest."

Instead of a stimulant, they tried a simple plan: earlier dinner, lights dim an hour before bed, no phone in bed, a consistent wake time — even on weekends — and a small dose of magnesium to support relaxation. (If you're considering supplements, check with your clinician.) Within a few weeks his mood steadied, focus sharpened, and sugar cravings fell. Two months later, his work was back. His boss asked, "You seem different — what changed?" Henry smiled. "I started treating sleep like part of my job."

Quick science

- Sleep loss impairs emotional regulation and decision-making, making you more impulsive, more irritable, and more likely to choose unhealthy foods and behaviors.
- Even a few nights of short sleep can worsen insulin sensitivity and raise blood pressure, nudging you toward diabetes and heart disease.
- Deep and REM sleep support memory consolidation, clearance of metabolic waste from the brain, immune function, and more ethical, prosocial choices the next day. [4]

Compass link: If you want the deeper "why" see Part III — The Compass Explained — Chapter 14: Sleep — The First Domino. *(Optional. Not required today.)*

Inspiration note

Sleep is not time taken from your life; it's the architect that shapes the quality of every waking hour.

Today's Invitation

One thing I will do for myself today:

- ☐ Wind-down alarm: Set a 60-minute wind-down alarm and follow it tonight.
- ☐ Screens out of bed: Keep screens out of bed tonight (phone charges across the room).
- ☐ Morning light: Get 5–10 minutes of outdoor light in the morning.

Action Step:
Choose the easiest one today. Do it now or set one reminder and do it when it best fits your schedule.

Reflection:
After I took the step today, I felt: ☐ calmer ☐ clearer ☐ steadier ☐ proud ☐ no change yet (effort still counts)

Bottom line

Sleep is the muse behind every strength, every insight, and every healthy choice.

Your lines

(write one thought, one insight, or rewrite one sentence that rang true)

_____

_____

_____

☐ Done for today

Why this matters

Writing just a few lines by hand locks the concept into memory and gently primes your subconscious mind to adopt and act on it, leading to better recall and follow-through.

DAY 5

"Well begun is half done."
— Aristotle

The way you begin often decides how you end.
A quiet, intentional morning is a force multiplier for the rest of your day.
Your first hour is the foundation under every other hour.

Reflection

Treat your first waking hour as your Golden Hour — the hour that belongs to you and no one else. Most people give it away for free. The alarm goes off, the phone comes up, and before you've even sat up you're reacting to other people's words, worries, and emergencies. Your day starts in someone else's story.

The first hour is when your nervous system is most impressionable. The tone you set there colors everything that follows. Begin with noise and urgency and you tilt the day toward stress. Begin with water, light, a little movement, and a clear intention, and you tell your body, "We are not prey today. We're in charge."

You don't need a perfect morning routine. You need a simple one you can repeat.

- Water: Drink a full glass of water before coffee. It's the cleanest first win you can give your body.
- Light: Step into daylight as soon as you reasonably can. (If it's dark, use bright indoor light.)
- Movement: Gently move — walk, stretch, or take the stairs once. Just enough to wake the engine.
- Attention: Keep your phone out of reach for the first 30 minutes. Let your mind arrive before the world does.
- Direction: Write 1–3 priorities and one sentence about why they matter. Give the day a shape before it gives you one.

If a whole hour feels impossible, start with 15 minutes. Protect that small corner like an appointment with someone important — because it is. The Golden Hour is not about waking earlier at all costs; if you're severely sleep-deprived, fix your night first (earlier, better sleep), then gently expand the morning once you're not starting in debt.

The goal isn't a perfect routine. It's a sane start. You can't control everything that happens once you step into the day, but you can shape the first minutes. Own that, and the rest of the day has something solid to stand on.

Real-life snapshot

Jasmine used to roll out of bed late, phone already in hand. Before her feet hit the floor, she'd already seen emails, news alerts, and three problems she couldn't fix yet. By breakfast, her mind already felt scattered and behind. The rest of the day followed that script.

On a friend's suggestion, she tried a small experiment: gift herself 20 phone-free minutes after waking. No phone. No inbox.

Her new Golden Hour seed looked like this: open curtains, stand by the window for a minute, and breathe; drink a full glass of water; do a few slow stretches; write one line of gratitude and one priority for the day. Only after that could she touch her phone.

The first few mornings felt strange — like she was "missing" something. After a week, she noticed she wasn't starting at a 7/10 stress level anymore. Her focus improved, and she felt less yanked around by the day.

"The tasks didn't change," she said. "The way I met them did. Owning that first little piece of the morning made everything else feel less like an ambush."

Quick science

- A consistent morning routine is linked with better mood and lower perceived stress.
- Morning light helps anchor your body clock, which supports sleep and daytime energy.
- Starting the day with low-stress inputs (light, movement, calm focus) reduces impulsive decisions later and supports clearer thinking.[5]

Inspiration note

You don't need a perfect morning — just one you own on purpose.

Today's Invitation

One thing I will do for myself today:

- ☐ Phone later: Keep your phone away for the first 15–30 minutes after waking.

- ☐ Light + water first: Step toward daylight, then drink a full glass of water.
- ☐ Wake the engine: Add 2–10 minutes of easy movement (walk, stretch, stairs).

Action Step:
Choose the easiest one today. Do it now or set one reminder and do it when it best fits your schedule.

Reflection:
After I took the step today, I felt: ☐ calmer ☐ clearer ☐ steadier ☐ proud ☐ no change yet (effort still counts)

Bottom line

Half the battle is how you begin. Protect your first hour, and the rest of the day gets lighter.

Your lines

(write one thought, one insight, or rewrite one sentence that rang true)

_____

_____

_____

☐ Done for today

Why this matters
Writing just a few lines by hand locks the concept into memory and gently primes your subconscious mind to adopt and act on it, leading to better recall and follow-through.

DAY 6

> **"Course correction counts more than perfection."**
> — A. Smyrlis, MD

Planes spend most of a flight slightly off course — thousands of tiny adjustments bring them home.
Health works the same way.
Drift is normal. Return is the skill.

Reflection

Life will always pull you off your plan. A sick child, a delayed train, a bad night of sleep, a stressful week — these are not failures. They're weather. A health plan that only works on perfect days is not a health plan; it's a fantasy.

What actually changes people over years is quieter: the ability to restart without drama. You don't fail when you drift. You fail when you decide the drift means, "I'm done."

A tiny correction — a 10-minute walk after a heavy meal, a real-food next meal after a detour, an earlier bedtime after a chaotic week — keeps your identity intact. You're not "off the rails." You're someone who comes back quickly. And that identity is gold.

Think of a compass. The needle trembles before it finds north — but it finds it. That's your job: don't panic when you wobble. Just return.

Here's the truth: your body doesn't need perfection. It needs your next honest step.

Real-life snapshot

Sara was doing well with her routine until life hit. A sick family member, a disrupted schedule, and two missed workouts later, she panicked. "I ruined my streak," she told her trainer.

He smiled and said, "Perfect streaks die. Flexible streaks live. Do a brisk 10-minute walk tonight — and the streak stays alive."

That night she walked. The next day she took her next honest step.
The win wasn't the workout. The win was the return.

Quick science

- Returning quickly ("never miss twice") keeps small slips from turning into full drop-offs.
- The brain rewards continuity and identity ("this is who I am") more than sporadic bursts of effort.
- Self-compassion — not self-punishment — predicts long-term habit adherence and emotional resilience.[6]

Inspiration note

Even the compass needle trembles before it finds north.

Today's Invitation

One thing I will do for myself today:

- ☐ Next cue reset: Choose your reset cue now (next meal, next hour, or tonight).
- ☐ Smallest version: Do the smallest version of the habit today (2 minutes counts).
- ☐ One correction: Make one tiny correction now (water, short walk, or lights down).

Action Step:
Choose the easiest one today. Do it now or set one reminder and do it when it best fits your schedule.

Reflection:
After I took the step today, I felt: ☐ calmer ☐ clearer ☐ steadier ☐ proud ☐ no change yet (effort still counts)

Bottom line

You don't fail when you drift — you only fail when you stop steering.

Your lines

(write one thought, one insight, or rewrite one sentence that rang true)

_____

_____

_____

☐ Done for today

Why this matters
Writing just a few lines by hand locks the concept into memory and gently primes your subconscious mind to adopt and act on it, leading to better recall and follow-through.

DAY 7

"A joyful heart is good medicine."
— Proverbs 17:22

Joy is not a luxury; it's one of your body's clearest signals that you are safe. A single real laugh can soften the sharp edges of an entire day. Protecting joy isn't childish — it's protecting your physiology.

Reflection

Choose joy on purpose. Joy isn't fluff; it's physiology. A real laugh loosens the jaw, lengthens the exhale, and tilts your chemistry toward health — lower stress signals, a quick lift in your natural painkillers (endorphins), and a steadier immune tone. In research settings, even short bursts of comedy — one funny clip or a few minutes of live laughter — have been linked with higher pain tolerance, which researchers often interpret as consistent with endorphin activity. Heartfelt laughter can lower perceived stress and may support healthier immune balance over time. It's also one of the fastest ways to tell your nervous system, "We can exhale." A looser body, a calmer edge, and an easier slide into sleep can follow.

Think of joy as sunlight through a window. The furniture doesn't move. The bills aren't paid. The diagnosis hasn't changed. But the light shifts the room — edges soften, colors return, and your body stops bracing quite so hard. That small shift is medicine: muscles uncoil, appetite steadies, sleep comes easier, and patience comes back online. Joy doesn't deny hardship; it simply refuses to let hardship be the only voice in the room.

Evenings are especially important. What you feed your nervous system after sunset sets the tone for sleep. Negative news at night primes fight-or-flight and raises stress hormones; your brain tries to sleep with the alarm still ringing. Swap that last hit of drama for something light — a bit of comedy, a warm conversation, a gentle show, a few minutes with a pet — and you give your system a softer landing into the night. Joy is not about pretending everything is fine. It's about giving your heart and nervous system a chance to breathe, so you have strength for whatever is real.

Real-life snapshot

Margaret was caring for her mom with dementia during a long, exhausting season. Meds. Appointments. Paperwork. Worry that never fully shut off. By night, she was so tired she couldn't relax — she just scrolled, stared, and replayed the day.

A friend gave her a simple rule: "One small dose of joy every evening. Five minutes. That's it."

So Margaret picked one tiny ritual: while the kettle heated, she watched one short comedy clip — nothing heavy, nothing dramatic. Some nights she didn't even laugh out loud. She just felt her shoulders drop a notch.

After a week, she noticed something surprising: her chest felt less tight at bedtime. Her sleep wasn't perfect, but it wasn't as brittle. And the next day, she had a little more patience — not because life got easier, but because her body stopped bracing every second.

Quick science

- Genuine laughter reduces stress hormones like cortisol and adrenaline while increasing endorphins, your body's natural pain-relieving and feel-good chemicals.
- Positive emotions briefly "broaden" attention, helping you think more flexibly and build emotional resilience over time.
- Evening emotional input strongly shapes sleep quality — lighter, warmer content supports better rest, while intense or negative input can delay sleep and fragment deep rest.[7]

Inspiration note

Joy doesn't fix everything — it helps you face everything.

Today's Invitation

One thing I will do for myself today:

- ☐ Tiny joy: Do 10 minutes of something light and fun (music, hobby, silly clip, game).
- ☐ Share warmth: Send one kind text/voice note or share one quick laugh.
- ☐ Smile on purpose: Watch one short funny clip and actually let yourself laugh.

Action Step:
Choose the easiest one today. Do it now or set one reminder and do it when it best fits your schedule.

Reflection:
After I took the step today, I felt: ☐ calmer ☐ clearer ☐ steadier ☐ proud ☐ no change yet (effort still counts)

Bottom line

A joyful heart doesn't ignore reality — it strengthens you to walk through it.

Your lines

(write one thought, one insight, or rewrite one sentence that rang true)

_____

_____

_____

☐ Done for today

Why this matters
Writing just a few lines by hand locks the concept into memory and gently primes your subconscious mind to adopt and act on it, leading to better recall and follow-through.

DAY 8

> "A man too busy to take care of his health is like a mechanic too busy to take care of his tools."
> — Spanish Proverb

Your body is the tool that builds every part of your life — guard it.
Neglect is cumulative; so is care.
Maintenance today prevents breakdown tomorrow.

Reflection

We clean and polish the car, mow the lawn, service the furnace, update the phone — yet often neglect the one tool that makes all of it possible: the body. Many people truly believe they are "too busy" for a walk, too stretched for an unhurried meal, too wired for sleep. But health does not pause because the calendar is full. The deeper truth is simple and uncomfortable: When you neglect the body long enough, it starts asking for attention in louder ways — not to punish you, but to protect you.

There is a painful unfairness here. Most people were never really shown the "owner's manual" for their body. No one explained why deep sleep is foundational repair time, how packaged and ultra-processed foods can add wear over time, or how something as ordinary as walking can support steadier blood sugar, a calmer mind, and a stronger heart. So when illness shows up and someone says, "Well, you haven't been doing X…," of course there is anger. In many cases, it was not conscious neglect. It was missing information mixed with modern busyness.

Still, the body quietly keeps score. Illness rarely appears out of nowhere. The cereal-or-bagel breakfast turns into years of blood sugar spikes and crashes. An ignored ache in the back becomes chronic pain. Late nights and shallow sleep accumulate into mood swings, memory lapses, and a brain that never feels fully "on." Small, daily wounds add up until one day the system finally says, "No more," and forces a stop. The hours we thought we saved show up later as waiting rooms, scan appointments, and pharmacy lines.

The hope is that maintenance takes far less time and drama than repair. Twenty minutes of daily movement and gentle stretching loosen stiff joints and oil the "hinges." A protein-rich, healthy-fat breakfast steadies blood sugar and appetite for hours. Even an extra hour of sleep can lower stress signaling and support clearer thinking and immune function. Small, faithful care compounds over time. Well-maintained tools last for decades. So do well-maintained bodies.

Real-life snapshot

Carlos and Stefan started a small lawn-care business together. Same clients, same equipment, same weather, same town. The only real difference was how they treated their tools — and themselves.

Carlos had a simple routine. At the end of each day he brushed grass off the mowers, wiped the blades, and checked for nicks. Once a week he sharpened blades, checked oil, and topped off fluids. His machines cut cleanly, started easily, and used less fuel. Jobs finished on time. Customers were happy. At some point, he noticed the parallel with his own body and quietly added a few "maintenance" steps: a 15-minute walk most days, a real breakfast, a bottle of water he actually finished, and a set bedtime on work nights.

Stefan was "too busy" for all that. He parked the mowers at the end of the day and left them caked with wet grass. He didn't check oil unless something smoked. Blades dulled and engines strained. Breakdowns began happening in the middle of jobs. Repairs and replacements ate into their profits. The stress from constant stop–start spilled into his habits: drive-thru meals, energy drinks, and late-night TV to "unwind." Sleep shrank. His back started to ache from wrestling half-broken machines around all day. He brushed it off and took more pills.

Ten years in, the contrast was stark. Carlos's equipment still ran smoothly, needing only routine service. His body held up — a bit older, but steady. Stefan's tools were constantly in the shop or being replaced. His blood pressure was up, his doctor was talking about prediabetes, and his back pain sometimes kept him off the job entirely.

"It's not fair," Stefan said once, looking at the bills on his desk. Carlos nodded gently. "It's not about fairness," he replied. "It's about maintenance. The tools you care for last. That includes us."

Quick science

- Your body responds to what you repeat. Small daily stressors (short sleep, sitting, ultra-processed food, chronic stress) add up into cumulative "wear and tear" — higher blood pressure, worse insulin sensitivity, and more inflammation over time.
- The maintenance levers can work surprisingly fast. Even small upgrades — a consistent sleep window, a short daily walk (especially after meals), and one real-food meal — can improve next-day energy and help flatten glucose spikes over time.

- Habits beat willpower. When a health action is attached to a cue ("after dinner, I walk 10 minutes"), the brain runs it more automatically, reducing decision fatigue and increasing follow-through.[93]

Inspiration note

The world sees the performance; your body remembers the maintenance.

Today's Invitation

One thing I will do for myself today:

- ☐ One small maintenance: Do one quick care task today (stretch, floss, or prep a real meal).
- ☐ Move the hinges: Take 10 minutes to move your joints (walk, mobility, or gentle strength).
- ☐ Prevent future hassle: Schedule one prevention step (refill, checkup, or a future appointment).

Action Step:
Choose the easiest one today. Do it now or set one reminder and do it when it best fits your schedule.

Reflection:
After I took the step today, I felt: ☐ calmer ☐ clearer ☐ steadier ☐ proud ☐ no change yet (effort still counts)

Bottom line

Maintain your body the way you maintain what you depend on — because you depend on it most.

Your lines

(write one thought, one insight, or rewrite one sentence that rang true)

_____

_____

_____

☐ Done for today

Why this matters
Writing just a few lines by hand locks the concept into memory and gently primes your subconscious mind to adopt and act on it, leading to better recall and follow-through.

DAY 9

"Hydration is the secret edge."
— A. Smyrlis, MD

Dehydration disguises itself as fatigue, fog, and cravings.
Water is the cheapest performance enhancer you'll ever use.
Tiny sips, repeated often, quietly change your whole day.

Reflection

We underestimate water because it is simple. It has no label, no hype, and no flavor — so we assume it can't be the missing piece. But many of the things you want from a day — clear thinking, a steadier mood, better workouts, and calmer cravings — depend on whether your cells are well hydrated.

Dehydration doesn't always look dramatic. It often feels like small things: a heavy head, "tip-of-the-tongue" word searching, irritability, mid-afternoon yawns, a workout that never quite lifts off, an odd pull toward sugar or coffee you can't explain. The fix isn't another stimulant or snack. Most of the time, it's water — clean, consistent, enough.

How much is "enough"? There's no perfect number for everyone. A simple starting point for many adults is about 6–8 cups of water per day, then adjust based on thirst, heat/exercise, and urine color (aim for pale yellow). If you've been told to limit fluids (for example, in heart failure or kidney disease), follow your clinician's plan.

One glass matters more than the rest, though: the **first** one after you wake. Overnight you lose water through your breath and skin. Drinking before email, before coffee, before anything else is like priming the pump for the whole day.

Purity matters too. Tap quality varies. If possible, choose natural spring water or use a good filter — and change the filters on time. Carry water in glass or stainless steel rather than plastic, especially away from heat. If plain water feels boring, brighten it with lemon, cucumber, or herbal tea.

Spread your intake through the day; chugging a huge amount at once mostly sends you to the restroom while your cells stay thirsty. Hydration isn't a one-time event; it's a quiet rhythm.

Real-life snapshot

Naomi and Jess were college teammates on the same soccer team. Same practices, same travel, same classes. By mid-season, they felt very different.

Naomi was talented but dragging. By afternoon she fought heavy eyelids in lecture, grabbed vending-machine sugar, and hit practice already depleted. Halfway through drills her legs felt like wet cement. She kept telling herself she needed a stronger pre-workout — or more willpower.

Jess wasn't perfect, but she was steady. She recovered faster after games and stayed sharper in class. On a long bus ride to an away match, Naomi finally asked, "Okay — what are you taking? What's the secret?"

Jess laughed and tapped the big stainless-steel bottle at her feet. "Honestly? Mostly this. Coach told me freshman year: 'You can't play well if you're dried out.' So I started treating water like part of training."

Her system was simple: one full glass on waking, one bottle finished by lunch, another by late afternoon, and a small glass with dinner. No fancy powders. Just steady sips.

Naomi copied it for two weeks. The change surprised her. Afternoon headaches eased. Cravings softened. Practice stopped feeling like she was fighting her own body.

"I kept trying to upgrade everything," she said later—"my gear, my supplements, my snacks. The real upgrade was water, on purpose."

Quick science

- Even mild dehydration (1–2% loss of body weight in water) can impair attention, memory, and mood — you feel more tired, scattered, and irritable.
- Adequate hydration supports blood volume and circulation, helps regulate body temperature during activity, and reduces perceived exertion in workouts.
- Staying well hydrated supports kidney function, helps regulate blood pressure, and assists the body's natural detox and repair processes.[9]

Inspiration note

Hydration is a quiet habit with loud benefits.

Today's Invitation

One thing I will do for myself today:

- ☐ First glass: Drink a full glass of water soon after waking.
- ☐ Make it visible: Put a bottle where you'll see it and finish it by midday.
- ☐ Simple cue: Drink a glass of water before one meal today.

Action Step:
Choose the easiest one today. Do it now or set one reminder and do it when it best fits your schedule.

Reflection:
After I took the step today, I felt: ☐ calmer ☐ clearer ☐ steadier ☐ proud ☐ no change yet (effort still counts)

Bottom line

Sometimes the missing upgrade is just a glass of water.

Your lines

(write one thought, one insight, or rewrite one sentence that rang true)

_____

_____

_____

☐ Done for today

Why this matters

Writing just a few lines by hand locks the concept into memory and gently primes your subconscious mind to adopt and act on it, leading to better recall and follow-through.

DAY 10

> **"Simplicity is the ultimate sophistication."**
> — Leonardo da Vinci

Clarity grows when you remove what drains you.
Simplicity frees the mind to notice what actually matters.
The body performs best when the signals are few and clear.

Reflection

Simplicity is not small; it is sharp. Your body thrives on clear signals: real food, deep rest, honest work, warm connection. Complexity scatters attention and frays the nerves. Simplicity gathers your strength and points it in one direction.

Imagine each day as a single circle. The upper half is output: hours of action, service, focus. The lower half is restoration: sleep, nourishment, quiet, unhurried joy and relaxation. When the top half steals from the bottom — late nights, extra tasks, constant scrolling — tomorrow shows up underpowered. When the halves meet cleanly, your days start to feel strong instead of scrambled. Sophistication is often subtraction. Remove the extras and what remains is signal — meals that look like ingredients, work with a clear finish line, evenings that dim on purpose. Keep the rhythm simple: fill up, pour out, refill. In my view, living your days in these simple circles is the hidden operating system of health — work, recover, repeat. And if you're a high performer, the very same pattern is what makes true, sustainable performance possible — not one more hack or push, but a cleaner rhythm of work and restoration.

So cut to the core. Do the vital few, protect the nightly half, and let the circle repeat. Over time, simplicity stops feeling like sacrifice and starts feeling like strength.

Real-life snapshot

Rhea lived in constant overwhelm — crowded calendar, full inbox, chaotic meals, late nights. She was trying to "do it all," and felt like she was failing at all of it. Her therapist gave her a simple assignment: subtract one thing each day.

First she deleted late-night scrolling and plugged her phone in across the room. Then she simplified breakfast to the same easy, balanced meal every morning. She dimmed lights after sunset, set a rough 12/12 rhythm — about 12 hours 'on,' and 12 hours winding down and sleeping — and stopped saying yes to every evening plan.

Within two weeks she felt calmer, slept deeper, and stopped craving sugar at night. Her to-do list was still real, but no longer endless. "Life didn't suddenly get easier," she said. "It just got simpler — and that made it feel lighter."

Quick science

- Reducing mental and digital clutter lowers stress hormones like cortisol and can improve focus and decision-making.
- Predictable daily rhythms (similar wake, eat, and sleep times) strengthen your circadian clock, which supports energy, mood, and hormones.
- Light patterns matter: bright light in the morning and dim, warm light at night strongly influence sleep quality and timing.[10]

Inspiration note

Simplicity is strength without noise.

Today's Invitation

One thing I will do for myself today:

- ☐ One Big Thing: Write your One Big Thing for today on paper.
- ☐ Park the phone: Put your phone in one place for a set window (first 30 minutes or one meal).
- ☐ 5-minute reset: Clear one small surface and prep one "tomorrow helper" (water/clothes/breakfast).

Action Step:
Choose the easiest one today. Do it now or set one reminder and do it when it best fits your schedule.

Reflection:
After I took the step today, I felt: ☐ calmer ☐ clearer ☐ steadier ☐ proud ☐ no change yet (effort still counts)

Bottom line

Simplify the day, and your biology quietly follows.

Your lines

(write one thought, one insight, or rewrite one sentence that rang true)

_____

_____

_____

☐ Done for today

Why this matters
Writing just a few lines by hand locks the concept into memory and gently primes your subconscious mind to adopt and act on it, leading to better recall and follow-through.

DAY 11

"What gets measured gets improved."
— A. Smyrlis, MD

A streak turns hope into momentum.
What you see, you shape.
The right numbers become a compass, not a cage.

Reflection

An athlete would never try to compete without tracking performance. They count laps, log splits, measure strength, time recovery. Not because they're obsessive, but because feedback tells them what's working. Your health is no different.

Most of us guess. We tell ourselves, "I sleep okay. I move enough. I don't work that much." Then a week of honest numbers lands, and the story changes. Sleep turns out to be closer to six hours than eight. Steps drift closer to three thousand than ten. Work stretches to ten or eleven hours, not eight. The reality may not be what you hoped for, but at least it's solid ground.

You don't need to track everything. In fact, you shouldn't. A handful of well-chosen numbers is plenty. For some people, that's counting steps or minutes of movement. For others, it's noticing how many hours they're actually in bed, or checking blood pressure at home a few times a week. If blood sugar is an issue, an occasional reading before and after certain meals can be enough to see a pattern. Even something as simple as jotting down weekly work hours can reveal why your body feels the way it does.

Think of numbers as mirrors, not judges. The goal isn't perfection; it's awareness. Once you see the pattern, you can change it — and your doctor can help you adjust treatment based on reality, not guesswork or one rushed reading in the office.

Then there are streaks. Scoreboards change behavior. When the score is visible, effort improves. A streak turns "I should" into "I do." One small action, one visible mark, repeated. The chain becomes something you can feel.

Keep your streak tiny and winnable. Choose one keystone habit — the kind of change that quietly supports everything else. It might be a fixed wake time. It might be a ten-minute walk after your largest meal. It might be a protein-anchored breakfast that steadies your day, or taking your home blood pressure at the same time on several days of the week. Make the version so small you can do it even on your worst day. Winnable is sustainable.

Once you've chosen it, give it a simple scoreboard. A pen and paper grid on the fridge. A tiny calendar by your bed. Every checked box is a vote for a new identity: "I'm someone who does this, every day." Over time, the streak gathers gravity. On days when motivation is thin, the chain itself pulls you forward.

Start small. Measure what matters. Make it visible. Protect the chain.

Real-life snapshot

Lena's blood pressure was "always high" at the doctor's office. Every visit, the cuff reading crept up. Her medication dose went up too. At home, she often felt weak, lightheaded, and more tired than before treatment.

One clinician finally asked, "Do you ever check it at home?" She didn't. They suggested a good home monitor and a simple plan: measure at the same times on several days — sitting, relaxed, no caffeine right before — and write the numbers down.

The pattern surprised her. Most mornings and evenings at home, her blood pressure was close to normal. But the day after takeout Chinese food, her reading jumped by ~10–20 points. The same thing happened after a night out with friends and several drinks. She hadn't seen the link because she was only looking at office readings and vague memories. The numbers told a clearer story.

She made two changes: she cut way back on salty takeout and heavy restaurant meals, and she reduced alcohol. Then she brought three weeks of home readings to her next appointment. With real data in front of them, her doctor saw that her pressure was often overtreated between visits. They safely lowered her medication dose and focused more on lifestyle.

Within weeks, the dizziness and fatigue eased. Her blood pressure stayed in a healthier range most days — without feeling like she was walking through mud.

"It wasn't just the medicine," she said. "It was finally measuring the right things and seeing what my choices actually did."

Quick science

- Visible tracking increases follow-through because progress is motivating.
- Home blood pressure monitoring, when done correctly, improves diagnosis and management of hypertension and helps avoid both under- and overtreatment.

- Small, repeated actions build neural efficiency and strengthen identity-linked behavior ("I'm someone who walks / measures / cares for my health"), making future healthy choices easier.[11]

Inspiration note

Consistency is built one honest square — and one honest number — at a time.

Today's Invitation

One thing I will do for myself today:

- ☐ Track one thing: Track one simple marker today (sleep window, steps, or a habit streak).
- ☐ Keep it simple: Log one quick note that helps you learn (mood/energy after a meal or walk).
- ☐ Mark the chain: Add one check mark to your streak grid today.

Action Step:
Choose the easiest one today. Do it now or set one reminder and do it when it best fits your schedule.

Reflection:
After I took the step today, I felt: ☐ calmer ☐ clearer ☐ steadier ☐ proud ☐ no change yet (effort still counts)

Bottom line

Small wins stack. Visible wins stick. Measure what matters, protect the chain, and the chain will start to protect you.

Your lines

(write one thought, one insight, or rewrite one sentence that rang true)

_____
_____
_____

☐ Done for today

Why this matters
Writing just a few lines by hand locks the concept into memory and gently primes your subconscious mind to adopt and act on it, leading to better recall and follow-through.

DAY 12

> **"No man is an island, entire of itself."**
> — John Donne

True connection is not a bonus — it's basic human infrastructure. Your body relaxes when you know you don't carry life alone. Community turns "getting through the day" into "being held in it."

Reflection

In the longest-lived communities on earth — the so-called "Blue Zones" of Okinawa, Ikaria, Sardinia, Nicoya, and Loma Linda — people don't just eat differently or move more. They belong differently. Neighbors check on each other. Meals are shared. Elders are woven into family life instead of left on the margins. Problems still exist — money worries, health scares, disagreements — but underneath them runs a steady current: I am not alone in this.

That sense of "I am held here" is not sentimental; it is biological. Strong social connection consistently lowers the risk of death and serious illness. Loneliness and isolation, by contrast, are linked to higher rates of heart disease, stroke, depression, dementia, and earlier death. Some researchers estimate that lacking social connection can carry a mortality impact comparable to smoking up to 15 cigarettes a day.

For most of human history, multigenerational families and tightly knit villages were the norm. You grew up with grandparents in the house or nearby. You knew who to call when something broke — or when you did. Modern life has given us more freedom and more options, but it has also scattered us. Many of us have networks, not communities — dozens of contacts and followers, but very few people who know our story well enough to notice when we go quiet. That gap shows up in the body as tension, hypervigilance, and a background hum of "I'm on my own."

Rebuilding connection doesn't mean surrounding yourself with people 24/7. Healthy connection is always balanced with healthy solitude. It means having a small circle you can rely on and spaces where you belong: a faith community, a book club, a walking group, a choir, a volunteer team, a neighborhood dinner, even a regular table at the same café where people know your name. In some places, such circles are formalized — like the Okinawan moai, small groups that meet regularly and support each other for life. You can create your own modern version.

Connection does not erase your responsibilities or solve every problem. But it spreads the weight. It turns "my burden" into "our burden." Your nervous system feels the difference. In a connected life, you still face storms, but there are more hands on the ropes.

Real-life snapshot

When Elena turned 62, her lab results weren't terrible — just "borderline" in too many areas: blood pressure a little high, blood sugar drifting up, sleep light and broken. What bothered her most wasn't the numbers; it was the emptiness. Her children lived in other states. Her days were quiet. Most of her conversations were with cashiers and the TV.

Her clinician asked a simple question: "Who do you feel you belong with?" The answer made her throat tighten: "No one, really." Together they made a different kind of plan — not another supplement, but community as medicine. She tried three small steps: she stayed for coffee at a local church, joined a weekly library book club, and invited a neighbor for tea once a month.

The first few weeks felt awkward. She almost didn't go. But she kept showing up. People at church started greeting her by name. The book club gave structure to her week and something to look forward to. Her neighbor turned out to love gardening, and they began trading seeds and stories.

Six months later, her repeat labs had improved modestly. More striking was how she described her days: "I still have my own problems," she said, "but I don't feel like I'm carrying them alone. There are people who would notice if I didn't show up. That changes how I sleep at night."

Quick science

- Strong social connection and community involvement are linked with lower risk of death from many causes and better heart health.
- Feelings of belonging and being cared for reduce stress hormones and support better immune function.
- Loneliness and social isolation increase risk for depression, anxiety, cognitive decline, and early death — as harmful as some major physical risk factors when they are chronic.[12]

Inspiration note

Belonging is a nutrient — a small, steady circle can feed a very long life.

Today's Invitation

One thing I will do for myself today:

- ☐ Reach out: Contact one person today (text, call, or voice note).
- ☐ Shared space: Take one small step toward a place you belong (pick it, look it up, or RSVP).
- ☐ One together moment: Share one meal or one walk with someone (or schedule it).

Action Step:
Choose the easiest one today. Do it now or set one reminder and do it when it best fits your schedule.

Reflection:
After I took the step today, I felt: ☐ calmer ☐ clearer ☐ steadier ☐ proud ☐ no change yet (effort still counts)

Bottom line

Isolation is a real health risk. You don't need a crowd — you need a few people and a place where you truly belong.

Your lines

(write one thought, one insight, or rewrite one sentence that rang true)

_____

_____

_____

☐ Done for today

Why this matters
Writing just a few lines by hand locks the concept into memory and gently primes your subconscious mind to adopt and act on it, leading to better recall and follow-through.

DAY 13

"Only the dose makes the poison."
— Paracelsus

Almost nothing in health is all good or all bad — context is everything. Dose, timing, and quality decide whether something heals or harms. Wisdom is learning to ask, "What's the net effect for me?"

Reflection

Think in net positive. Most people think in labels: "This food is good." "That habit is bad." It feels simple, but it's not how biology works. Your body thinks in dose, frequency, timing, quality, and you. The same thing can be medicine at one dose and poison at another.

Take fruit. Whole fruit comes packaged with fiber and water — for most people, net positive. But when fruit turns into an all-day sugar stream (giant bowls of very sweet fruit, juice, and dried fruit), the math can flip. For many, 2–3 servings of whole fruit a day — with berries and lower-sugar options most often — is a strong middle.

Caffeine is another example. In the right dose, it can sharpen focus and lift mood — net positive. In the wrong dose, or too late in the day, it can flip: more anxiety, a racing mind, lighter sleep. For many people, caffeine works best earlier, in a modest amount, and after some food — not as an all-day drip.

Movement follows the same law. Regular, moderate exercise is profoundly net positive: lower blood pressure, better mood and sleep, stronger bones and brain, better metabolic health. Too much, too hard, too often, with too little recovery, can go net negative — think fractures, overtraining, stubborn insomnia, and crashes. The "right" amount isn't what looks good on paper; it's what you can recover from consistently.

Here's the lens for almost any health decision: How much? How often? When? What form? And how does my body respond right now?

Flexible thinkers stay healthier longer. Nothing is only upside or only downside. The art is in the net.

Real-life snapshot

Sophie had decided that "carbs are bad." She cut them almost completely. No bread, no rice, no fruit, no potatoes. At first the scale moved, and she felt proud. But as weeks turned into months, something cracked. She was constantly exhausted, craving sugar at night, and "falling off" on weekends — eating big bowls of sweets and ultra-processed snacks in secret, then swinging back to restriction on Monday.

Her clinician invited her to use a different lens. "Let's stop calling carbs 'good' or 'bad' for a moment," she said. "Let's ask: When, how much, and which kinds help your body — and when do they hurt it?"

They made a new plan. She brought back whole-food carbohydrates — oats, beans, lentils, quinoa, potatoes, and fruit — in small to moderate portions. She placed most of them after real effort, like a workout or long walk, when her body could use them well. Refined sweets became occasional treats instead of nightly coping. And she anchored each meal with protein and fiber to steady her blood sugar. She didn't go "high-carb." She went targeted-carb.

Within a few weeks, her evening binges faded. Her energy stabilized. Her workouts felt stronger. Lab work showed better fasting glucose and more stable lipids. "It wasn't the carbs," she said. "It was the dose, the timing, and the type. Once I stopped fearing all of them and used them wisely, everything got easier."

Quick science

- Many essential substances — including water, vitamins, and minerals — have a therapeutic window: too little causes deficiency, too much causes toxicity.
- Exercise often follows a J-shaped curve: too little or too much both increase risk; consistent, moderate-to-vigorous activity in the middle zone is protective.
- Toxicity from many environmental and dietary exposures is often a function of dose × chronicity — not mere existence. A small, rare exposure may be trivial; small doses every day for years are where problems arise.[13]

Inspiration note

Balance is less about avoiding things and more about asking better questions.

Today's Invitation

One thing I will do for myself today:

- ☐ Choose one dial: Keep one thing moderate today (portion, caffeine, screens, or intensity).
- ☐ Ask before: Before you do it, ask: how much — and how often?
- ☐ Adjust for today: Match the dose to your current sleep/stress/energy (smaller still counts).

Action Step:
Choose the easiest one today. Do it now or set one reminder and do it when it best fits your schedule.

Reflection:
After I took the step today, I felt: ☐ calmer ☐ clearer ☐ steadier ☐ proud ☐ no change yet (effort still counts)

Bottom line

Whether something is poison or medicine often lies not in what it is, but in how — and how much — you use it.

Your lines

(write one thought, one insight, or rewrite one sentence that rang true)

_____

_____

_____

☐ Done for today

Why this matters

Writing just a few lines by hand locks the concept into memory and gently primes your subconscious mind to adopt and act on it, leading to better recall and follow-through.

DAY 14

"Every human being is the author of his own health or disease."
— Swami Sivananda

You're holding the pen, whether you realize it or not.
Every choice is a sentence in the story of your health.
When you change the script, your body rewrites the ending.

Reflection

It's a hard truth to swallow — especially when you're already struggling. We inherit genes. We face real stress. And many things happen that we did not choose. But within all of that, we still have real influence over how we respond day after day. Some circumstances are not chosen, and this is never about shame — it's about reclaiming the small levers you still have.

It's often not the stressful event itself that does the most damage; it's the chain reaction that follows. After a hard moment, do you step outside for a 10-minute walk and a few slow breaths — or do you reach for a cigarette, a sugary snack, or a double drink? When you're tired, do you push bedtime later and scroll — or do you protect sleep so tomorrow has a chance? Each response is a sentence in the story of your health.

Genes aren't a fixed sentence. They're more like a script with many possible directions. Epigenetics shows that sleep, food, stress, and movement can turn certain genes up or down. You may have inherited higher risk for diabetes, heart disease, or depression — but you also inherited patterns of living: a bread-and-pasta table, a culture of no movement, a habit of ignoring sleep. Often it's the shared habits, not just the shared DNA, that carry the bigger weight.

This is not about blame. It is about power. To know you are the author means you can revise the story. The plate can hold vegetables, protein, and healthy fats instead of crackers and sweets. The evening can close with a wind-down routine instead of endless scrolling. The morning can begin with water and a short walk instead of a frantic rush.

Most outcomes build quietly. One choice won't save you or sink you. But repeated choices become chapters. The pen is in your hand. The question is not whether you're writing — but what kind of story your days are writing now.

Real-life snapshot

Carlos grew up in a family "doomed" to diabetes and heart disease. The story was told at every holiday: "In this family, everyone ends up on meds." His uncle had a heart attack in his 50s, his mother took insulin, and his older cousin was already on three blood pressure pills.

By 45, Carlos's labs began to match the family script: rising fasting glucose, higher A1c, borderline blood pressure, triglycerides climbing. His cousin shrugged and said, "See? It's in our genes. Nothing you can do." He accepted more medications as just "the way it is," while keeping the same habits: big plates of white rice and bread, no real exercise, late-night snacking, and very little sleep. Over the next few years his doses went up, his waist grew, and his energy fell. The story continued, line by line.

Carlos felt the same fear, but something in him rebelled against the idea that nothing could change. At one appointment, his clinician said, "Your genes may load the gun, but your daily choices decide how often the trigger gets pulled." That image stuck.

He decided to co-author a new chapter. Nothing extreme — just a different script, repeated: a 20-minute walk most days (especially after dinner), swapping most white bread, rice, and sugary drinks for whole foods and water, earlier bedtimes with a simple wind-down routine, and a weekly grocery list so he wasn't living off last-minute takeout.

One year later, his follow-up told a different story: his blood sugar had moved toward normal, his blood pressure had improved, his triglycerides were down, and his energy was back. With his clinician's guidance, some medications were able to be reduced instead of increased.

Quick science

- Epigenetic mechanisms (like DNA methylation and histone modification) respond to lifestyle inputs — sleep, food, stress, and movement can literally change how certain genes are expressed.
- Consistent changes in diet and activity may reverse early insulin resistance in many people (even with a strong family history) and improve lipid patterns, reducing the risk of type 2 diabetes and heart disease.
- Regular movement and balanced nutrition lower the risk of many so-called "genetic" diseases by shifting gene expression and reducing chronic inflammation.[14]

Inspiration note

You don't need a new life. You need a new line. One small choice today is a pen stroke — and pen strokes become chapters. Keep writing. Your body will follow the story you repeat.

Today's Invitation

One thing I will do for myself today:

- ☐ One better default: Take 5 slow breaths before you react to stress today.
- ☐ One body vote: Do one simple action (10-minute walk, 10 minutes strength, or a real-food meal).
- ☐ One input upgrade: Improve one input today (earlier dinner, fewer late screens, or more water).

Action Step:
Choose the easiest one today. Do it now or set one reminder and do it when it best fits your schedule.

Reflection:
After I took the step today, I felt: ☐ calmer ☐ clearer ☐ steadier ☐ proud ☐ no change yet (effort still counts)

Bottom line

You are not stuck with the script you inherited — you are still writing.

Your lines

(write one thought, one insight, or rewrite one sentence that rang true)

_____

_____

_____

☐ Done for today

Why this matters
Writing just a few lines by hand locks the concept into memory and gently primes your subconscious mind to adopt and act on it, leading to better recall and follow-through.

DAY 15

"Slow fuels carry you; fast fuels drop you."
— A. Smyrlis, MD

Your fuel sets your rhythm.
Slow inputs steady the day; fast inputs steal it back in crashes.
Build your day on foods that last, not foods that lunge.

Reflection

Your brain is a demanding organ. It burns a lot of energy and is picky about how it receives it. Food isn't just fuel and building blocks — it's instruction. Every bite tells your body how quickly to burn, how steadily to focus, and how evenly to feel. Your brain and adrenals work best on slow, steady signals: protein for the brain chemicals that support focus and mood, and for steadier stress signals; fiber and intact carbohydrates for gradual, even glucose; natural fats to keep energy and mood from swinging.

Fast fuels — coffee latte on an empty stomach, pastries, sugary cereals, juice, candy "energy" bars, instant oats — hit hard and drop fast. You feel sharp, then shaky. Motivated, then moody. Hungry again long before you should be. The brain gets a sugar-and-adrenaline blast, then fumes. That pattern doesn't just harm long-term health; it sabotages your day. It trains your biology to crave constant stimulation instead of learning how to sustain itself.

Slow fuels tell a different story.

A protein-anchored breakfast with fiber and color sends a message of stability: a gentler rise in blood sugar, a slower, smoother fall, fewer cravings and less 10 a.m. desperation. Think: eggs, Greek yogurt, nuts or seeds, steel-cut oats, berries, vegetables, whole-grain toast with nut butter — plus tea or moderate coffee with food, not as your only intake. Less fireworks. More sunrise. Gradual, even, reliable. Your brain loves steady fuel. Your mood loves it even more.

Real-life snapshot

Dan started most days with an espresso and a pastry on the way to work. By 10 a.m., his brain felt like a pinball machine — racing thoughts, sugar cravings, and a shorter fuse in meetings. By 3 p.m., he was wiped out and hunting for snacks, then somehow wired again at night.

On his clinician's suggestion, he ran a simple "slow-fuel" experiment for one week. He ate a real breakfast — eggs with oats and berries — and had his caffeine with food, not as his only intake. At lunch, he chose protein and fiber (chicken and salad, or beans and vegetables) instead of a grab-and-go slice and soda. And after lunch, he took a 10-minute walk.

The first few days felt strange — fewer fireworks. But within a week he noticed something new: his focus lasted longer, his email tone softened, the 3 p.m. crash faded, and he didn't need as much coffee.

"Same job, same hours," he said. "Different fuel. It's like my brain finally had a steady power line instead of a series of surges."

Quick science

- Protein and healthy fats slow stomach emptying, which smooths the rise and fall of blood sugar and provides amino acids for neurotransmitters (brain chemicals) that regulate mood and focus.
- Refined sugars and ultra-processed breakfast foods (cereals, pastries, bars, juices) spike blood glucose quickly, followed by a crash that drives cravings, brain fog, and irritability.
- Tea's L-theanine can soften the edges of caffeine and support calm alertness compared with high-dose coffee on an empty stomach.[15]

Inspiration note

Marathoners don't win on candy — they win on pacing. Slow fuels don't slow you down. They help you last.

Today's Invitation

One thing I will do for myself today:

- ☐ Build a steady breakfast: Add a real protein anchor (eggs, yogurt, beans, or leftovers).
- ☐ Caffeine after calories: Have your coffee/tea after you've eaten something.
- ☐ Color + fiber add-on: Add one handful of berries or veggies to a meal today.

Action Step:
Choose the easiest one today. Do it now or set one reminder and do it when it best fits your schedule.

Reflection:
After I took the step today, I felt: ☐ calmer ☐ clearer ☐ steadier ☐ proud ☐ no change yet (effort still counts)

Bottom line

Build your day on slow inputs if you want steady, stable output. Change the fuel, and your brain's rhythm will follow.

Your lines

(write one thought, one insight, or rewrite one sentence that rang true)

_____
_____
_____

☐ Done for today

Why this matters
Writing just a few lines by hand locks the concept into memory and gently primes your subconscious mind to adopt and act on it, leading to better recall and follow-through.

DAY 16

"Stuck? Downshift with your breath."
— A. Smyrlis, MD

A restless mind needs a gentler gear.
Slow breath is that gear.
Shift down, and the whole system follows.

Reflection

When your mind feels jammed — anxious, overwhelmed, spinning in place — the instinct is usually to push harder. It's like a car stuck in mud: you slam the gas, the wheels spin faster, and you only dig in deeper. The real move isn't more force; it's a downshift. Ease off, drop into a lower gear, rock gently, and suddenly the car climbs free.

Your breath is that lower gear. Fast, shallow breathing is like flooring the accelerator: heart rate climbs, muscles tighten, thoughts scatter. Slow, nasal breathing with a longer exhale is the brake — the parasympathetic cue that says, "You're safe. You can think again." This isn't philosophy; it's wiring. Your breath talks directly to your brain.

One minute of intentional breathing can change your internal weather. Muscles soften. Vision widens. Thoughts line up. Emotions regain their edges instead of spilling everywhere. You haven't solved every problem — but you've changed the state of the driver.

Babies do this instinctively. Watch a baby self-soothe — two small inhales, one long, sighing exhale. That "physiological sigh" is built into us from birth. We're born knowing the brake; adulthood just buries it under noise.

Breathing is not a "soft" skill. It is a high-performance skill — a lever for clarity, focus, safety, and sleep. Learn your gears, and the road feels different.

Real-life snapshot

On most mornings, Elena sat in her car outside the clinic, heart already racing. She'd scroll her email, feel her chest tighten, then walk in braced for the day. By noon, she was snappy with staff and patients, then guilty on the drive home.

One colleague mentioned a one-minute "breathing stoplight" she used before walking through the door. Elena tried it: park, phone face-down, inhale for 4 seconds, exhale for 6, repeat until one minute passed. No fixing the whole day, just arriving differently.

Within a week, she noticed she wasn't exploding at small delays. Her voice sounded calmer on the phone. She started using the same pattern before difficult conversations and again before bed. "The problems didn't vanish," she said, "but I finally had a way to turn down the volume inside before I walked into them."

Quick science

- Longer exhales increase vagal tone and help downshift the fight-or-flight response.
- Slow, nasal breathing can raise heart rate variability (HRV) — a marker of resilience — and sharpen focus.
- The "physiological sigh" (two inhales followed by one long exhale) has been shown to quickly reduce anxiety and ease shortness of breath.[16]

Inspiration note

Your body comes with a built-in brake — you just have to use it.

Today's Invitation

One thing I will do for myself today:

- ☐ One minute downshift: Do one minute of slow nasal breathing with longer exhales.
- ☐ Three sighs: Do 3 physiological sighs when you feel tense (two inhales, one long exhale).
- ☐ Use it before: Do it before bed or before one hard conversation (state first, then words).

Action Step:
Choose the easiest one today. Do it now or set one reminder and do it when it best fits your schedule.

Reflection:
After I took the step today, I felt: ☐ calmer ☐ clearer ☐ steadier ☐ proud ☐ no change yet (effort still counts)

Bottom line

Breathe on purpose. Your breath is a steering wheel — choose the gear your moment needs.

Your lines

(write one thought, one insight, or rewrite one sentence that rang true)

_____

_____

_____

☐ Done for today

Why this matters
Writing just a few lines by hand locks the concept into memory and gently primes your subconscious mind to adopt and act on it, leading to better recall and follow-through.

DAY 17

"Hold the line; loosen the grip."
— A. Smyrlis, MD

Strength is not rigidity — it's flexibility with direction.
When life pulls, you can bend without breaking.
You don't have to abandon the goal to adjust the plan.

Reflection

Rigid things snap. Elastic things hold. A lot of people don't fail because their goal was wrong. They fail because their plan was too rigid. They grip so tightly to one version of success that the first disruption — a sick child, a late shift, a trip, a stressful week — shatters the whole routine.

All-or-nothing thinking sounds like this: "I missed a day, so the week is ruined." "I'm traveling, so I'll restart next month." "I couldn't do the full workout, so I did nothing." Real life never matches the script. But goals don't need perfect scripts — they need elastic systems.

Think of fishing: you don't land a strong fish by yanking the line. You keep steady tension, play the pull, give when it surges, reel when it softens. Too tight, and the line snaps. Too loose, and the fish is gone. The art is in the balance.

Your habits need the same give-and-take. Flexibility is not weakness — it is durability. It's the difference between someone who exercises for three weeks and someone who exercises for thirty years. It's the skill of staying in motion when life gets inconvenient, messy, or unpredictable.

Flexibility doesn't mean "anything goes." It means the direction stays, even if the route changes. You keep faith with the goal — better sleep, stronger body, calmer mind — while letting the daily plan bend to reality instead of breaking against it.

Real-life snapshot

Ravi aimed for five workouts a week. Then travel blew up his schedule. Instead of throwing the whole month away, he shifted to an elastic plan: three full sessions when home; on the road, short hotel circuits and brisk walks. Six weeks later, he had more total workouts than before — because flexibility kept him in the game.

Ana, a new parent, watched her old routine evaporate. Instead of collapsing into frustration, she wrote her A/B/C list:

- Plan A: 40-minute lift.
- Plan B: 20-minute kettlebell session + a short walk.
- Plan C: 2-minute micros — a stroller loop, five wall push-ups while coffee brews, two stretches while rocking the baby.

She adopted the 85% rule: good enough counts. Eight weeks later, she hadn't lost strength — she'd gained consistency.

Both Ravi and Ana stayed on track not by being rigid, but by refusing to quit when life pulled them sideways. Their identity stayed intact because their plans could bend.

Quick science

- Psychological flexibility is linked to lower distress, better health behaviors, and higher persistence.
- Self-compassion after slips increases adherence far more than self-criticism.
- "If–then" backup plans (Plan B, Plan C) keep habits alive in unpredictable weeks.[17]

Inspiration note

You don't need perfect conditions — you need an elastic strategy that survives real life.

Today's Invitation

One thing I will do for myself today:

- ☐ Plan B now: Choose your Plan B version (the shortened version that still counts).
- ☐ Keep it alive: Do a 2–10 minute "some is better than none" version today.
- ☐ One kind reset line: Say it once after a slip: Back on track at the next cue.

Action Step:
Choose the easiest one today. Do it now or set one reminder and do it when it best fits your schedule.

Reflection:
After I took the step today, I felt: ☐ calmer ☐ clearer ☐ steadier ☐ proud ☐ no change yet (effort still counts)

Bottom line

Bend so you don't break. Flexibility keeps the goal alive when life changes the weather.

Your lines

(write one thought, one insight, or rewrite one sentence that rang true)

_____
_____
_____

☐ Done for today

Why this matters
Writing just a few lines by hand locks the concept into memory and gently primes your subconscious mind to adopt and act on it, leading to better recall and follow-through.

DAY 18

> "Overdrive feels powerful — until the engine runs dry."
> — A. Smyrlis, MD

Hustle can look like strength while it quietly empties you.
Your body keeps a score your résumé can't hide.
Real power is effort with rhythm, not effort without rest.

Reflection

Overdrive feels heroic at first. Early alarms, late emails, workouts squeezed into the edges. People admire the grind, and for a while, you admire it too. It feels like proof of discipline, proof of worth, proof that you can take on more than the next person.

But inside the body, a different story begins to unfold.

Running hot all the time keeps your nervous system in a constant state of readiness. Cortisol stops rising and falling in waves and becomes more of a steady pour. Your pulse never fully settles. Sleep becomes lighter, shorter, or more fragile. Mornings lose their clarity. Joy thins out. Focus scatters. The body starts whispering warnings long before the mind listens.

The truth is simple: nothing built to last is built to run at redline.

Even steel warps under constant heat. Engines fail not from effort, but from never cooling down. Humans are no different. Strength isn't found in constant throttle — it's found in knowing when to surge and when to coast, when to push and when to pit for fuel, repairs, and recalibration.

Modern life rewards the performance but hides the cost. "Always on" becomes an identity. Productivity becomes the measure of a day. But the grind that gets you ahead in the short term quietly wears you down in the long term. The difference between burnout and brilliance isn't talent — it's timing.

Real strength is rhythm: effort and ease, acceleration and glide, drive and recovery.

Think of your body as a race car — built for power, but only if it respects the pit stops. Great drivers win because they know exactly when to pull in — before the engine strains, before the tires thin, before the fuel hits zero. The pause is not a delay. The pause is the strategy. Without it, no race can be finished — let alone won.

Real-life snapshot

Evan lived in the red for years. Five a.m. workouts. Midnight emails. A schedule with no edges. He called it discipline. His colleagues called him unstoppable. His body, meanwhile, was keeping score: first migraines, then nights where sleep never landed deeply, then labs showing cortisol triple the normal range.

His doctor didn't give him more tools; he gave him less. Slower mornings instead of hitting the ground at a sprint. Real meals instead of skipped breakfasts and desk lunches. A lights-down hour before bed with screens off and lights dim.

One week later, his pulse softened. Two weeks later, the migraines loosened. Four weeks later, he woke with clarity instead of static.

Quick science

- Chronic sympathetic overdrive raises blood pressure, tightens blood vessels, and blunts immune function.
- Excess cortisol suppresses hormones that support vitality — including testosterone, thyroid hormones, and growth and repair signals.
- Deep recovery shifts the body back toward parasympathetic dominance, improving emotional regulation, metabolism, and cognitive performance.[18]

Inspiration note

Even a race car wins because of its pit strategy — not its speed alone.

Today's Invitation

One thing I will do for myself today:

- ☐ Recovery block: Schedule one recovery block today (even 15 minutes).
- ☐ One focus sprint: Do one 25-minute focus sprint, then take a real break.
- ☐ Night shutdown: Choose a clear shutdown cue tonight (lights down, screens off, bed on time).

Action Step:
Choose the easiest one today. Do it now or set one reminder and do it when it best fits your schedule.

Reflection:
After I took the step today, I felt: ☐ calmer ☐ clearer ☐ steadier ☐ proud ☐ no change yet (effort still counts)

Bottom line

Fatigue disguised as discipline is still fatigue. The goal of a healthy life is not to burn at full brightness for a short time, but to burn long and steady.

Your lines

(write one thought, one insight, or rewrite one sentence that rang true)

_____

_____

_____

☐ Done for today

Why this matters
Writing just a few lines by hand locks the concept into memory and gently primes your subconscious mind to adopt and act on it, leading to better recall and follow-through.

DAY 19

> "What you call weakness might just be wisdom asking for a pause."
> — A. Smyrlis, MD

The body whispers before it screams.
Fatigue and soreness are not failure; they're feedback.
Wisdom often wears the mask of weakness.

Reflection

Every living system has a language for "slow down." A tree drops its leaves before winter. Animals grow quiet and retreat before winter. Your body does something similar. Long before it breaks, it whispers.

That whisper can feel like heaviness, low drive, strange soreness, or the foggy sense of "I can't push today." Most people mislabel it: lazy, weak, losing it. But biology has no moral vocabulary. It doesn't shame you. It guides you.

Often, what you call weakness is wisdom protecting you — asking for a pause before the scream. And the signal is almost always some version of: less load, more rest, better fuel, a gentler rhythm.

Ignoring these signals doesn't make you stronger; it makes you brittle. Respecting them doesn't make you fragile; it makes you durable. When you treat "off days" as calibration rather than character flaws, the whole system softens. Sleep comes easier. Muscles repair. Stress signals settle. Mood breathes again. The nervous system stops bracing for war and begins shifting back into repair.

Strength is not the absence of limits. Strength is the humility to respond when limits appear. The pros in every field — elite athletes, master craftsmen, world-class thinkers — all learn this lesson: you don't push through red lights. You pause, reset, repair, and return with more accuracy, more power, and more longevity. Amateurs interpret fatigue as failure. Masters interpret it as data. Your body isn't trying to block your progress. It's trying to protect it.

Real-life snapshot

Daniel called himself "weak" when his morning lifts felt heavy. A mentor told him, "Don't judge your body on a low-sleep day."

His friend Ravi tried to grind through the same week on four hours of sleep and tweaked his shoulder — same goal, different choice.

He took two lighter days, added an early night, and even let himself nap. By the weekend, his strength returned like a tide rising back to shore.

Quick science

- Low motivation and heavier fatigue can reflect overload and stress physiology — not personal weakness.
- Short deloads and real recovery can support performance and resilience better than constant pushing.
- Training or working through deep fatigue dramatically raises the risk of injury and burnout.[19]

Inspiration note

Even trees shed leaves to survive winter; slowing down isn't dying — it's design.

Today's Invitation

One thing I will do for myself today:

- ☐ Quick check-in: Note energy + mood + tension once today.
- ☐ One deload move: Choose one gentler move (smaller workload, easier pace, or earlier bedtime).
- ☐ One-minute brake: Do one minute of slow breathing to reset.

Action Step:
Choose the easiest one today. Do it now or set one reminder and do it when it best fits your schedule.

Reflection:
After I took the step today, I felt: ☐ calmer ☐ clearer ☐ steadier ☐ proud ☐ no change yet (effort still counts)

Bottom line

Your body's feedback is the map, not the mistake.

Your lines

(write one thought, one insight, or rewrite one sentence that rang true)

_____

_____

_____

☐ Done for today

Why this matters
Writing just a few lines by hand locks the concept into memory and gently primes your subconscious mind to adopt and act on it, leading to better recall and follow-through.

DAY 20

> "Play is health work."
> — A. Smyrlis, MD

Play is pure oxygen for your nervous system.
Creativity is exercise for your brain and soul.
When you stop playing, life becomes dull and heavy.

Reflection

Somewhere along the way, many adults quietly decide that play is for children. The schedule fills with work, errands, obligations, and "serious" things. Hobbies get pushed to "when everything else is done" — which means almost never.

But your nervous system didn't get that memo. Your body and brain still respond to play and creativity as essential inputs. Play loosens the grip of stress. It gives the mind safe room to experiment and improvise. It reminds your system that life is not only threat, duty, and survival.

Think of play as a pressure valve and a tuner. When you sketch, play music, dance, throw a ball, garden, tinker, joke, or build something just because you want to, your body hears a different message:

I'm not only a problem-solver — I'm a maker. Life isn't only heavy. My body is allowed to move with joy, not just obligation.

These moments aren't frivolous. They lower stress, support bonding, and give your brain the novelty it uses to stay flexible. People who play — even a little — often sleep better, cope better, and bounce back faster.

Play and creativity also reconnect you with meaning when the health journey starts to feel like a grind. Eating differently, walking more, sleeping earlier — all of that is work. Play reminds you what you're protecting: the part of you that laughs, imagines, creates, and enjoys being alive.

You don't need talent. You don't need an audience. You don't need to monetize it. In fact, it's better if you don't. This is the one area of life that doesn't owe anyone productivity. It only owes your nervous system a little space to breathe.

Real-life snapshot

Mark used to play guitar for hours in college. Then residency, career, and kids arrived, and the instrument moved into a closet. His life became work–commute–family–collapse–scroll–sleep. He ate better and walked more, but something still felt flat.

One day, cleaning the garage, he found his old guitar case. On a whim, he tuned it and played for 10 minutes. His fingers were clumsy; his timing off. But something in him lit up.

He made a small rule: 10 minutes of guitar, three nights a week, after the kids went to bed and before any screens. No goals, no recordings, no "improving," just playing songs he loved.

Within a few weeks, he noticed that his evenings felt less like a dead zone and more like a small gift. Sleep came easier after those nights. His patience at work improved because he had one corner of life that wasn't about performance.

Quick science

- Play and creative activities can reduce perceived stress and improve mood by engaging brain circuits tied to reward, curiosity, and exploration.
- Light, enjoyable movement and creative focus support parasympathetic activity (the "rest and digest" branch), which helps counterbalance chronic stress.
- Engaging in hobbies has been linked to better mental health, lower rates of depression, and even improved cognitive health as we age.[20]

Inspiration note

You're not just here to survive — you're here to live with joy.

Today's Invitation

One thing I will do for myself today:

- ☐ Ten minutes of play: Do 10 minutes of something just for fun.
- ☐ Joyful movement: Move in a way that feels good today (not a workout, just motion).
- ☐ Invite someone: Share one light moment (game, silly text, shared laugh).

Action Step:
Choose the easiest one today. Do it now or set one reminder and do it when it best fits your schedule.

Reflection:
After I took the step today, I felt: ☐ calmer ☐ clearer ☐ steadier ☐ proud ☐ no change yet (effort still counts)

Bottom line

Play and creativity are not extra — they're part of real health. Give your nervous system a little room to breathe and remember who you are beyond your problems and your plan.

Your lines

(write one thought, one insight, or rewrite one sentence that rang true)

_____

_____

_____

☐ Done for today

Why this matters
Writing just a few lines by hand locks the concept into memory and gently primes your subconscious mind to adopt and act on it, leading to better recall and follow-through.

DAY 21

> "I never found the companion that was so companionable as solitude."
> — Henry David Thoreau

Solitude is not loneliness; it's space to hear yourself again.
Time alone is where reflection becomes possible.
Without reflection, it's hard to notice what you actually need.

Reflection

Connection is essential — and so is solitude. If connection is the medicine of belonging, solitude is the medicine of clarity.

Solitude is not the absence of love. It's the presence of listening to yourself. When you're alone on purpose, your nervous system settles. Your mind stops performing. Your body starts sending cleaner signals. You notice what you've been ignoring: tension in your shoulders, a tiredness you've been masking, an emotion you keep outrunning, a truth you keep postponing.

This is why time alone is a skill. If you never practice being with yourself, then being alone only happens when life forces it — travel, loss, a change in relationships, an empty house, a new season. And when it's not chosen, it can feel heavy and stressful. But when you train it gently, solitude becomes a place you can enter without panic. You can be alone without feeling abandoned.

Solitude doesn't need a cabin in the woods. It lives in small, repeatable moments: a few minutes early in the morning before anyone wakes up, part of the drive in silence, or a short walk outside — especially in nature.

The goal is not to withdraw from life. The goal is to return to life more centered, more steady, and more aware of what you actually need.

Real-life snapshot

Two coworkers, Priya and Ben, were both overwhelmed and exhausted — but they treated "alone time" differently.

Priya filled every quiet gap with input. Podcasts on the commute. Scrolling in the parking lot before she walked in. TV running as background noise while she cooked, cleaned, and "unwound." Silence felt like a room with the lights off — so she kept turning the noise up. But the more noise she added, the louder her mind felt when she finally stopped. When her head hit the pillow, her thoughts surged in.

Ben did the opposite. Not a retreat. A practice. Five minutes in the morning with no phone. Two silent commutes a week — just hands on the wheel and breath in his body. One short walk outside without earbuds, letting his mind roam and settle. It felt almost boring at first. Then it started to feel like relief.

Over a month, Priya felt more reactive and tired-but-wired — braced, edgy, always "caught up" on content but never caught up with herself. Ben felt steadier — not because his life got easier, but because he rebuilt the skill of being with himself without needing constant noise to numb the day.

Quick science

- Quiet, reflective time can help your nervous system downshift and settle.
- Uninterrupted "mind-wandering" time may support integration — memory, meaning-making, and problem-solving often improve after a pause.
- Regular, chosen solitude can make being alone feel more familiar and less stressful over time.[21]

Inspiration note

Solitude is a meeting with yourself — and a chance to come back clear.

Today's Invitation

One thing I will do for myself today:

- ☐ Morning quiet: Take 5 minutes alone before anyone wakes (no phone, no input).
- ☐ Silent commute: Do part of the drive in silence (no radio, no podcast).
- ☐ No-earbuds walk: Take a short walk outside and let your mind settle.

Action Step:
Choose the easiest one today. Do it now or set one reminder and do it when it best fits your schedule.

Reflection:
After I took the step today, I felt: ☐ calmer ☐ clearer ☐ steadier ☐ proud ☐ no change yet (effort still counts)

Bottom line

Solitude is a skill — and practicing it turns alone time into clarity instead of stress.

Your lines

(write one thought, one insight, or rewrite one sentence that rang true)

_____
_____
_____

☐ Done for today

Why this matters
Writing just a few lines by hand locks the concept into memory and gently primes your subconscious mind to adopt and act on it, leading to better recall and follow-through.

DAY 22

> **"What you do speaks so loudly that I cannot hear what you say."**
> — attributed to Ralph Waldo Emerson

Most people don't want a lecture — they watch your life.
Arguments don't often change habits; experience does.
Quiet action is often the strongest persuasion.

Reflection

When you decide to change your health, you expect resistance from yourself. You don't always expect it from the people you love. But it often comes in little comments: "Gluten-free? Yeah, we'll see how long that lasts." "Gym membership? Remember the last time?" "Organic? Pesticides? What's wrong with you now?"

It stings more when it comes from people who truly care. And humans are generally resistant to change — especially change that makes them feel judged, left behind, or uncertain about their own habits.

Here's the trap: when we get fired up about a new insight or plan, we want to talk about it endlessly. We try to convince everyone: spouse, kids, friends, coworkers. We give them articles, podcasts, and lectures they didn't ask for. Sometimes we're really trying to convince ourselves.

Early motivation is fragile. Exposing it to constant debate is like pulling a seed out of the soil every day to "check on it." It doesn't grow; it withers.

For the first season of change, treat your plan like a small flame. Protect it. Don't argue. Don't announce every detail. Don't try to drag anyone with you. Smile. Say less. Do more.

If you know in your bones that a path is right — better food, less alcohol, earlier nights, walks after dinner, gluten-free, fewer chemicals — walk it. Let your choices quietly accumulate. Let your body start to show the difference: clearer eyes, steadier mood, better sleep, steadier energy.

People are rarely persuaded by being told they are wrong. They are often persuaded by watching someone they trust become calmer, stronger, and kinder over time.

If you want your spouse, children, or friends to come along, resist the urge to preach or pressure. Lectures increase resistance. Quiet conviction invites curiosity. When they ask, share simply and humbly — what you changed, how it feels in your body, why it matters to you. Then go back to walking.

Be the change you hope to see in your home. Let them be drawn by what they can see and feel, not by what they're forced to hear.

Real-life snapshot

When Eli first decided to overhaul his eating, he told everyone. He announced he was "done with sugar," "never touching gluten again," and "getting shredded this year." His wife rolled her eyes. His friends made jokes. Every slip became a public failure. Within a month, he'd dropped the plan and felt worse than before.

A year later, after a serious health scare, he tried again — but differently. This time, he said almost nothing. He just started going to bed earlier. He took a 15-minute walk most evenings. He swapped his weekday lunches for simple meals he brought from home. He quietly stopped drinking on weeknights.

When his wife asked, "Are you on another diet?" he just said, "I'm trying a few things to feel better." No lecture. No rules for her. Months passed. His energy improved. He was less irritable in the evenings. Even his numbers started trending in a better direction.

One night his wife said, "You seem…different. Calmer. What are you doing?"

He listed three things. Earlier sleep. A walk most evenings. Simple meals.

The next day she left her shoes by the door and said, "Don't go without me tonight."

That was the beginning.

Quick science

- Telling people what they "must" do often triggers psychological reactance — a defensive pushback that makes them less likely to change.
- Modeling behavior (quietly doing the new habit yourself) is a strong form of social influence; people copy what they see more than what they're told.
- Autonomy — feeling a change is self-chosen — helps habits stick and supports well-being.[22]

Inspiration note

The most powerful argument for change is a life that's quietly getting better.

Today's Invitation

One thing I will do for myself today:

☐ Do it quietly: Complete the habit today without announcing it.
☐ One calm line: If questioned, use: I'm trying this for my health.
☐ Track it privately: One small check mark that only you need to see.

Action Step:
Choose the easiest one today. Do it now or set one reminder and do it when it best fits your schedule.

Reflection:
After I took the step today, I felt: ☐ calmer ☐ clearer ☐ steadier ☐ proud ☐ no change yet (effort still counts)

Bottom line

You don't have to convince anyone with words. Walk the path, protect your flame, and let your life make the case.

Your lines

(write one thought, one insight, or rewrite one sentence that rang true)

_____

_____

_____

☐ Done for today

Why this matters
Writing just a few lines by hand locks the concept into memory and gently primes your subconscious mind to adopt and act on it, leading to better recall and follow-through.

DAY 23

"Walking is the best medicine we have."
— attributed to Hippocrates

Movement is the body's reset button — simple, free, and immediately effective. Every step sends medicine through your bloodstream. Walking is not extra exercise; it is daily repair work your body depends on.

Reflection

Imagine a pill that could lower your risk of heart attack and stroke, cut your chance of dying early, protect your brain from dementia, ease depression and anxiety, improve blood sugar, reduce blood pressure, help with weight, and sharpen your thinking. No serious side effects. Works at any age. Pairs well with every other treatment.

That pill exists. It's called walking.

Modern studies validate what Hippocrates saw centuries ago: regular walking is real medicine for body, mind, and spirit. When people move from very low daily activity into a consistent walking routine, large observational studies often show a substantially lower risk of early death compared with staying sedentary.

The brain gets its own special benefit. In large studies higher step counts are linked with a lower risk of depression and dementia. In a large study with step trackers, about 10,000 steps a day was associated with roughly half the risk of dementia compared with very low activity (under 2,000 steps). In other words, every ordinary walk you take is sending a message to your brain to stay younger, more flexible, and more resilient.

Walking isn't just "burning calories." It's a whole-body signal: circulation improves, joints stay oiled, the mind unclenches, and the stress system quiets. Sugar is pulled out of the bloodstream into working muscle. Most people never see walking this way. They think it's optional — something you do only if there's time left. But your body was built on the assumption that you would walk a lot. When walking disappears, everything that depends on it starts to rust: mood, metabolism, blood pressure, sleep, even how clearly you think.

You don't have to become a step-obsessed robot. Start tiny. Ten minutes after one meal is enough to change the character of a day. The magic isn't one heroic walk — it's hundreds of ordinary walks stacked quietly over months and years.

Real-life snapshot

George, a 52-year-old accountant, spent most of his day seated — desk, car, couch. His weight had crept up, his blood pressure was rising, and his labs were drifting into the "we should watch this" zone. His doctor started talking about adding more medication. George felt old, tired, and trapped. "I barely have time to sleep," he said. "There's no way I can live at the gym."

Instead of a complex program, his doctor suggested one rule: walk after meals. Ten minutes, most days — especially after lunch or dinner. No special clothes. No stopwatch. Just out the door.

The first week he mostly trudged, but he noticed one thing: the afternoon crash softened. Over the next few months, he made it a ritual — a short loop after lunch, and a calmer after-dinner walk when he could.

At follow-up, the story was different. He'd lost some weight, his blood pressure and blood sugar had improved, his mood felt steadier, and the "add another med" conversation got quieter. "I thought I needed a new prescription," he said. "Turns out, I needed a sidewalk."

Quick science

- Higher daily step counts are consistently associated with lower all-cause and cardiovascular mortality.
- Brief walks after meals can reduce post-meal glucose spikes and improve glucose control.
- Walking is associated with better mood, and higher activity levels are linked with better brain aging outcomes. [23]

Compass link: If you want the deeper "why," see Part III — The Compass Explained — Chapter 15: Movement — Your Daily Dose. *(Optional. Not required today.)*

Inspiration note

When the mind feels stuck, the feet often know the way.

Today's Invitation

One thing I will do for myself today:

- ☐ After-meal walk: Walk 10 minutes after one meal today.
- ☐ Add steps once: Add steps on purpose once today (park farther, stairs, walking call).
- ☐ Choose the time: Pick your next walk time and set shoes where you'll see them.

Action Step:
Choose the easiest one today. Do it now or set one reminder and do it when it best fits your schedule.

Reflection:
After I took the step today, I felt: ☐ calmer ☐ clearer ☐ steadier ☐ proud ☐ no change yet (effort still counts)

Bottom line

Walking is medicine you can take anytime, anywhere — and the dose is steps.

Your lines

(write one thought, one insight, or rewrite one sentence that rang true)

_____

_____

_____

☐ Done for today

Why this matters

Writing just a few lines by hand locks the concept into memory and gently primes your subconscious mind to adopt and act on it, leading to better recall and follow-through.

DAY 24

> "The doctor of the future will give no medicine, but will interest his patients in the care of the human frame, in diet and in the cause and prevention of disease."
> — attributed to Thomas Edison

Lasting health isn't built in clinics — it's built in kitchens, bedrooms, and daily routines.
Medications can be an important bridge, but habits determine whether you keep needing the bridge.
When you fix the root, symptoms stop having so much power.

Reflection

Edison saw something coming that modern science keeps validating: the most powerful medicine is not in a bottle — it's in how you live. Prevention, nutrition, movement, sleep, and stress patterns are the real engines of long-term health. A doctor can prescribe, operate, and rescue. But what you eat, how you sleep, how often you move, and what you're exposed to each day quietly decide whether you stay well — or keep bouncing back into the system.

This is the heart of integrative, root-cause medicine: don't just silence symptoms — go looking for why they showed up. When reflux flares, do we reach first for an acid-suppressing medicine, or do we pause and listen — late dinners, hurried meals, and screens that keep the body from truly settling? When blood pressure rises, is it only genetics — or is it also sleep debt, salt-heavy processed food, constant sitting, tight shoulders, and stress that never lets up?

Medications and procedures save lives; they are often necessary and wise. But without addressing the habits and environments driving the problem, you're bailing water out of a boat without patching the hole.

Here's the pivot: instead of waiting for a pill to repair what daily habits are breaking, you build a life that needs fewer pills over time. The strongest part of your healthcare plan is not your insurance card; it's your daily rhythm. Real food more often. A consistent bedtime more often. Walks and movement whenever you can. Time outside, not only fluorescent light. Boundaries on stress instead of saying yes to everything.

None of this has to be perfect. Foundations are slow medicine. They work quietly, day after day, below the surface. Over years, they can redraw lab values, shift risk, and change how you feel when you wake up. Roots you cultivate at home will do more for your future than any one prescription written in a rush.

Real-life snapshot

Kathy struggled with reflux for years. Medication helped for a while, but the burn always returned. Over time, she started to believe she was "just someone who will need pills forever."

At one visit, her new doctor asked different questions: "What time do you eat?" "How fast do you eat?" "What does your last hour before bed look like?" Kathy realized the pattern was almost always the same: late, heavy dinners, eating while stressed, and collapsing into bed with her phone.

They ran a simple experiment — without stopping her medication at first. Dinner moved earlier and lighter. She took a short walk after her evening meal. Screens stayed out of bed, and lights went down earlier so her nervous system could settle.

Within a few weeks, the nightly burn faded to an occasional whisper. Two months later, she was using medication as needed instead of by default.

Quick science

- Lifestyle changes (nutrition, movement, weight loss, alcohol reduction, and stress management) can meaningfully improve blood pressure, blood sugar, and cholesterol — and for some people can be comparable to first-line medications, especially when combined.
- Earlier, lighter dinners and short walks after eating improve digestion and lower nighttime reflux by reducing stomach pressure and supporting better gastric emptying.
- Whole, minimally processed foods provide vitamins, minerals, and phytonutrients that support immune function, hormone balance, detox pathways, and repair — things medications often can't replace.[24]

Inspiration note

The roots no one sees determine how strong your health can stand when life gets windy.

Today's Invitation

One thing I will do for myself today:

- ☐ Name the root: Name the one pattern you're working on (sleep/food/movement/stress/screens).
- ☐ Do one foundation: Do one foundation action today (10-minute walk, real meal, or lights down earlier).
- ☐ Add an "instead": Choose one simple instead rule (when stressed → walk/breathe, not scroll).

Action Step:
Choose the easiest one today. Do it now or set one reminder and do it when it best fits your schedule.

Reflection:
After I took the step today, I felt: ☐ calmer ☐ clearer ☐ steadier ☐ proud ☐ no change yet (effort still counts)

Bottom line

Foundations are slow medicine — but they are the strongest medicine you'll ever have.

Your lines

(write one thought, one insight, or rewrite one sentence that rang true)

_____

_____

_____

☐ Done for today

Why this matters
Writing just a few lines by hand locks the concept into memory and gently primes your subconscious mind to adopt and act on it, leading to better recall and follow-through.

DAY 25

> "So many people spend their health gaining wealth, and then have to spend their wealth to regain their health."
> — A.J. Reb Materi

Wealth without health becomes a burden, not a blessing.
Every trade you make shapes the body that has to carry your life.
Protect your engine before you ask it for more miles.

Reflection

A quiet tragedy of modern life is how easily we bargain away our bodies in the chase for money. We skip cooking and grab whatever is fastest because "time is money." We sleep less, take on more, and call it progress. Some work nights for higher pay, not realizing it steals from the body's deepest repair. Others save dollars with ultra-processed convenience, while their cells quietly pay the difference. We brag about never taking vacations while stress chemistry stays high and recovery gets thinner.

The trap is the time lag. Trouble doesn't arrive like food poisoning — sudden and obvious. It behaves more like slow rust or credit card debt. You can run on 5–6 hours of sleep, sit all day, and eat convenience food for years and feel "fine enough." Meanwhile, blood pressure inches up, blood sugar drifts, cholesterol thickens, and plaque quietly builds. By the time the bill arrives — a diagnosis, a scare, a hospital visit — the interest feels brutal.

Wealth is not the enemy. Money can buy options and safety. But the mind, body, and spirit that create wealth must be protected if you want to enjoy what you build. The wiser path is not to reject ambition, but to pair it with boundaries: guard your sleep, your food, your movement, and your peace while you build your career. Otherwise, you risk trading the very thing you wanted money for: a life you can actually live.

Real-life snapshot

John prided himself on being "the guy who never stopped." In his 40s he was working 70-hour weeks to get ahead — early emails, late meetings, constant travel. Most meals came from drive-thrus, airports, or takeout. He slept 5–6 hours on a good night and told himself he'd "catch up on vacation," a vacation he never took.

One morning, a tightness in his chest spread into his jaw on the way to work. In the ER, he heard words he never expected: "You're having a heart attack." A stent opened a blocked artery. The pain eased. He lay there stunned. "I don't understand," he told his cardiologist. "I had no warning signs."

His doctor drew a simple picture. "This is the inner lining of your artery — the endothelium," she said. "When it's healthy, it's smooth and flexible. Modern life can irritate it little by little: high blood pressure, high sugar, smoking, stress, poor sleep, and ultra-processed food. Tiny injuries form under the surface. Cholesterol and inflammation collect there quietly as plaque."

She pointed to the drawing. "For years, plaque can grow with no pain. Then one day, a soft spot cracks. Your body tries to heal it — like it heals a cut — and forms a clot. On your skin, that's helpful. In a heart artery, a clot can block blood flow. That's your heart attack."

Then she looked up and said, "Here's the good news: the same daily habits that irritate this lining can be replaced with habits that protect it — more real food, better sleep, regular walking, and less constant stress. It's one of the strongest protections we have."

Quick science

- Chronic sleep debt (regularly <6–7 hours per night) raises insulin resistance, blood pressure, and inflammation, all of which damage the endothelium and increase cardiovascular risk.
- High, unrelieved stress activates the sympathetic nervous system and stress hormones, accelerating arterial plaque formation and making plaque more unstable.
- Diets high in ultra-processed foods, refined carbs, and processed meats injure the endothelium, while diets rich in vegetables, fruits, fiber, healthy fats, and omega-3s improve endothelial function and help protect against heart attacks and strokes.[25]

Inspiration note

Success that costs your health is failure in disguise.

Today's Invitation

One thing I will do for myself today:

- ☐ Protect one non-negotiable: Choose one (real meal, walk break, or on-time bedtime).
- ☐ Say one no: Say no to one optional task that would steal sleep or recovery.
- ☐ One clean choice: Make one clean choice today (real food, movement, or early wind-down).

Action Step:
Choose the easiest one today. Do it now or set one reminder and do it when it best fits your schedule.

Reflection:
After I took the step today, I felt: ☐ calmer ☐ clearer ☐ steadier ☐ proud ☐ no change yet (effort still counts)

Bottom line

Health is the capital that makes all other wealth usable.

Your lines

(write one thought, one insight, or rewrite one sentence that rang true)

_____

_____

_____

☐ Done for today

Why this matters
Writing just a few lines by hand locks the concept into memory and gently primes your subconscious mind to adopt and act on it, leading to better recall and follow-through.

DAY 26

"He who has a why to live can bear almost any how."
— Friedrich Nietzsche

A strong why can carry you through almost any how.
When your purpose is clear, effort feels less like struggle and more like devotion.
Meaning turns hard choices into aligned ones.

Reflection

Meaning fuels effort. A clear Why outlasts a hard How. Your Why is the compass; your How is the road. When the compass is true, even a rough road still moves you in the right direction. When the compass is missing, even "perfect" habits eventually fall apart — you can only muscle your way through health for so long.

When your goal has a heartbeat, effort feels different. You're not "exercising"; you're staying strong so you can carry a sleepy toddler, climb stairs without wheezing, or walk with someone you love. You're not "eating clean"; you're clearing brain fog so you can do work that matters and still have energy and patience left when you come home. You're not "going to rehab"; you're voting for a birthday, a graduation, a trip you refuse to miss.

You see this everywhere: the person in cardiac rehab who walks a little farther because they want to dance at their child's wedding; the parent who keeps lacing up because they want to model health; the student who studies early because they want a brain that serves their future. A heartfelt Why doesn't erase the hard, but it makes the hard worth doing.

You can find your Why with a simple ladder: say your goal, then add "so that..." two or three times until you reach the real reason.

Example: "Walk every morning... so that I get daylight... so that my sleep resets... so that I'm present and kind at home."

Keep it short enough to remember when you're tired. Put a real face in it. Let it be personal.

Let your Why steer your day. Put it where you'll see it — mirror, fridge, lock screen — and choose one small daily action that matches it: protect sleep, eat one real-food meal, take a walk, or reach out to someone you love. These aren't rules. They're daily ways of saying "yes" to your Why.

Guardrails matter. If your Why regularly costs your sleep, health, or integrity, it may need adjusting. The right Why strengthens your foundations — sleep, movement, real food, and connection — and gives you staying power when willpower is thin.

Real-life snapshot

After his heart attack, Marcos was terrified — and unmotivated. Cardiac rehab felt like punishment: treadmills, wires, other people watching him struggle. His doctor talked about risk; the nurse talked about diet. None of it reached his heart.

Then his granddaughter, age six, climbed onto his lap and asked, "Will you dance with me at my wedding someday?"

That sentence became his Why.

Suddenly, every treadmill step was not just "exercise." It was rehearsal for that dance. Every time he chose fish and vegetables instead of fast food, it was a vote for that future moment. Every early bedtime, every skipped cigarette, every walk around the block when he didn't feel like it became a quiet way of saying, "Yes, I want to be there." "The rehab didn't get easier," he said. "It got meaningful. Once I had her in my mind, the 'how' stopped feeling like punishment and started feeling like a promise."

Quick science

- A strong sense of purpose is linked with lower all-cause mortality and better cardiovascular outcomes.
- Framing difficult behaviors (like rehab, exercise, or dietary change) around personal values and purpose increases adherence and long-term consistency.
- Meaning-driven goals activate motivation and reward circuits more effectively than external pressure, fear, or vague "shoulds."[26]

Inspiration note

A powerful why doesn't erase the hard — it makes the hard worth doing.

Today's Invitation

One thing I will do for myself today:

- ☐ Write the why: Write one sentence with a name: I'm getting healthy for ___ so I can ___.
- ☐ One why-step: Take one step today (10-minute walk, real-food meal, or lights-down 30 minutes earlier).
- ☐ Remove one thief: Remove one thief today (late scroll, extra drink, or unnecessary yes).

Action Step:
Choose the easiest one today. Do it now or set one reminder and do it when it best fits your schedule.

Reflection:
After I took the step today, I felt: ☐ calmer ☐ clearer ☐ steadier ☐ proud ☐ no change yet (effort still counts)

Bottom line

When your Why is strong, your How becomes possible — especially on the hard days.

Your lines

(write one thought, one insight, or rewrite one sentence that rang true)

_____

_____

_____

☐ Done for today

Why this matters
Writing just a few lines by hand locks the concept into memory and gently primes your subconscious mind to adopt and act on it, leading to better recall and follow-through.

DAY 27

"An apple a day keeps the doctor away."
— English Proverb

Whole fruit speaks the body's language; juice speaks too loudly.
Fiber is the brake your metabolism depends on.
Small, steady choices protect you more than dramatic ones.

Reflection

The line survives because it's true in the ways that matter. An apple carries its own brakes: soluble fiber (pectin) that slows sugar, polyphenols that calm inflammation, and vitamin C for repair. Its low glycemic load means a gentler rise in blood sugar — more whisper than shout — especially compared with sweet snacks or juices.

But fruit isn't a free pass. How much you eat and how you eat it matters. Berries are everyday heroes: rich in fiber, light on sugar. Apples, pears, citrus, and kiwi usually behave well too when portions stay modest. At the other end of the spectrum are sugar-dense fruits like pineapple, grapes, mango, ripe banana, figs — and anything dried or juiced. Those act more like dessert; enjoy them as treats, not all-day habits. Many people drift into blood-sugar trouble not from "junk food" alone, but from huge smoothie bowls, juices, and giant fruit plates with very little fiber or protein to slow things down.

In nature, carbohydrates almost never arrive alone. They come packaged with fiber, water, and often a mix of vitamins, minerals, and plant chemicals that slow the impact. An apple is not "just sugar"; it's sugar wrapped in pectin, water, and phytonutrients such as quercetin and catechins. Beans are starch wrapped in fiber and protein. Even a potato in its skin carries more than carbs alone. When we create food, it's wise to copy this pattern.

A simple sequence helps: fiber first, then protein and healthy fats, and only then a small portion of starch or fruit.

A few bites of salad or non-starchy vegetables, followed by protein and fat, with carbs coming last, is like putting cushions around the impact. Fiber, protein, fat — and even a little acid (like vinegar or lemon) — can flatten the sugar curve and help your body handle it more gracefully.

Cookies, juice, or energy bars on an empty stomach are carbs with no brakes — naked sugar, fast to hit and fast to crash. Dress your carbs wisely: more fiber, more color, a little protein or fat, maybe a splash of vinegar. Choose the varieties that serve your health, and set a gentle limit — enough to nourish, not enough to push your metabolism beyond what it can gracefully handle.

Real-life snapshot

Two friends, Rosa and Carla, worked in the same office and ate about the same number of calories — and roughly the same grams of carbs — most days. But their carb dressing could not have been more different.

Rosa started lunch with a small salad, then ate a simple plate: chicken or beans, vegetables, and a modest scoop of rice or potatoes. If she wanted something sweet, she finished with a small bowl of berries or half an apple. She drank water or sparkling water.

Carla usually skipped breakfast, then grabbed "quick energy" through the day: a muffin here, a granola bar there, a big cup of juice, a handful of gummies, a late-afternoon cookie. By dinner she was starving and often ordered takeout with a sugary drink. Most of her carbs arrived naked — no fiber first, very little protein, and no real pause.

Ten years later, their numbers told two different stories. Rosa's waist was stable, her A1c and triglycerides sat in the healthy range, and she felt steady after meals. Carla's waist had thickened, her A1c had crept into the prediabetic zone, and her energy spiked and crashed all day.

"But we eat about the same," Carla said, looking at their food logs. Rosa's clinician pointed to the pattern gently: "You're living on carbs without brakes. The carbs aren't just *how much* — they're *how*."

Quick science

- Soluble fiber (like the pectin in apples and the fiber in berries) slows glucose absorption and feeds healthy gut bacteria.
- Eating carbs with "dressing" — fiber, protein, fats, and acids like vinegar — flattens glucose spikes, improves insulin response, and reduces cravings.
- Fructose-heavy drinks and fruit sugars without much fiber (juice, sugary drinks, lots of dried fruit) are absorbed quickly and, over time, can raise triglycerides and metabolic strain. [27]

Compass link: If you want the deeper "why," see Part III — The Compass Explained — Chapter 16: Food — Instructions for Your Brain, Energy, and Sleep. *(Optional. Not required today.)*

Inspiration note

Nature packaged fruit with its own safety system: fiber. Trust the package.

Today's Invitation

One thing I will do for myself today:

- ☐ Fiber first: Start one meal with a fiber buffer (raw/cooked veggies or veggie soup).
- ☐ Whole fruit only: Choose whole fruit/berries today (skip juice/sweet drinks).
- ☐ Dress the carbs: Pair starch/fruit with protein or healthy fat (keep portion modest).

Action Step:
Choose the easiest one today. Do it now or set one reminder and do it when it best fits your schedule.

Reflection:
After I took the step today, I felt: ☐ calmer ☐ clearer ☐ steadier ☐ proud ☐ no change yet (effort still counts)

Bottom line

Whole fruit nourishes; fruit sugar without brakes overwhelms.

Your lines

(write one thought, one insight, or rewrite one sentence that rang true)

_____

_____

☐ Done for today

Why this matters

Writing just a few lines by hand locks the concept into memory and gently primes your subconscious mind to adopt and act on it, leading to better recall and follow-through.

DAY 28

> **"The time will come when men will be amazed that they did not know how to regulate the day and the night."**
> — Hippocrates

Your body's deepest healing depends on light and dark arriving on time.
Rhythm isn't optional — it's biology.
Align the clocks, and the whole system begins to sing again.

Reflection

Everything in nature moves in cycles — the planets above you, the tides and trees around you, and the organs within you. Your body is a symphony of clocks. Every cell keeps time, while the brain's master clock — the SCN — conducts the score. When those cycles line up with day and night, energy, focus, digestion, and sleep rise and fall in harmony.

When day–night signals blur — late screens, irregular meals, lingering caffeine — the clocks fall out of sync. Morning clarity turns to fog. Afternoons sag into exhaustion. Nights unravel into restless tossing. You start to feel "tired and wired" at the wrong times.

The trap is the lag. One late night doesn't wreck you. One 10 p.m. dinner doesn't collapse your health. But repeat them, and the body pays on delay. Days later the fog feels normal, afternoons crash, and nights turn shallow. Small timing errors compound until your inner clocks keep the wrong time. Fatigue, cravings, and low mood become your new time zone. The bells of the body are still ringing — just at the wrong hours.

The answer is not exotic. It is as old as sunrise. Step into morning light and let your eyes drink the day — it's one of the most powerful ways to reset your master clock. Keep meals steady so your organs know the rhythm. Use movement, temperature, and supplements as gentle "time-givers" instead of random events. Dim your home at dusk so the body senses that night has come. Eat earlier so digestion can rest before sleep.

When you honor these ancient cues, the orchestra retunes itself — and life begins to play in harmony again.

Real-life snapshot

Patricia struggled with chronic fatigue and nightly insomnia. Her labs were "fine," but her rhythm wasn't: bedtime bounced between 10 p.m. and 1 a.m., dinner often landed late, caffeine drifted into the afternoon, and her phone stayed bright until the moment she tried to sleep.

At her visit, her doctor said, "Your problem isn't just sleep — it's timing. Your body listens to time-givers — little cues that tell every clock in you what time it is." Then she offered Patricia a one-month **Time-Giver Challenge**. No perfection. Just a few repeatable cues:

Morning: step outside for light soon after waking, even for a few minutes.

Midday: move a little before noon — a short walk counts.

Caffeine: keep it to the morning so it doesn't blur the night signal.

Meals: aim for steadier times, and finish dinner earlier with a clear buffer before bed.

Evening: set a lights-down time — dim the house, dim screens, and let the night arrive.

The shift wasn't instant, but it was steady. By week three, Patricia fell asleep faster and woke up fewer times. By six weeks her mornings felt clearer, her cravings eased, and her mood stopped swinging so hard.

Quick science

- Morning outdoor light helps entrain the brain's master clock (the suprachiasmatic nucleus, SCN), synchronizing circadian rhythm and supporting energy, mood, and hormone timing.
- Earlier, consistent eating (especially less late-night eating) supports metabolic health and is linked with better sleep.
- Evening bright/blue-rich light suppresses melatonin and delays sleep onset; dim, warm light helps natural sleepiness arrive. [28]

Inspiration note

The sun is your oldest medicine — and the cheapest.

Today's Invitation

One thing I will do for myself today:

- ☐ Morning light: Step outside for 5–10 minutes soon after waking.
- ☐ Earlier finish: End eating earlier tonight (skip late-night snacking).

☐ Lights-down: Set a lights-down time and make the last hour dim and calm.

Action Step:
Choose the easiest one today. Do it now or set one reminder and do it when it best fits your schedule.

Reflection:
After I took the step today, I felt: ☐ calmer ☐ clearer ☐ steadier ☐ proud ☐ no change yet (effort still counts)

Bottom line

Let sunrise start your day — and let sunset end it.

Your lines

(write one thought, one insight, or rewrite one sentence that rang true)

_____

_____

_____

☐ Done for today

Why this matters
Writing just a few lines by hand locks the concept into memory and gently primes your subconscious mind to adopt and act on it, leading to better recall and follow-through.

DAY 29

"Nothing can bring you peace but yourself."
— Ralph Waldo Emerson

Peace isn't delivered from the outside — it's built from the inside out. Your nervous system can be trained; what you practice becomes your default. When you choose quiet on purpose, your whole body exhales.

Reflection

Peace is not a place; it is a practice. You can change jobs, homes, even relationships, and still carry the same storm inside you. For years, many of us have waited for life to "finally calm down" so we can feel okay — as if peace will appear only after the last task is done and the last fire is put out. It almost never works that way. Real peace begins when you learn to downshift your own nervous system on purpose, even while life is still imperfect and noisy.

Think of your body like a ship at sea. You can't control the weather, but you can learn how to lower the sails, steady the rudder, and ride the waves differently. At first, those skills feel clumsy. You forget what to do. You practice three breaths and your mind runs away again. That doesn't mean you're bad at peace; it means you're new at it. Nobody is born knowing how to relax on command. Calm people aren't magically "zen" — they have simply practiced certain moves so many times that their bodies recognize them as signals to soften.

With repetition, small choices start to add up: shoulders that don't live by your ears, a jaw that spends more time unclenched, a heart that doesn't slam with every email, a bedtime that arrives with less fight, mornings that feel less like being thrown into a sprint. The signs of progress aren't mystical. They're ordinary and bodily: you fall asleep a bit faster, you feel a little less tight in your chest, and you don't snap as quickly at people you love.

Peace doesn't mean nothing hard is happening. It means your system is no longer locked at a 10/10 alarm level all day. The world may still storm — but inside, you are slowly becoming someone who knows how to steady the ship.

Real-life snapshot

After years of constant stress, Lila kept telling herself, "I'll feel better once things finally calm down." They never did. There was always another deadline, another family issue, another late-night problem to solve. She fell into bed scrolling the news and woke up feeling like she hadn't rested at all.

On a friend's suggestion, she tried something that felt almost too simple: a nightly relaxation drill. Each evening, she put her phone in another room, dimmed the lights, and played a short head-to-toe muscle relaxation video on YouTube. She followed along, noticing each part of her body and inviting it to release. Then she breathed slowly — in for four, out for six — until the audio ended. After 8 p.m., she avoided bright screens (or used blue-light-filtering glasses) and chose only light, kind input — a book, a gentle show, or a warm phone call, never heavy news.

Within a week, she was falling asleep faster. Within a month, her mornings felt less jagged. Her problems hadn't disappeared, but her body was no longer living at a constant red alert.

"Life didn't get easier," she said. "But I stopped fighting myself. That alone made everything feel a little lighter."

Quick science

- Paced breathing — especially with longer exhales (for example, in for 4 seconds, out for 6) —can increase parasympathetic activity (vagal tone) and help the body downshift; over time it may support lower resting heart rate and blood pressure.
- Progressive muscle relaxation and body scan practices have been shown to reduce anxiety, ease physical tension, and improve sleep onset when practiced regularly.
- Repeating the same calming cues (like a specific breathing pattern or guided relaxation each night) conditions the nervous system to associate those cues with safety, making it easier to shift out of fight-or-flight and into rest-and-digest.[29]

Inspiration note

You may not control the storm — but you can practice, daily, how to steady the ship.

Today's Invitation

One thing I will do for myself today:

- ☐ One minute breath: Do paced breathing for one minute (longer exhale).
- ☐ Soften one place: Unclench one area (jaw, shoulders, walking pace).

☐ Night cue: Dim lights and do one low-input activity for 10 minutes tonight.

Action Step:
Choose the easiest one today. Do it now or set one reminder and do it when it best fits your schedule.

Reflection:
After I took the step today, I felt: ☐ calmer ☐ clearer ☐ steadier ☐ proud ☐ no change yet (effort still counts)

Bottom line

Peace is not found; it is trained — one simple, repeatable practice at a time.

Your lines

(write one thought, one insight, or rewrite one sentence that rang true)

_____

_____

☐ Done for today

Why this matters
Writing just a few lines by hand locks the concept into memory and gently primes your subconscious mind to adopt and act on it, leading to better recall and follow-through.

DAY 30

"If you chase two rabbits, you catch neither."
— Proverb

Chasing everything guarantees you finish nothing.
Focus is how you turn effort into results.
Scattered attention is expensive fuel burned in the wrong gear.

Reflection

Split focus splits results. One target, one effort, then switch. Most people never learn that focus isn't just a productivity trick — it's a health practice. Your brain runs on a limited daily budget of cognitive energy. Every time you jump from one task to another, your mind has to unload the old task, load the new one, and rebuild the mental map. That "reload tax" feels tiny in the moment. Repeated all day, it becomes a real drain.

Every switch is a micro-stressor. You have to re-orient, working memory thins, reaction time slows, and irritability rises. Errors creep in. Decision fatigue accelerates. Over time, this can feel like brain fog, emotional reactivity, chronic burnout, and the wired-but-tired pattern that makes sleep harder than it should be.

The opposite of multitasking is flow — the quiet power of monotasking. In flow, attention converges into a single stream. Distractions fade. Time bends. Athletes call it "the zone." Musicians say the instrument "plays them." Writers say the page "opens." Deep focus often improves the quality and efficiency of your work — not because you're straining harder, but because your brain is finally doing what it was designed to do: work on one meaningful thing at a time, whole and unbroken.

Protecting your focus is protecting your health. Choose your One Big Thing for the day. Clear the deck by closing extra tabs and putting your phone out of reach. Then set a timer and let yourself sink in. When stray ideas pop up, jot them on a "parking lot" card instead of chasing them. When the timer ends, take one breath, save your work, and write the next tiny step so tomorrow's re-entry is easy. One honest session of monotasking often lifts the entire rest of the day.

Less spread, more speed. Focus is a quiet accelerator — and a form of self-respect.

Real-life snapshot

Leah prided herself on multitasking: email, messages, charts, and news all open at once. Her day was a blur of half-finished tasks. By 6 p.m. she felt drained, yet oddly unfinished. "I'm busy all day," she said, "but nothing really moves."

On a mentor's suggestion, she tried one change: a single 45-minute focus block each day on her most important task. Phone in another room, notifications off, one tab only.

At first she felt itchy, like she was "missing something." After a week, she noticed two things: more real progress on the work that actually mattered, and more energy left at the end of the day.

Quick science

- Task switching carries measurable "switch costs" — it slows thinking, increases errors, and raises subjective fatigue.
- Deep, focused work promotes neural efficiency and better learning by letting the brain build and strengthen a single network instead of fragmenting across many.
- Consistent monotasking reduces stress load and supports long-term cognitive health, in part by lowering chronic mental overload and decision fatigue.[30]

Inspiration note

You don't need more hours — you need more wholeness in the ones you already have.

Today's Invitation

One thing I will do for myself today:

- [ ] One task: Do one 25-minute monotask block (one task, no switching).
- [ ] Remove one splitter: Close extra tabs and put the phone out of reach.
- [ ] Reset after: Take a real 5-minute reset (stand, breathe, or walk).

Action Step:
Choose the easiest one today. Do it now or set one reminder and do it when it best fits your schedule.

Reflection:
After I took the step today, I felt: ☐ calmer ☐ clearer ☐ steadier ☐ proud ☐ no change yet (effort still counts)

Bottom line

Catch one rabbit at a time — that's how real progress is made.

Your lines

(write one thought, one insight, or rewrite one sentence that rang true)

_____

_____

_____

☐ Done for today

Why this matters
Writing just a few lines by hand locks the concept into memory and gently primes your subconscious mind to adopt and act on it, leading to better recall and follow-through.

DAY 31

> "Poison rarely arrives with a skull and crossbones; it hides in convenience, fragrance, and habit."
> — A. Smyrlis, MD

The most dangerous exposures are often the ones you barely notice. Tiny doses, repeated daily, are what quietly shape long-term risk. You don't need fear — you need wiser defaults.

Reflection

Across many countries, cancer and chronic illness in people in their 20s–40s have been rising, and many are asking why. There isn't a single smoking gun. But many of the clues sit in plain sight — woven into our morning routines, our kitchens, our air, and our water. The answers are, quite literally, right in front of us.

Before sunrise, the day quietly loads our bodies with exposures. Dust from synthetic mattresses and carpets. Residues from "fresh scent" detergents. Fumes from scented candles and air fresheners. VOCs — gases that can off-gas from new furniture and finishes. In the shower, warm water increases what you inhale; if the water isn't filtered, chlorine/chloramine and other contaminants can become part of what you breathe in with the mist. Hot coffee pushed through plastic pods may add unwanted plastic-related chemicals. Some common foods can carry pesticide residues. None of this looks dramatic. That's the point. A little from the bed, a little from the air, a little from the water, a little from the cup — layer upon layer, day after day.

History repeats the same pattern: discovery → denial → delay → damage → late admission. Lead in gasoline and paint. Asbestos in buildings. Tobacco in every pocket. Today's cast includes PFAS, phthalates (often hiding under the word "fragrance"), and various VOCs. Convenience and marketing move faster than caution.

Awareness isn't paranoia; it's sight. You don't need perfection; you need direction. Small upgrades matter. Filter the water you drink — and, if you can, the water you bathe in with a showerhead or whole house filter. Retire single-serve plastic brewers; use glass, stainless steel, or a simple pour-over. Store food in glass or stainless instead of hot plastic. Choose unscented basics instead of "ocean breeze." Buy organic or low-spray where it matters most (start with high-residue produce and common grains). Run a bedroom air purifier if possible.

You don't have to scrub your life of every chemical. But you can turn down the daily "drip" that your liver, kidneys, and immune system have to manage. A kinder environment is one that quietly harms you less, so your body can spend more energy healing — not just defending.

Real-life snapshot

Hannah worked as a cashier at a busy store. She loved beautiful scents — her home was full of perfumed candles, plug-in air fresheners, and a rotating collection of perfumes on her dresser. At work, she handled hundreds of thermal-paper receipts each day. Over time, she began having thyroid-related symptoms, chronic headaches, and stubborn fatigue. Her standard lab work was mostly "normal," but she felt nowhere near well.

At a longer appointment, her doctor asked a different kind of question: "What do you touch, breathe, and put on your skin every day?" As they talked, a pattern appeared — constant contact with receipt paper, heavy daily fragrance use, scented detergents and softeners, plastic-lidded hot drinks, unfiltered tap water. None of these things alone were "the cause," but together they were a steady stream of extra work for her body.

Hannah decided to make changes that felt doable, not perfect. She switched to unscented laundry detergent and skipped fabric softener. She cut back on daily perfume, saving it for special occasions instead of all day, every day. She swapped most scented candles and plug-ins for beeswax candles and fresh air. She replaced her plastic coffee maker with a stainless steel setup. She started using a basic water filter for drinking and cooking and began asking customers if they wanted a receipt instead of printing automatically, trying to touch receipts less when she did.

Within about three months, her headaches became rare instead of daily, her energy felt steadier, and her sleep improved.

Quick science

- Chemicals like PFAS, phthalates, and certain VOCs can act as endocrine disruptors and immune irritants, subtly influencing hormones, inflammation, and metabolism over time.
- For many environmental toxins, it's chronic low-level exposure, not a single high dose, that drives long-term risk.
- Reducing your overall "toxic load" — by choosing cleaner water, air, food, and everyday products — can lower what your body has to process each day, leaving more bandwidth for steady repair and resilience. [31]

Compass link: If you want the deeper "why," see Part III — The Compass Explained — Chapter 19: Hidden Saboteurs. *(Optional. Not required today.)*

Inspiration note

Clean up what surrounds you, and your body can finally exhale.

Today's Invitation

One thing I will do for myself today:

- ☐ Fragrance-free swap: Switch one everyday product to fragrance-free today (soap, detergent, lotion, or cleaner).
- ☐ Fresh air: Air out one room for 10 minutes (open a window or run a vent/fan).
- ☐ Hot in glass: Keep hot food/drinks out of plastic today (use glass, ceramic, or stainless).

Action Step:
Choose the easiest one today. Do it now or set one reminder and do it when it best fits your schedule.

Reflection:
After I took the step today, I felt: ☐ calmer ☐ clearer ☐ steadier ☐ proud ☐ no change yet (effort still counts)

Bottom line

You don't need a perfect environment — just a kinder one that drips less harm into your system.

Your lines

(write one thought, one insight, or rewrite one sentence that rang true)

_____
_____
_____

☐ Done for today

Why this matters
Writing just a few lines by hand locks the concept into memory and gently primes your subconscious mind to adopt and act on it, leading to better recall and follow-through.

DAY 32

> "The best time to plant a tree was twenty years ago. The second best time is now."
> — Chinese Proverb

Yesterday is gone — today is fertile ground.
Growth begins with a single planted habit.
What you tend each day shapes who you become each year.

Reflection

Health habits are trees. Like anything living, they take time to root and longer to bear fruit. When they finally ripen, they feed mind, body, and spirit. The best time to plant them was years ago — before fatigue, weight gain, or disease took hold. The second best time is today. No regret required. You didn't know. Now you do.

Many people feel crushed when they finally see the cost of neglect. They look at their numbers, their symptoms, their reflection, and think, "It's too late." From that place, shortcuts look tempting: crash diets, detox kits, miracle gadgets, triple-shot caffeine, "30 days to a new you." But your body — like a garden — obeys the laws of growth, not marketing. Quick fixes don't grow roots.

The hopeful news is that the soil is still alive. Muscles can strengthen. Sleep can return. Blood sugar can steady. Nervous systems can calm. If you plant now and keep tending, months and years from now there can still be shade and fruit where there is only dry ground today.

Beware the fake forest. Hacks without roots are like cut-stem wedding flowers: beautiful for a night, wilted by morning. Plastic plants and fake lawns look green and never change — but they never deepen either. Energy drinks, crash diets, all-nighters, and "on/off" health kicks can mimic vitality for a moment. They do not build it.

The path back is quieter and simpler than most people think. Pick one seed and plant it today: a 10-minute walk after dinner, a vegetable added to each meal, lights out 30 minutes earlier, a glass of water on waking, three slow breaths before opening your email. Plant it at roughly the same time each day. Protect it from being bumped off the schedule. Let it be small enough that you can keep it, even on hard days.

Once it starts to feel natural — like part of who you are — plant the next seed. In the end, a life that looks "lucky" or "disciplined" from the outside is usually just a well-tended habit garden.

Real-life snapshot

Luis and his younger brother grew up in the same house, eating the same mostly home-cooked meals. Their father had one simple ritual: every morning, he went for a run. When they were little, both boys sometimes joined him — shuffling along beside his steady pace. Their dad kept this rhythm well into his late 70s and enjoyed good health into his 80s.

Life scattered the brothers in different directions. The younger brother kept a version of the morning habit, even through college, work, and kids: sometimes a run, sometimes a brisk walk, sometimes a short strength routine, but always something most mornings. He wasn't perfect, but the "movement tree" stayed planted. He mostly stuck with the family pattern of simple, whole-food meals.

Luis told himself he'd "get back in shape later." Early on, work felt more urgent: long days, late nights, quick takeout, skipped workouts. Fast food saved time and money. He pushed annual checkups off because nothing felt "that bad." Years passed. A bigger belly, tighter belts, more heartburn.

When he finally went to the doctor because he was getting up five times a night to urinate, he was stunned. His A1c was in the diabetic range. His blood pressure and cholesterol were high enough that he left with three prescriptions. "How did this happen so quickly?" he asked. His doctor gently pointed out that it hadn't been quick at all — it had just been quiet.

Later that year, at a family gathering, Luis watched his father — now in his late 80s — walking calmly around the yard, and his younger brother returning from a morning jog, flushed but relaxed. In that moment he saw it: those small daily choices, planted early and tended over decades, had grown into shade trees. His own soil was not ruined, but it was underplanted.

With support, Luis started small instead of trying to overhaul everything. He committed to a 10–15 minute walk after dinner most nights, packing one simple whole-food lunch instead of fast food, and keeping a consistent bedtime at least five nights a week. The changes felt tiny compared with years of drift. But within months, he was sleeping better, waking less often at night, feeling steadier, and watching his numbers begin to move in the right direction.

Quick science

- Repeating a small behavior in the same context (same time, same cue) strengthens neural pathways in the basal ganglia, turning effortful actions into easier, automatic habits.
- Even 10 minutes of movement — like a brisk walk — helps muscles pull more glucose from the blood and can blunt post-meal blood sugar spikes.
- Over time, simple, consistent habits (regular movement, not smoking, basic sleep hygiene, mostly whole foods) are strongly linked with lower cardiovascular and metabolic risk compared with sporadic, intense "health kicks."[32]

Inspiration note

A forest begins with one seed — and so does a new life.

Today's Invitation

One thing I will do for myself today:

- ☐ Plant one seed: Pick one tiny habit for today (2–10 minutes).
- ☐ Attach it to a cue: Decide when it happens (after breakfast / after dinner / when I get home).
- ☐ Make it easy: Set it up now (shoes out, water ready, reminder set).

Action Step:
Choose the easiest one today. Do it now or set one reminder and do it when it best fits your schedule.

Reflection:
After I took the step today, I felt: ☐ calmer ☐ clearer ☐ steadier ☐ proud ☐ no change yet (effort still counts)

Bottom line

You can't change yesterday — but you can plant a better tomorrow.

Your lines

(write one thought, one insight, or rewrite one sentence that rang true)

_____

_____

_____

☐ Done for today

Why this matters
Writing just a few lines by hand locks the concept into memory and gently primes your subconscious mind to adopt and act on it, leading to better recall and follow-through.

DAY 33

> "Early to bed and early to rise makes a man healthy, wealthy, and wise."
> — Benjamin Franklin

Your strongest sleep happens early — and it determines tomorrow's clarity. Protect the first half of the night and the whole body repairs better. Early rhythms are ancient, powerful, and biologically non-negotiable.

Reflection

Franklin's proverb is repeated so often it risks sounding quaint, yet modern sleep science keeps circling back to the same point: when you protect your night, your body repairs more effectively. In the first half of the night — often the first 3–4 hours after you fall asleep — slow-wave (deep) sleep is typically strongest. This is prime maintenance time: the brain's glymphatic "rinse" helps clear metabolic waste, and the body shifts toward repair and immune housekeeping.

Miss that early window — bright lights on, screens glowing, meals late, bedtime drifting — and the peaks often flatten. The work still happens, but it becomes thinner and delayed. You can wake up feeling like you showed up for the night shift after the best crew already clocked out.

We like to imagine lost sleep can be "caught up" on weekends. But the body doesn't keep books that way. Over years, late nights, irregular sleep, heavy evening eating, and rotating schedules can quietly wear on the system. The bill tends to arrive later: more insulin resistance, higher blood pressure, lower mood and resilience. In studies, chronic sleep loss is also linked with weaker resistance to infections, and long-term sleep/circadian disruption has been associated with higher risk of some cancers — most clearly in settings like night shift work (an association, not a verdict, and not proof of direct cause).

The tragedy is that the cost is hidden until it's heavy. Many risks build quietly, without a dramatic alarm bell. The good news is that protection can build quietly too.

Like a compass, the body still points home if you will follow. Aligning with a more natural light–dark cycle helps restore steadier rhythm — better mood, more stable appetite and blood sugar, more usable energy. It doesn't require perfection or a 9 p.m. bedtime forever. One earlier bedtime, one week of consistent wake times, one evening without screens or heavy food can be enough to feel the reset begin. Each small adjustment is a deposit into strength, clarity, and long-term protection.

Real-life snapshot

Theo always called himself a "night owl." He stayed up later than everyone else and still woke early "to get a jump on the day." Midnight was normal; 1 a.m. was common. Nights were a mix of Netflix, emails, and late snacks. For years, his performance was "good enough" — until it wasn't.

By his late 30s, he woke foggy, craved sugar mid-morning, and dragged through afternoons. His temper shortened. Coffee cups multiplied on his desk. His labs were edging the wrong way: rising blood pressure, creeping A1c. "But I'm sleeping the same number of hours," he told his doctor. "Isn't that what matters?"

His doctor drew a simple graph on the exam table paper. "Total sleep matters," she said, "but when you sleep matters too. Your deepest, most restorative sleep — slow-wave sleep — tends to be front-loaded, strongest in the first few hours after you fall asleep, when cortisol is typically near its nightly low. If you're asleep by around 10, that 'front of the movie' often lands roughly between 10 and 2 — but the key is early in your sleep window, not the clock. You've been skipping the front of the movie and only watching the middle and end."

She offered him an experiment, not a lecture: keep about the same number of hours, but slide the whole block earlier by 60–90 minutes. He moved dinner earlier and kept it lighter. He set a screens-dim time about an hour before bed. He aimed for lights-down around 10 p.m. instead of starting a new show. And he kept his wake time steady — even on weekends — for one month.

Theo agreed, skeptical but tired enough to try. The first week felt strange; he missed the late-night "free time." By week two, something shifted. He fell asleep faster. He stopped waking at 3 a.m. His mornings felt less like wading through mud. After a month, his cravings eased, his mood steadied, and his focus at work sharpened.

Quick science

- Slow-wave sleep (SWS) — the deepest, most physically restorative stage — peaks in the first half of the night and is crucial for metabolic repair, immune function, and hormone balance.
- Evening screen light and bright indoor light can delay melatonin release by 1–2 hours, pushing deep sleep later and shrinking its total amount.

- Going to bed earlier and keeping a consistent sleep window is associated with better blood sugar control, more efficient immune surveillance, and sharper cognitive performance during the day.[33]

Inspiration note

Give your body the early night it was built for, and it will pay you back all day long.

Today's Invitation

One thing I will do for myself today:

- ☐ Lights-down alarm: Set a 60-minute lights-down alarm for tonight.
- ☐ Caffeine earlier: Keep caffeine to the morning (or use a 2 p.m. cutoff).
- ☐ Sleep cave: Make the room cooler, darker, and quieter (or use an eye mask/white noise).

Action Step:
Choose the easiest one today. Do it now or set one reminder and do it when it best fits your schedule.

Reflection:
After I took the step today, I felt: ☐ calmer ☐ clearer ☐ steadier ☐ proud ☐ no change yet (effort still counts)

Bottom line

Protect the early night, and your body protects you back.

Your lines

(write one thought, one insight, or rewrite one sentence that rang true)

_____

_____

_____

☐ Done for today

Why this matters
Writing just a few lines by hand locks the concept into memory and gently primes your subconscious mind to adopt and act on it, leading to better recall and follow-through.

DAY 34

> "A man's health can be judged by which he takes two at a time — pills or stairs."
> — Joan Welsh

Every stair is a small prescription for your future self.
Strong legs today mean more freedom tomorrow.
Movement doesn't just prevent disease — it builds capacity.

Reflection

We've been conditioned to outsource what the body wants to do itself. We sit for hours, take the elevator, circle for the closest parking space, and don't notice we're quietly rehearsing for a future built on more pills and less strength. Pills have a place; they were never meant to carry the full load of health.

A short stair climb raises heart rate just enough to train elasticity in your arteries. Repeat that dose across the day and those mini-spikes teach blood pressure to settle lower at rest. Working muscle acts like a sponge for glucose, pulling sugar out of the bloodstream and lowering the burden on your pancreas. Even a few minutes of movement can lift endorphins and dopamine, boosting your mood, often faster than a snack or a scroll. Your legs are a key to your own pharmacy.

Every time you climb, squat, or walk, you trigger compounds your body makes on demand. Stairs are a tiny prescription your body writes, fills, and benefits from in the same minute. Do this most days and you build the two things that predict healthy aging: legs that can carry you and lungs that can keep up.

We aren't lazy; we're busy and heavily marketed to. Convenience sells you thirty seconds now and steals capacity later. Elevators, escalators, delivery everything — each trade saves a moment and quietly taxes your future strength. The bill arrives as breathlessness on a small hill, sore knees after a short stand, or a wobble on the stairs that didn't used to be there.

Stairs are the perfect dose: no outfit, no membership, no app. Two flights after a call. One flight at every bathroom break. Take the long way once; the short way next time. Every decision is a message to your body. Stairs say, "Stay strong."

Real-life snapshot

Elias and Tom worked in the same office, same floor, same age, same long meetings. The building had both an elevator and a big central stairwell.

Elias almost always took the elevator. "Why waste energy?" he'd joke, coffee in hand. A short walk from the parking lot left him slightly winded. By mid-afternoon he felt heavy and foggy, and the idea of exercising after work seemed impossible.

Tom, starting in his early 40s, made a different quiet rule: "If I can take the stairs, I do." No fanfare. No fitness tracker posts. Just a simple line in his head. Up two flights in the morning, down and up again at lunch, once more at the end of the day. On calls, he'd sometimes pace the hallway instead of sinking deeper into his chair.

At a routine checkup, Elias's blood pressure ticked into the "borderline high" range. His doctor mentioned exercise. Later that week, Tom caught him waiting for the elevator to go up one floor. "Come on," Tom said, nodding toward the stairs. "Train for stairs, not for the couch." Elias laughed — and then, slightly embarrassed, followed.

He decided to try a simple experiment for three months: never skip stairs if he had the choice, and add one extra trip up and down during the day when time allowed. No gym, no big program — just this one rule.

At first, he was breathing hard after a single flight. But the days stacked up. After a few weeks, two flights felt normal. After three months, he could walk up three floors without stopping, felt less winded from the parking lot, and noticed his energy dipping less in the afternoon. At his next appointment, his blood pressure had dropped into a healthier range.

Quick science

- Regular stair climbing in short bouts improves cardiovascular fitness and VO2 max, even when total exercise time is modest.
- Repeated short bursts of exertion, like taking the stairs, improve endothelial function (the health of blood vessel linings) and can help lower blood pressure over time.
- Leg strength and the ability to rise, walk, and climb independently are strong predictors of mobility and longevity in older age.[34]

Inspiration note

The smallest hill you climb today prevents the mountain you can't climb later.

Today's Invitation

One thing I will do for myself today:

- ☐ One stair choice: Take the stairs once today (even one flight counts).
- ☐ Leg snack: Do 2 minutes of leg work (sit-to-stands, step-ups, or stairs).
- ☐ Add one extra effort: Park farther or take the long way once today.

Action Step:
Choose the easiest one today. Do it now or set one reminder and do it when it best fits your schedule.

Reflection:
After I took the step today, I felt: ☐ calmer ☐ clearer ☐ steadier ☐ proud ☐ no change yet (effort still counts)

Bottom line

Choosing stairs today is choosing strength, circulation, and independence for your future self.

Your lines

(write one thought, one insight, or rewrite one sentence that rang true)

_____

_____

_____

☐ Done for today

Why this matters
Writing just a few lines by hand locks the concept into memory and gently primes your subconscious mind to adopt and act on it, leading to better recall and follow-through.

DAY 35

> "He who takes medicine and neglects his
> diet wastes the skill of his doctors."
> — Chinese Proverb

Food can heal what medicine can only manage.
Your diet is the daily prescription your body listens to most.
When you nourish the root, symptoms lose their grip.

Reflection

Pounds of poor-quality food will often overpower milligrams of medication. When prescriptions for blood pressure, cholesterol, and blood sugar keep rising — more pills, higher doses — it often signals a deeper mismatch: daily inputs (food, sleep, movement) are pushing one way while your doctor is trying to pull the other.

The harm is usually quiet and routine. Day after day, common foods work against the body's design. Bread, pasta, cereal, crackers, chips, and cookies are easy to overeat and are rapidly absorbed as sugar. Over time, that pattern pulls the body toward insulin resistance and diabetes. A few milligrams of a diabetes pill may struggle to balance pounds of processed carbohydrates. Medicine helps; habits decide.

When food quality improves — more single-ingredient foods, fiber, protein, and healthy fats; fewer refined starches and sugars — the "dose of life" that once demanded more medication often demands less.

The same is true for blood pressure and chronic pain. Milligrams of a blood pressure pill are an unfair match for daily meals built around salty takeout, highly processed meats (containing nitrates and nitrosamines), and refined carbs that spike insulin. High insulin tells the kidneys to hold onto salt and water and keeps blood vessels tense — pushing pressure up all day long. And with back or joint pain, daily ibuprofen can dull the ache for a while, but if most days are still spent sitting for hours, under-moving, and eating ultra-processed foods low in fiber and vegetables, the fire under the pain keeps burning. The pill turns down the volume on the signal; it doesn't repair the reasons your pressure or your joints are inflamed in the first place.

Medicine without diet is like painting over a wall stained with mold while a pipe still leaks behind it. For a while, things look better, but the damage continues

— and returns. Pills can support, but food should be the foundation. Clinicians can guide, but the plate sustains. Many doctors were not deeply trained in nutrition, and many simply don't have the time to teach it. That's frustrating for both sides.

The aim here is not guilt, but clarity and power: understand what processed foods do, replace them — bit by bit — with real nourishment, and let biology start working for you instead of against you. See medication as a bridge when needed, not a license to keep pouring in what harms you.

Real-life snapshot

Daniel was told his blood pressure was "a little high" for years before it suddenly wasn't little anymore. By his 40s he was on two medications — one to lower pressure, another to protect his kidneys. His numbers looked better on paper, but he still had headaches, felt wiped out after work, and his lab slip quietly showed the pattern underneath: rising A1c, higher triglycerides, and a growing waist.

At a follow-up visit, his doctor paused and said, "The meds are doing their job — but your daily life is still pushing in the other direction. If we change the inputs, we may be able to use less medicine, not more." Together they chose a few simple anchors. Daniel would crowd his plate with vegetables at lunch and dinner, swap most processed meats and cold cuts for real protein like fish, chicken, or beans, cut back on salty takeout, and tame white bread, pasta, and sugary snacks. He also tried a gentle 16:8 rhythm most days — eating within an eight-hour window, finishing dinner earlier, skipping late-night grazing, and keeping a clear buffer before bed.

To help his body use food better, he built movement into the day instead of "saving it" for the gym. He walked after meals, took the stairs when he could, and gradually moved toward a steady daily step goal. With his clinician's guidance, he added magnesium in the evening and protected a real wind-down routine at night.

The first few weeks were clumsy, but he stuck with "good enough," not perfect. At his three-month check, his blood pressure had dropped enough to safely lower one medication dose. Six months in, something more striking showed up: his A1c had returned to the normal range, his triglycerides had fallen, his HDL had inched up, and his waistline had shrunk.

Quick science
- Real food changes signals. Meals higher in fiber, protein, and unsaturated fats tend to flatten glucose spikes, improve satiety, and reduce inflammatory stress on blood vessels (endothelial function).

- Late eating raises strain. Eating close to bedtime and frequent refined-carb intake can worsen insulin resistance and keep the sympathetic "on" signal higher; earlier, lighter dinners and fewer nighttime snacks often improve next-day glucose control and blood pressure.
- Insulin and pressure are linked. Higher insulin levels can increase kidney sodium retention and vascular tone, which is one reason metabolic dysfunction often travels with rising blood pressure — and why improving food quality and timing can move both in the right direction.[35]

Inspiration note

Pills can steady the numbers; only your daily choices can heal the system that creates them.

Today's Invitation

One thing I will do for myself today:

- ☐ Real-food plate: Build one plate today (protein + vegetables + healthy fat).
- ☐ Earlier dinner: Finish dinner earlier and skip late-night snacking.
- ☐ After-meal walk: Walk 10–15 minutes after your biggest meal.

Action Step:
Choose the easiest one today. Do it now or set one reminder and do it when it best fits your schedule.

Reflection:
After I took the step today, I felt: ☐ calmer ☐ clearer ☐ steadier ☐ proud ☐ no change yet (effort still counts)

Bottom line

Medicine can stabilize — but only daily choices can truly transform.

Your lines

(write one thought, one insight, or rewrite one sentence that rang true)

_____

_____

_____

☐ Done for today

Why this matters
Writing just a few lines by hand locks the concept into memory and gently primes your subconscious mind to adopt and act on it, leading to better recall and follow-through.

DAY 36

"The greatest healing therapy is friendship and love."
— Hubert H. Humphrey

Your heart heals faster when it doesn't have to beat alone.
Love and friendship are not sentimental extras — they are biologic necessities.
Connection turns surviving into living.

Reflection

Let people close. Medicines can steady numbers and mend tissue, but love reaches the places no scan can see. A shared laugh, a hand on your shoulder, someone who remembers how you like your tea — these are quiet treatments that tell your nervous system, "You are not alone." Friendship is the unseen vitamin of health. People who feel cared for often recover better, cope longer, and find reasons to keep choosing life on the hard days.

Your body keeps a record of connection. After a warm conversation, stress hormones can ease, heart rate settles, breathing softens, and sleep comes more deeply. The opposite is just as real: chronic loneliness keeps the system on alert, like a smoke alarm that never turns off. You can have a full calendar and still feel alone; it's being known, not being busy, that calms the body.

Connection is not extra; it is protective. Letting even a few trusted people close is not weakness — it is one of the strongest health decisions you can make. You do not need a crowd. One or two people who see you, check on you, and care about your wellbeing can change the entire story your nervous system tells itself about the world: from "danger, handle everything alone" to "I have help; I can rest sometimes."

Real-life snapshot

After surgery, Martin went home with a folder of instructions and a bag of pills. His appetite was low, his mood flat, and the days blurred together. He did the basics, but he felt like he was drifting — sleeping late, picking at food, barely moving from his chair.

His neighbor, Mrs. Alvarez, noticed his lights were off most afternoons. She began stopping by for ten minutes — just to sit, ask how he was, and share a small story. Some days she brought soup. Other days she pointed out something blooming in the yard.

Within a few weeks, Martin was walking to the mailbox before she arrived, then around the block with her. His appetite started to return. He found himself looking forward to their talks. At a follow-up, his doctor was pleased with his recovery.

"The medicines mattered," Martin said, "but the visits did more than I expected. They reminded me I still mattered to someone. That's when I started wanting to get better, not just waiting to."

Quick science

- Social support improves health partly because it makes recovery behaviors easier to sustain (walks, meals, appointments, meds).
- Supportive relationships buffer stress reactivity — your body spends less time in "high alert" and more time in repair mode.
- Loneliness is not just being alone; it's feeling unsupported — and one steady, repeatable relationship can reduce that load.[36]

Inspiration note

Being deeply seen by even one person changes the nervous system's story from "danger" to "safe."

Today's Invitation

One thing I will do for myself today:

- ☐ Check-in text: Send one simple check-in to someone today.
- ☐ One true line: Share how you're really doing (one sentence) with someone you trust.
- ☐ Put it on the calendar: Schedule one connection (walk, call, or meal).

Action Step:
Choose the easiest one today. Do it now or set one reminder and do it when it best fits your schedule.

Reflection:
After I took the step today, I felt: ☐ calmer ☐ clearer ☐ steadier ☐ proud ☐ no change yet (effort still counts)

Bottom line

Friendship and love reach places no medication can — they are medicine in human form.

Your lines

(write one thought, one insight, or rewrite one sentence that rang true)

___

___

___

☐ Done for today

Why this matters
Writing just a few lines by hand locks the concept into memory and gently primes your subconscious mind to adopt and act on it, leading to better recall and follow-through.

DAY 37

> "It is health that is real wealth and not pieces of gold and silver."
> — attributed to Mahatma Gandhi

The richest life is one you are healthy enough to enjoy.
Every time you trade health for hurry, you spend what you can't get back.
True wealth is the capacity to show up fully — body, mind, and heart.

Reflection

Health is the treasure that makes every other joy possible. Without it, even riches lose their shine, because having energy, clarity of mind, and the freedom to move your body without pain or strain are the true luxuries of life. A healthy person can love more deeply, create more fully, and enjoy even the simplest pleasures. Illness, by contrast, makes the world feel narrow, no matter how much is in the bank. Each choice you make for your well-being is a quiet investment in your future strength.

Here's the common trap: we trade health for small coins. We cut sleep to "gain" an hour. We skip cooking and grab fast food to save time. We buy the cheapest calories and call it a bargain. We take jobs that keep us sitting all day — or flip night and day — and tell ourselves it's only temporary. Each trade looks minor, but together they drain energy, mood, and years. It's like drawing from your real bank account without checking the balance.

If you stepped back and let a stranger read your calendar and your last week of days, what would they say your "real wealth" is? Work? Screens? Other people's priorities? Or your own health, relationships, and inner life? This isn't about blame; it's an invitation to gently compare the list in your heart with the way your time is actually spent — and begin to bring them closer together.

If shift work, caregiving, or tight budgets are your reality, the answer isn't shame — it's extra protection. Defend sleep where you can. Plan simple home-cooked meals when possible. Seek daylight. Move your body in small, steady ways. You may not control every circumstance, but you can begin treating health as something you're responsible for protecting, not something left over when everything else is done.

Real-life snapshot

Angela poured herself into her career and savings, telling herself she'd "live later." By 55, she had the money but also hypertension, prediabetes, and chronic fatigue. When her doctor asked, "What good is wealth if you can't walk the beach you dreamed of?" it broke something inside her open.

She began investing differently: sleep first, daily walks, simple home meals, and protected time with loved ones. Over time, her labs improved, her mood lifted, and the world felt bigger again. "I still have my retirement account," she said. "But now I value even more the health to enjoy it."

Quick science

- After basic financial security is met, additional income tends to bring smaller gains in day-to-day well-being.
- Using money to buy time (time-saving services) is linked to greater happiness/life satisfaction than spending the same money on material purchases — largely because it reduces time pressure.
- Chronic stress and short sleep accelerate biological wear-and-tear (blood pressure, insulin resistance, inflammation), which is one reason "hurry" can quietly spend health.[37]

Inspiration note

Money buys options — but only health lets you use them.

Today's Invitation

One thing I will do for myself today:

- ☐ Buy time back: Use one time-saver today (delivery/pickup/shortcut) and spend that time on sleep or a walk.
- ☐ End on time once: Finish work on time once today (or set a hard stop).
- ☐ One delayed appointment: Schedule one basic visit you've been delaying (dental/physical/etc.).

Action Step:
Choose the easiest one today. Do it now or set one reminder and do it when it best fits your schedule.

Reflection:
After I took the step today, I felt: ☐ calmer ☐ clearer ☐ steadier ☐ proud ☐ no change yet (effort still counts)

Bottom line

Treat health like your most valuable asset — because it is.

Your lines

(write one thought, one insight, or rewrite one sentence that rang true)

_____
_____
_____

☐ Done for today

Why this matters

Writing just a few lines by hand locks the concept into memory and gently primes your subconscious mind to adopt and act on it, leading to better recall and follow-through.

DAY 38

> "If a man does not keep pace with his companions,
> perhaps it is because he hears a different drummer.
> Let him step to the music which he hears,
> however measured or far away."
> — Henry David Thoreau

The crowd is loud. Your body is quieter and truer.
When you chase someone else's pace, you pay in stress, injury, and burnout.
Today, trust your own drummer.

Reflection

There is a compass inside you. It is quiet, but exact. At the table, it knows when you are satisfied even if your plate isn't empty. Your hunger is not your neighbor's. The marathoner at your left is burning a furnace; you might be tending a candle today. Eat to *your* signal. Stop when the inner voice says "enough," not when the bowl is bare or the clock says so.

If you try to run another person's race or lift another person's bar, you borrow their injury. Progress comes like sunrise — steady, brightening minute by minute — when you honor your limit and then nudge it forward.

But the inner drummer doesn't just speak in the gym or at the table. It speaks in your rest: that tug to go to bed instead of watching one more episode. It speaks in your work: the sense that you've hit your focus limit and need a short break before the next task. It speaks in your relationships: the quiet knowing that you need a night in, or that a certain "yes" will cost you too much. When you ignore that voice, life becomes a cycle of overcommitting and crashing.

When your compass is calibrated, you stop chasing the crowd. You can be calm and confident because you know what honest effort feels like *for you* today. That calm is power. Records fall and lives change not from frenzy, but from fidelity: show up, do your best for this season, recover, repeat.

So tune to your drummer; measure by your truth; progress by respectful inches.

Real-life snapshot

Sam and David were training partners and close friends in their 40s. Same season of life, same starting mile pace, same dream: "be in the best shape of our lives." They both signed up for races, followed fitness influencers, and compared every workout.

Sam pushed hardest whenever he saw someone faster. If a friend added miles, he added more. If a coworker posted a personal record, he doubled his training the next week. Soreness and fatigue were badges of honor. Twice he ran through sharp knee pain "to keep up." Each time, he landed in physical therapy, stopped completely, lost ground, then started over. His efforts became a cycle: ramp up, get hurt, stop, repeat.

David quietly took a different path. He used others' progress as inspiration, not a stopwatch. On good days, he leaned in. On tired days, he dialed back. He listened when his body said, "Today, shorter," or "Today, walk instead of run." He applied the same rule to life: leaving gatherings when his social battery emptied, taking one true day off each week, stopping email at a set time even when others kept going.

Years later, Sam had a drawer full of race bibs — and a knee that hurt on stairs, a shoulder that ached at night, and a sense that he was always "starting over." David's times were never flashy, but his curve was smooth: fewer injuries, steady strength, better sleep, and a quiet confidence in his body.

"Your pace is so much slower than what you could do," Sam teased once. David smiled. "Maybe," he said. "But it's a pace I can keep for decades."

Quick science

- Matching pace to current capacity lowers injury risk and burnout, and helps you keep going long enough to improve.
- Interoceptive awareness — noticing internal cues like hunger, fatigue, and tension — supports better self-regulation and steadier choices.
- Self-paced routines tend to be more consistent and sustainable than routines driven mainly by comparison.[38]

Inspiration note

Your rhythm is your power — no one else can set it for you.

Today's Invitation

One thing I will do for myself today:

- ☐ Mid-meal pause: Pause for 10 seconds mid-meal and stop at satisfied.
- ☐ Train at your pace: End movement one rep or one minute before form breaks.
- ☐ Follow the sleepy wave: Use a lights-down cue tonight and go with the first sleepy wave.

Action Step:
Choose the easiest one today. Do it now or set one reminder and do it when it best fits your schedule.

Reflection:
After I took the step today, I felt: ☐ calmer ☐ clearer ☐ steadier ☐ proud ☐ no change yet (effort still counts)

Bottom line

Your best results come from listening inward, not chasing outward.

Your lines

(write one thought, one insight, or rewrite one sentence that rang true)

_____

_____

☐ Done for today

Why this matters
Writing just a few lines by hand locks the concept into memory and gently primes your subconscious mind to adopt and act on it, leading to better recall and follow-through.

DAY 39

"We can't live without eating, but we don't live to eat."
— Ben Franklin

Your body thrives on "enough," not excess.
Eating lightly earlier in the day builds energy instead of draining it.
Real nourishment comes from rhythm, not volume.

Reflection

Food is fuel first, not entertainment. Too little food harms health. Too much food does, too. Studies in humans and animals suggest that modest calorie reduction — without malnutrition — is linked with healthier aging and better metabolic markers, and in some settings may lower the risk of chronic disease (like diabetes, heart disease, and some cancers).

Why this makes sense: digesting and processing food is work. Every bite asks your body to break down, absorb, transport, and store nutrients, then clean up the leftovers. More than your body needs means more metabolic "wear and tear." Eating closer to enough — but not extra — lightens the load.

Long-lived cultures live this way. In traditional Okinawa (a Blue Zone), where people commonly live into their 90s and beyond, many practiced *hara hachi bu* — "eat until 80% full" — and historically ate fewer calories than Americans, mostly from plants and sweet potatoes. They didn't starve; they stopped just short of full.

A few simple guardrails help avoid overeating:

- **Fewer eating windows, not constant grazing.** Many people do well with three meals and no snacks. A time-restricted pattern (for example, eating within 8–10 hours and finishing earlier in the evening) can help some people keep structure, especially with an earlier eating window.
- **Fiber first.** Start meals with salad or vegetables. Fiber has almost no calories, fills you up, and makes overeating less likely.
- **No "automatic" snacking.** If it's not one of your meals, pause and ask: *Am I truly hungry, or just bored, stressed, or tired?*
- **Protect sleep and walking.** Both reduce appetite swings and stress-eating, making "enough" much easier to feel.

The goal isn't to eat tiny amounts or live in fear of food. It's to eat to support life — not to stuff discomfort. Enough is a place; learning to recognize it is one of the deepest skills in nutrition.

Real-life snapshot

Miguel constantly felt bloated and tired after meals. At first it was just a little heaviness. Then the classic pattern showed up: burning in his chest after dinner, a sour taste in his throat at night, propping himself up on extra pillows to sleep. Late-night pizza, big portions, and "just one more snack" before bed were part of the routine. He started keeping antacids in his car, his desk, and his nightstand.

When the burning became a near-nightly visitor, he went to his doctor asking for a prescription acid-blocking pill "to fix the acid." The doctor could have simply written the script and moved on, but instead he slowed down and explained the bigger picture. Stomach acid wasn't Miguel's enemy; his habits were. Acid-suppressing medicines can help short term, but long-term use can carry tradeoffs: reduced absorption of nutrients like magnesium and vitamin B12, higher risk of certain infections, and associations with bone-thinning/fracture risk in some studies.

So they tried a different path. For six weeks, Miguel made three simple shifts. He ate within an eight-hour window, with his last meal in the early evening. He stopped food at least three hours before bed. And he leaned on mostly whole, simple meals instead of heavy late-night snacks and fast food.

He still ate enough — he just stopped eating right up until bedtime and dropped the "entertainment" extras.

By the end of week two, the burning had eased from nightly to occasional. By week four, he wasn't reaching for antacids out of habit. By six weeks, his reflux and heartburn were essentially gone. His stomach felt calmer, his head clearer, and his sleep deeper.

Quick science

- Eating to comfortable satisfaction (often described as ~70–80% full) can improve post-meal glucose control and may reduce markers of oxidative stress.
- Earlier, time-restricted eating can improve metabolic flexibility and better align digestion with your natural circadian rhythm.
- Fiber-first meals blunt glucose spikes, smooth energy, and reduce downstream cravings. [39]

Compass link: If you want the deeper "why," see Part III — The Compass Explained — Chapter 17: Gut Health — Soil Before Seeds.

Inspiration note

Satisfaction is a signal — fullness is a warning.

Today's Invitation

One thing I will do for myself today:

- ☐ Screen-free meal: Eat one meal seated and without screens.
- ☐ Practice enough: Pause mid-meal and stop at satisfied (not stuffed).
- ☐ Evening food stop: Choose a stop time for food tonight (aim for 2–3 hours before bed if you can).

Action Step:
Choose the easiest one today. Do it now or set one reminder and do it when it best fits your schedule.

Reflection:
After I took the step today, I felt: ☐ calmer ☐ clearer ☐ steadier ☐ proud ☐ no change yet (effort still counts)

Bottom line

Eat to fuel your life — not just to fill your stomach.

Your lines

(write one thought, one insight, or rewrite one sentence that rang true)

_____

_____

_____

☐ Done for today

Why this matters
Writing just a few lines by hand locks the concept into memory and gently primes your subconscious mind to adopt and act on it, leading to better recall and follow-through.

DAY 40

> "Discipline is remembering what you want."
> — David Campbell

Discipline is not punishment; it's memory in action.
When your why stays visible, your choices stop feeling random.
A clear daily structure turns vague wishes into real change.

Reflection

If you're trying to restore your health — lift brain fog, ease persistent fatigue, sleep more deeply, steady your mood— you don't just need more "willpower." You need a structure that helps you remember what you want before the day sweeps you away.

Most people actually know what they want: "I want my brain back." "I want to wake up with energy." "I want to be here, fully, for my family." The problem isn't desire; it's drift. The alarm goes off, notifications hit, demands pile up, and by noon the only thing you're remembering is the next urgent task. Health becomes a vague background wish you hope to "get to" later.

Discipline, in this light, is not white-knuckling your way through one more perfect day. It's simply remembering what you truly want — and organizing your time and environment so your actions match it more often than not. When your aim is written where you see it morning and night, when your calendar shows a small, protected block for health work, when your phone nudges you with reminders that feel like encouragement instead of nagging, choices get easier. You're not starting from scratch each day; you're following a map you drew for yourself.

This is how identity shifts. At first you feel like someone "trying to be healthy." Over time, with repeated structure, you begin to feel like someone who *is* the kind of person who protects their sleep, moves daily, eats for their future brain, and says no to what drains them. The inner argument quiets. You stop asking, "Should I do this?" and start saying, "This is what I do because this is what I want."

If your goal is big — healing fatigue, improving metabolic strain, improving sleep — it deserves more than a passing thought. It deserves a system: words in front of your eyes, a block on your calendar, a tiny daily checklist. You are not being rigid; you are being kind to your future self.

Real-life snapshot

Two coworkers, Nina and Carla, both hit a wall in their early 40s. Same office, same long hours, same complaints: brain fog, poor sleep, stubborn weight, creeping labs. Both said, "I just want to feel like myself again."

Nina kept her goal mostly in her head. On inspired days she would walk, cook, or go to bed earlier. On stressful days she would fall back into old patterns. Her weeks swung between "on" and "off." Every Monday felt like a fresh start — and by Thursday her plan had disappeared under emails and errands. At follow-up visits, her symptoms bobbed up and down, but nothing really changed. "I guess I'm just not disciplined enough," she said.

Carla decided to treat her health goal like a real project. At her doctor's suggestion, she wrote a single sentence on an index card:

"I want my brain clear and my energy steady so I can enjoy my life and show up fully for the people I love."

She put it in three places: her phone lock screen, her bathroom mirror, and the top of her digital calendar. Then she blocked one 45-minute "Health Block" on weekdays. That block could be used only for three things: movement, meal prep and planning, or sleep systems (like wind-down routines, light management, or journaling).

It didn't look dramatic on paper: some mornings a 20-minute walk and quick breakfast prep, some nights a firm phone cut-off and earlier lights down. But it was consistent. Her Why was in her face every day, and her calendar had a place where that Why lived.

A year later, both women still had busy lives. But their trajectories had split. Nina felt like she was always "trying," with very little to show for it. Carla's brain fog had eased, her sleep had improved, her labs had shifted in the right direction, and, quietly, her identity had changed.

"I don't think I became more disciplined," Carla said. "I just stopped leaving my health to chance. I wrote down what I want, and I gave it a real place in my day."

Quick science

- Writing down a clear goal and seeing it often (on a card, screen, or wall) "primes" the brain — making choices that match that goal easier and more automatic.
- Creating a specific plan — what you'll do, when, and where — is called an *implementation intention* and has been shown to meaningfully increase follow-through compared with vague intentions.

- Time-blocking a small, regular window for health behaviors (even 20–30 minutes) reduces decision fatigue and helps move habits from effortful to more automatic over time.[40]

Inspiration note

Discipline is just your future self, brought into today.

Today's Invitation

One thing I will do for myself today:

- ☐ One-line why: Write one sentence: What I want most is _____.
- ☐ Schedule it: Put one small health block on your calendar today.
- ☐ Visible cue: Place your why where you'll see it (mirror, lock screen, or a note).

Action Step:
Choose the easiest one today. Do it now or set one reminder and do it when it best fits your schedule.

Reflection:
After I took the step today, I felt: ☐ calmer ☐ clearer ☐ steadier ☐ proud ☐ no change yet (effort still counts)

Bottom line

Discipline is not about being harsh with yourself. It's about remembering what you truly want — and giving it a real place in your day.

Your lines

(write one thought, one insight, or rewrite one sentence that rang true)

_____

_____

☐ Done for today

Why this matters
Writing just a few lines by hand locks the concept into memory and gently primes your subconscious mind to adopt and act on it, leading to better recall and follow-through.

DAY 41

> "For everything there is a season, and a time for every matter under heaven."
> — Ecclesiastes 3:1

Your body was built to live in seasons — not one endless sprint.
There is a time to push and a time to repair.
When you honor your seasons, strength stops feeling like an accident.

Reflection

Nature never runs at full blast all year. There are planting seasons and harvest seasons, long bright days and long quiet nights, growth spurts and dormancy. Your body is built the same way. Muscles, hormones, nerves, and mood do best when life has seasons: times of effort, and times of recovery.

Modern life sells one setting: "on." Same workload in January as in June. Same training intensity every week. Same social pace every month. No true off-season, no downshift. It looks productive on paper, but biology reads it as one long stress signal. At first, you can push through. Then sleep thins, injuries linger, cravings rise, patience shrinks, and ordinary tasks start to feel heavy.

Athletes learned this a long time ago. The best don't train hard at the same level every day of the year. They periodize: build, peak, then back off so the body can adapt. You can borrow this idea for real life, even if you never step on a track. There can be seasons where you lean in — improving sleep, building strength, tightening nutrition — and seasons where you mostly maintain what you've built. There can be weeks you ask more of yourself at work, and weeks you deliberately protect recovery.

Living in seasons can be simple:

- One lighter week every month where you protect sleep and keep workouts easy.
- One true rest day each week where health is supported, but productivity is not the goal.
- A winter rhythm that leans toward restoration, and a spring/summer rhythm that leans toward building.

You don't need a perfect plan. You need permission to stop treating your body like a machine that never deserves a downshift. When you honor seasons — effort, then ease — you stop burning out and start cycling forward. Strength, clarity, and emotional resilience grow not just from what you do, but from what you let sink in.

Real-life snapshot

Maya prided herself on being "consistent." Same intense workouts year-round, same long workdays, same full weekends. No breaks. For a while, it worked — she felt strong and admired. Then small cracks appeared: a knee that always ached, colds that kept returning, and a dread before workouts she used to love. Her sleep shortened and her joy faded.

One day her trainer said, "You're living in peak season all year." He offered a simple rhythm: three months of building, then a lighter month where she still trained but dropped intensity and volume. One weekly rest day that really was rest. Slightly earlier nights during heavy work weeks. No guilt — just seasons.

At first, easing off felt like failure. Then something surprising happened: the injuries stopped piling up. After the lighter weeks, her runs felt smoother and her strength climbed. Her mood steadied. She realized consistency wasn't doing the maximum every day — it was showing up in a way her body could sustain for years.

Quick science

- Bodies adapt best to cycles of stress and recovery. Constant high stress without rest drives allostatic load — the wear-and-tear of never turning off — which is linked to fatigue, depression, and chronic disease.
- Exercise studies show that periodized training (planned lighter phases) produces better gains and fewer injuries than pushing hard at the same level continuously.
- Rest days and lower-intensity periods are associated with lower burnout and better performance when you return to normal effort; some studies also link regular recovery time with better cardiovascular risk profiles.[41]

Inspiration note

You are not meant to live in harvest season all year.

Today's Invitation

One thing I will do for myself today:

- ☐ I live in seasons today by choosing one true recovery block (a real rest hour or a gentler evening).
- ☐ I match my body's season by doing low-intensity movement (easy walk, mobility, or light strength).
- ☐ I protect overnight repair by setting an earlier lights-down cue and following it.

Action Step:
Choose the easiest one today. Do it now or set one reminder and do it when it best fits your schedule.

Reflection:
After I took the step today, I felt: ☐ calmer ☐ clearer ☐ steadier ☐ proud ☐ no change yet (effort still counts)

Bottom line

Health thrives when your internal seasons are distinct, respected, and allowed to change.

Your lines

(write one thought, one insight, or rewrite one sentence that rang true)

_____

_____

_____

☐ Done for today

Why this matters
Writing just a few lines by hand locks the concept into memory and gently primes your subconscious mind to adopt and act on it, leading to better recall and follow-through.

DAY 42

> **"The wound is the place where the Light enters you."**
> — attributed to Rumi

Pain is not proof that you're broken — it's proof that you're alive.
Your deepest wounds can become your deepest sources of wisdom.
Light often enters through the places you wish didn't exist.

Reflection

When something breaks in your life — your health, your heart, your plans — it can feel like proof that you have failed. But often, that is the moment a different kind of knowing begins. Our wounds humble us. They strip away the illusion that we can control everything, and they open a small door for compassion — for ourselves, and for others who hurt in similar ways.

Healing is rarely a straight line, and it is almost never only physical. The body must mend, but so must the heart and mind. When light meets the broken place — through kindness, honesty, or support — the goal is not to erase what happened. It is to integrate it. This is how wisdom forms: hardship carves channels where love and insight can finally flow. Over time, the scar becomes proof that light entered — and stayed.

Mercy toward yourself is oxygen. Shame says, "You deserved this," or "You should be over this by now," and slams the door on healing. Self-compassion says, "This hurts, and I am still worthy," and the door cracks open again. Beginning again is not weakness; it is the mercy offered to every living being who wakes up to a new day.

Let the wound teach you. Instead of asking, "Why is this happening to me?" try asking, "What is this asking me to learn or change?" To rest instead of overdrive. To set a boundary instead of saying yes to everything. To forgive yourself for being human. To strengthen a part of you that has been neglected. Your wound is not your identity; it is an invitation to become truer — more honest, more compassionate, and more aligned with what matters.

Real-life snapshot

After a painful breakup, Nadia went quiet. She kept functioning, but she stopped sleeping well and replayed every conversation like a courtroom trial. Her friend

Jason went the other way after his own loss — nonstop distractions, more work, more scrolling, more noise. Both looked "fine," but both were bleeding inside.

Nadia started a small practice: hand on heart, one line — "This hurts, and I'm still worthy." Jason finally told one trusted friend the truth: "I'm not okay." Neither moment was dramatic. But both were doors. Over time, Nadia stopped chasing people who made her feel small. Jason slept better once he stopped carrying it alone. Their pain didn't vanish. It changed shape — from a trap into a teacher.

Quick science

- Self-compassion practices (kind self-talk, hand-over-heart) are associated with lower shame and anxiety, and greater emotional resilience.
- Processing emotions instead of suppressing them lowers sympathetic arousal (fight-or-flight) and can improve heart-rate variability (HRV), a marker of nervous system flexibility and recovery.
- Meaning-making and reframing can strengthen coping and improve long-term adaptation after stress.[42]

Inspiration note

Scars don't erase your story — they prove you survived and kept walking.

Today's Invitation

One thing I will do for myself today:

- ☐ I practice self-kindness by speaking to myself the way I would speak to a good friend today.
- ☐ I treat myself with kindness by calming my body first with 2 minutes of slow breathing.
- ☐ I respond to myself with compassion by reaching out for support (a text, a call, or scheduling help) instead of carrying it alone.

Action Step:
Choose the easiest one today. Do it now or set one reminder and do it when it best fits your schedule.

Reflection:
After I took the step today, I felt: ☐ calmer ☐ clearer ☐ steadier ☐ proud ☐ no change yet (effort still counts)

Bottom line

Your wound is not who you are — it's where the light is trying to enter.

Your lines

(write one thought, one insight, or rewrite one sentence that rang true)

_____

_____

_____

☐ Done for today

Why this matters
Writing just a few lines by hand locks the concept into memory and gently primes your subconscious mind to adopt and act on it, leading to better recall and follow-through.

DAY 43

"Slow is smooth, smooth is fast"
— Proverb

Real power isn't just speed — it's having all your gears.
High gear lets you perform; low gear lets you heal.
Master both, and you stop being dragged by your day and start driving it.

Reflection

Most people are lopsided in how they use their nervous system. Some live almost entirely in high gear: fast thinking, fast talking, constant problem-solving, adrenaline on tap. They're excellent in a crisis, but terrible at turning off. Others get stuck in low gear: hard to start, overwhelmed by decisions, always "tired but wired."

A healthy human needs both gears — and the skill to shift between them on purpose.

High gear looks like focused work, quick decisions, intense workouts, being fully "on" for a patient, a meeting, or a family situation. It's sympathetic activation — the part of your system built for action. You want this gear when you need performance.

Low gear looks like slower breathing, a relaxed jaw, softer shoulders, walking instead of rushing, eating without multitasking, letting the mind idle, connecting with someone you trust. It's parasympathetic — the part of your system built for digestion, repair, and integration. You want this gear when you need to absorb life, not fight it.

Modern life trains high gear and neglects low. Energy drinks, endless notifications, "one more thing," caffeine late in the day — all gas, no brakes. Then, when people finally feel like they can't stand it anymore, they try to force low gear with shortcuts: alcohol, sedatives, or heavy food. Those can take the edge off temporarily, but they don't teach your nervous system the skill. Over time, they can blunt your natural gears — fragmenting sleep, dulling mood, and making calm harder to reach without them.

Skillful shifting is simpler than it sounds. You don't slam into high gear right after a heavy meal. You don't do your hardest thinking at midnight with blue light in your face. And you don't rely on wine or benzos as your main "off switch."

Instead, you use high gear when your body can support it — morning and mid-day for deep work, training, and problem-solving. You use low gear around meals and in the evening — slower chewing, short walks, softer light, real conversation, a few minutes of breathing. You can nudge the gears with coffee, tea, chamomile, or magnesium — but the real shift comes from attention, boundaries, and practiced cues.

No one is born good at this. Calm people aren't magically "chill." High performers who don't burn out aren't superhuman. They're people who learned — often the hard way — that knowing when to go fast and when to go slow is as important as knowing how to go at all.

Real-life snapshot

Elliot prided himself on being "always on." His mornings started with emails in bed and strong coffee. From there it was back-to-back calls, fast lunches at his desk, high-intensity workouts squeezed between meetings, and late-night laptop time to "catch up." High gear from the moment he woke until he dropped into bed — wired and exhausted.

For a while, it worked: promotions, praise, productivity. Then the cracks appeared — a racing heart out of nowhere, trouble falling asleep, 3 a.m. wake-ups, cravings for sugar and more caffeine, a chest that never fully relaxed. "I don't know how to stop," he admitted.

With coaching, he began to think in gears instead of just tasks. Together they redesigned his day: a 60–90 minute deep-work block after breakfast (no phone, no notifications), a 10-minute slow walk after lunch (no calls, no screens), a coffee cutoff with no new intense projects late in the day, and a true evening downshift — dim lights, no "just one more" email, and a short breathing or body-scan practice instead of scrolling.

He didn't stop working hard. He just stopped driving in the wrong gear all day.

Within weeks, the random pounding eased. Sleep came easier. His workouts felt strong again instead of desperate. "I didn't lower my standards," he said. "I learned how to use my engine. High gear is there when I need it. Low gear is how I make sure I'll still be here in 10 years."

Quick science

- High gear (sympathetic activation) is essential for focus and performance, but chronic overactivation without enough parasympathetic time is linked to hypertension, impaired immunity, and burnout.

- Shifting into low gear with non-chemical tools — slow breathing, body awareness, light reduction, gentle movement — improves heart-rate variability, sleep quality, and perceived calm.
- Heavy meals increase blood flow to the gut and can impair alertness for a time; intense high-gear demands immediately after heavy eating are associated with discomfort, poor focus and, in vulnerable people, more physiologic strain.[43]

Inspiration note

Real strength isn't staying in high gear — it's knowing how and when to shift.

Today's Invitation

One thing I will do for myself today:

☐ I downshift after one meal today with 5 minutes of low gear (slow chew or a gentle walk).
☐ I use high gear once on purpose with one focused work block when my brain is best (morning or mid-day).
☐ I protect low gear tonight: dim lights, slow breathing, and screens off early.

Action Step:
Choose the easiest one today. Do it now or set one reminder and do it when it best fits your schedule.

Reflection:
After I took the step today, I felt: ☐ calmer ☐ clearer ☐ steadier ☐ proud ☐ no change yet (effort still counts)

Bottom line

You were built with more than one speed. Mastering both, and choosing them consciously, is how you stay effective without breaking yourself.

Your lines

(write one thought, one insight, or rewrite one sentence that rang true)

_____
_____
_____

☐ Done for today

Why this matters
Writing just a few lines by hand locks the concept into memory and gently primes your subconscious mind to adopt and act on it, leading to better recall and follow-through.

DAY 44

"Nature itself is the best physician."
— Hippocrates

Time in nature is medicine you're meant to drink daily.
Your nervous system recognizes trees, sky, and wind as home.
Even small doses of green and blue can change how your body feels.

Reflection

Your body was not designed for a lifetime of walls, screens, and recycled air. It was designed for horizons. For light shifting across the sky. For the texture of bark under your hand, grass under your feet, wind on your face, waves or rain in your ears.

Hippocrates called nature "the best physician." Modern research keeps pointing the same direction. People who spend more time in green and blue spaces — parks, forests, gardens, lakes, the sea — tend to have lower blood pressure, better mood, less anxiety and depression, and lower risk of heart disease and early death. Even short visits to nature help: studies suggest that even 15–20 minutes a day in green space can improve mood and stress, and that around 2 hours per week is associated with higher self-reported wellbeing.

Time in forests and parks isn't just "relaxing." Forest-bathing (Shinrin-yoku) research shows measurable changes: lower cortisol, lower blood pressure and heart rate, increased natural killer (NK) cell activity, and changes in some immune markers. The body can shift into a more restorative state when surrounded by trees and natural sounds.

You might think, "That's nice, but I live in a city and work in a building." Good news: this is not about living in a cabin. It's about daily contact with nature in whatever ways are realistically available — a 10–15 minute walk through a park or tree-lined street, standing barefoot on grass or sand for a few minutes, sitting on a bench where you can see sky and leaves instead of only walls, opening a window to feel real air and listen to birds, taking a weekend walk along a river, lake, or the sea when possible.

And if you truly can't get out easily on some days, you can bring small pieces of nature inside. Keep a few real plants at home or on your desk at work. Even one plant changes the feel of a room and gives your eyes something living to rest on. If possible, choose your seat so you can see a tree, sky, or courtyard through a window. Use nature sounds — rain, waves, forest — instead of news or talk radio during a short break. Indoor plants and views of nature aren't just decoration. Studies show they can reduce stress, improve mood, and support attention and productivity. A plant is a tiny patch of forest that quietly reminds your nervous system: life exists outside this email.

You don't have to hike a mountain to get the dose. Let "nature time" be simple, repeatable, and phone-light: a walk, a sit, a few deep breaths under the sky, a moment with your hand on a leaf in your living room. Over time, your nervous system will start to expect this daily relief. It will begin to trust that, no matter how digital your work and home life are, your body hasn't been entirely forgotten.

Real-life snapshot

Jared lived on the 23rd floor of a glass tower and spent his days in front of multiple screens. From January to March, he joked that the only "outdoors" he saw was the parking garage. His blood pressure crept up, his sleep felt thin, and his mood flattened. "I'm not outdoorsy," he said. "I'm a city guy. Nature is for vacations."

His clinician disagreed. "Nature is for Tuesday," she said. They made a tiny, city-friendly plan: a 10–15 minute phone-free walk near trees on workdays, one longer riverfront walk on a weekend day, and a few real plants at home and on his desk.

At first it felt pointless. "I'm just looking at trees and a fern," he thought. But he kept the streak going.

Within a few weeks, he noticed his shoulders weren't always up by his ears. The knot in his chest softened after park walks. Glancing at the plant on his desk made him pause and exhale. Sleep improved. After a few months, his blood pressure readings edged down and he felt less like he was "buzzing" all the time.

"I used to think nature was a luxury," he said. "Now I treat it like my daily pill. The city is still loud — but at least my body gets to remember what quiet feels like."

Quick science

- Living in greener environments and spending time in parks and forests are associated with lower mortality, better mental health, and improved cardiovascular outcomes.

- Forest-bathing and time in natural environments lower cortisol and blood pressure, reduce stress, and increase natural killer (NK) cell activity and shift some immune markers.
- Even short daily exposures (about 15–20 minutes) to urban green spaces improve mood and reduce anxiety. Views of nature and indoor plants have been shown to reduce stress and support attention and productivity compared to bare, artificial environments.[44]

Inspiration note

Nature is not a backdrop; it's a treatment. Let it touch your skin, your eyes, your lungs, and your nervous system — outdoors or in miniature, on your windowsill.

Today's Invitation

One thing I will do for myself today:

- ☐ I let nature support me by spending 15–20 minutes outside today (even a city block or park counts).
- ☐ I reset in the outdoors by taking an easy walk and letting my eyes rest on something living.
- ☐ I bring nature closer by adding one "living cue" to my space (open window, sunlight, or a plant).

Action Step:
Choose the easiest one today. Do it now or set one reminder and do it when it best fits your schedule.

Reflection:
After I took the step today, I felt: ☐ calmer ☐ clearer ☐ steadier ☐ proud ☐ no change yet (effort still counts)

Bottom line

You don't have to move to the wilderness to let nature help you. A daily sip — a tree, a plant, a patch of sky, a bit of wind — is powerful medicine your body knows how to use.

Your lines

(write one thought, one insight, or rewrite one sentence that rang true)

_____

_____

_____

☐ Done for today

Why this matters
Writing just a few lines by hand locks the concept into memory and gently primes your subconscious mind to adopt and act on it, leading to better recall and follow-through.

DAY 45

> "Money you invest in your health is the highest-yield investment."
> — A. Smyrlis, MD

Health is not a cost center — it's your primary asset.
Every choice is either a deposit or a withdrawal.
What you invest in consistently becomes your baseline.

Reflection

Make the health deposits daily. Every day you place small bets with your time and money. A home-cooked meal is a deposit; ultra-processed convenience is a withdrawal. An early night pays you back with interest; "just one more episode" charges a hidden fee. A 20-minute walk compounds; another hour in the chair compounds too — just in the other direction.

We're used to treating health spending as "extra" — a gym membership, better groceries, therapy, a decent mattress, a water filter, quality shoes, a counseling session, a quiet weekend off. But zoom out: these aren't luxuries. They're investments in the only system you can't replace.

Treat your body like a junk bond and it eventually trades like one. Treat it like a blue-chip asset and, over time, it behaves differently.

Just like in finance, wise investments often look small and boring up close. One better meal. One regular checkup. One course of physical therapy. One set of blood work before things go off the rails instead of after. Years later, those choices often look wise: less medical chaos, fewer preventable setbacks, and more functional years to earn, love, travel, and serve.

Spend on what makes you strong: sleep, light, movement, real food, honest connection, a safer environment, emotional support. These are not indulgences. They are deposits in your future ability to play with your children and grandchildren, to still think clearly, to still walk unassisted, to still do work that matters to you. Neglect, not health, is the real expense.

Real-life snapshot

Two brothers, Daniel and Chris, earned roughly the same income for most of their lives. Both worked hard, both were smart with money — but they treated health spending very differently.

Daniel was the classic saver. He prided himself on driving his old car, skipping vacations, and avoiding "unnecessary" costs. Gym fees, massage, therapy, better groceries, high-quality shoes — all "too expensive." He bought the cheapest food, delayed dental work, ignored back pain, and saw checkups as optional. His bank account grew. His health account quietly emptied.

Chris saved too, but he treated a few things as non-negotiable investments: better groceries most weeks, a basic gym or walking plan with good shoes, early help when pain started whispering, support during stressful seasons, and a sleep setup he protected. On paper, Chris had less in his retirement accounts. In his body, he had more.

By their late 60s, the difference was stark. Daniel had a much larger nest egg — and a long list of diagnoses: heart disease, diabetes, severe arthritis. He was on multiple medications and spent significant time and money on injections for his knees and spine, specialist visits, and procedures to manage complications. Travel was difficult. Climbing stairs was painful. Much of his "extra" money went to trying to buy back function.

Chris's retirement savings were more modest, but his body still carried him. He walked daily, traveled with his partner, played with his grandkids, and spent far less on doctors and procedures. He still took a couple of medications, but his life was not built around them. "I'm not rich," he joked, "but I can carry my own bags. That feels like wealth."

The ideal is to have both financial security and health. But if you have to choose where to invest first, start with the asset you can't borrow, insure, or replace: the body that has to live every day of your life.

Quick science

- Preventive health behaviors — such as not smoking, regular movement, mostly whole-food eating, and adequate sleep — substantially reduce the risk of chronic diseases that are costly in both money and quality of life.
- Good sleep, exercise, and nutrition are linked to higher productivity, fewer missed workdays, better decision-making, and longer "healthspan," which can indirectly support earning potential and stability.
- Studies generally find that early investment in health (prevention and lifestyle change) reduces long-term healthcare expenditures and the need for intensive interventions later.[45]

Inspiration note

Investing in health is the rare choice that pays you back in every currency — time, energy, mood, and years.

Today's Invitation

One thing I will do for myself today:

- ☐ I make a health deposit by doing 10 minutes of simple strength today (sit-to-stand, wall push-ups, and a plank).
- ☐ I grow my health account by choosing one "ingredients meal" today (protein + plants), even if it's the simplest version.
- ☐ I invest in my future capacity by setting a hard stop on "one more episode/scroll" tonight and starting wind-down on time (dim lights, low input).

Action Step:
Choose the easiest one today. Do it now or set one reminder and do it when it best fits your schedule.

Reflection:
After I took the step today, I felt: ☐ calmer ☐ clearer ☐ steadier ☐ proud ☐ no change yet (effort still counts)

Bottom line

Treat health as your most important portfolio — and fund it daily.

Your lines

(write one thought, one insight, or rewrite one sentence that rang true)

_____

_____

_____

☐ Done for today

Why this matters
Writing just a few lines by hand locks the concept into memory and gently primes your subconscious mind to adopt and act on it, leading to better recall and follow-through.

DAY 46

"Nature does not hurry, yet everything is accomplished."
— Lao Tzu

Nature achieves everything through rhythm, repetition, and patience.
Slow does not mean weak — it means aligned with biology.
Healing accelerates when you stop rushing the things that must grow.

Reflection

An oak earns its rings one season at a time. A pearl forms — layer by layer — around a grain of sand. Wine deepens in the cask year by year. True health is built the same way. Natural healing and growth are slow crafts. Quick fixes flare and fade; patient work takes root and lasts.

Think in pictures that map to real change. High blood pressure, sugar, or cholesterol unwind like a tight knot. Gentle, repeated pulls — daily walks, simple whole-food, fiber-rich meals, earlier nights — loosen what a single yank never will. Broken sleep rhythm? Set a steady tempo: a consistent wake-up and wind-down time, dim lights after sunset, and finish dinner at least three hours before bed. In a few weeks, the rhythm begins to return and hold.

When you change your lifestyle to improve health, your job is not to keep checking the roots. Do not pluck the shoot to see how it's doing. Have faith in the process and keep tending it — day by day, week by week. The fruit is real health: deeper, steadier, and stronger than any pill, quick fix, or patch can offer.

Real-life snapshot

Two brothers were given the same diagnosis: metabolic syndrome — a warning sign that blood sugar, blood pressure, and cholesterol were drifting into the danger zone. Their doctor put it simply: "If nothing changes, you're on track for diabetes, high blood pressure, and cholesterol problems, with pills for each."

Same age, same genes, same plan: simpler meals, daily walks, earlier nights.

For six weeks they both showed up: fewer takeout dinners, more fiber, more steps. The younger brother grew impatient. The scale barely moved. His labs had only budged. "This is useless," he said, and asked his doctor for a weight-loss medication to speed things up. The weight came off faster, and at first it felt like proof that shortcuts were better.

The older brother was discouraged too, but he kept going. By the third month his waist had shrunk, his blood pressure and fasting sugar improved, and his energy felt steady instead of crashing every afternoon. His new routine started to feel normal, not heroic.

Three years later, the picture had flipped. The younger brother stopped the medication after side effects, and without new habits to hold him, his weight and numbers drifted back toward where they started. The older brother wasn't perfect, but his daily rhythm held. His metabolic markers had improved, and his labs stayed steadier.

"I almost quit at six weeks. I am so glad I didn't," he told his doctor.

Quick science

- Small, steady lifestyle changes — more walking, fiber-rich whole foods, earlier sleep — can start improving blood pressure, blood sugar, and triglycerides within a few months, even before the scale moves much.
- GLP-1 medicines can help with weight loss and blood sugar, but without habit change, weight and metabolic risk can creep back after medication is stopped.
- When healthy routines are repeated long enough to feel automatic, they can reshape metabolism: muscles handle sugar better, liver fat can decrease, and inflammation markers may improve.[46]

Inspiration note

The seasons never rush — and yet nothing is left undone.

Today's Invitation

One thing I will do for myself today:

- ☐ I choose one anchor time today: the same wake time tomorrow or a lights-down time tonight.
- ☐ I take a simple 10–15 minute walk after one meal, at an easy pace.
- ☐ I build one steady plate today: protein + vegetables + a fiber-rich whole-food carb (beans/lentils or similar).

Action Step:
Choose the easiest one today. Do it now or set one reminder and do it when it best fits your schedule.

Reflection:
After I took the step today, I felt: ☐ calmer ☐ clearer ☐ steadier ☐ proud ☐ no change yet (effort still counts)

Bottom line

Go at nature's pace — slow enough to grow, steady enough to last.

Your lines

(write one thought, one insight, or rewrite one sentence that rang true)

_____

_____

_____

☐ Done for today

Why this matters

Writing just a few lines by hand locks the concept into memory and gently primes your subconscious mind to adopt and act on it, leading to better recall and follow-through.

DAY 47

"The soul becomes dyed with the color of its thoughts."
— Marcus Aurelius

Your inner world is painted by whatever you repeatedly look at and listen to. If you don't choose your inputs, they will choose your mood. A few small shifts in what you consume can recolor your entire day.

Reflection

Guard your inputs. Your mind eats what your eyes and ears feed it.
 Inputs become moods.
 Moods become choices.
 Choices become your life.
What you consume colors what you feel and what you notice. If you let anything in, at any time, you get dyed by accident. If you choose on purpose, you start dyeing your life in colors you can live with.

Here's my clear stance: if you want to be healthy, limit doom-heavy media. Keep news in small, intentional doses. For your nervous system, it behaves more like a drama series than a calm briefing. It loops the 1% that's wrong with the world and can crowd out the 99% that's ordinary and good. That distortion can keep your body on high alert — more worry, lighter sleep, shorter fuse. You stay marinated in threat.

That doesn't mean "never be informed." It means change the format. A newspaper, a short article, or a weekly intentional digest is different: finite, slower, easier to put down. If you follow events, do it on purpose and on a schedule, not in a constant drip.

Give your mind a palette, not a firehose. Start and end the day with a simple "color correction":

- Three fast lines of gratitude — something you saw, someone you appreciate, something you did right.
- One small action that lines up with your values — a walk, a call, a boundary.

Run a quick "color check" during the day:

- Was that thought dark (doom, spite, helplessness) or bright (curiosity, kindness, agency)?
- If it's dark, don't shame it — redirect it. Name one small action you can take or one thing you're genuinely thankful for. Swap the ink.

Begin the day with signal, not noise: daylight, water, one minute of movement, one written priority. When your inputs improve, your thinking improves. When your thinking improves, calm and wise choices get easier.

Your life slowly takes on the color of what you repeatedly allow in.

Real-life snapshot

Evan woke up to breaking-news alerts and doom-heavy podcasts, then wondered why his chest felt tight by 9 a.m. "I'm just stressed," he told himself. Mornings started with fear; nights ended with scrolling. Sleep was light and his fuse was short.

On a friend's suggestion, he tried a two-week experiment: no news or social media for the first 15 minutes of the day. Instead, he:

- Drank a glass of water.
- Stood by the window and looked outside.
- Read one page of an uplifting book.
- Wrote down one simple priority for the day.

He still checked the news later — but on a schedule, not as a reflex.

By the end of two weeks, his mornings felt less jagged. The anxious edge softened. Falling asleep came easier because he stopped feeding his brain worst-case stories right before bed.

"I didn't realize how much my inputs were shaping me," he said. "I thought I was just 'stressed.' But changing the first 15 minutes changed the tone of the whole day."

Quick science

- High exposure to distressing media is associated with higher perceived stress and anxiety, and a more pessimistic view of the world.
- Gratitude and reflective writing practices are linked to better sleep, improved mood, and shifts in brain networks toward calm and agency.
- Intentional "input routines" — such as structured morning practices — reduce cognitive load and support emotional regulation throughout the day.[47]

Inspiration note

You are the artist of your attention — choose pigments that make you stronger.

Today's Invitation

One thing I will do for myself today:

- ☐ I guard my inputs by choosing one set window for news/social today (not all day).
- ☐ I set my mind in a better direction by starting or ending the day with three lines of gratitude instead of doom scrolling.
- ☐ I protect my attention by replacing one scroll with one nourishing input (walk, music, prayer, or a real conversation).

Action Step:
Choose the easiest one today. Do it now or set one reminder and do it when it best fits your schedule.

Reflection:
After I took the step today, I felt: ☐ calmer ☐ clearer ☐ steadier ☐ proud ☐ no change yet (effort still counts)

Bottom line

Guard your inputs, and your thoughts — and life — will change color.

Your lines

(write one thought, one insight, or rewrite one sentence that rang true)

_____

_____

_____

☐ Done for today

Why this matters
Writing just a few lines by hand locks the concept into memory and gently primes your subconscious mind to adopt and act on it, leading to better recall and follow-through.

DAY 48

> **"Wealth consists not in having great possessions, but in having few wants."**
> — Epictetus

Money stress is a health stress.
Chasing "more" at all costs can quietly cost you everything that matters.
Enough + wisdom beats excess + anxiety every time.

Reflection

Money worries don't live only in your bank app. They live in your chest and your blood pressure and your sleep. They show up as 3 a.m. staring at the ceiling, grinding your teeth about bills, comparing your life to the neighbor's new car or bigger house. Financial stress is not just a "life problem." It's a physiological load.

Studies repeatedly show that once basic needs and a modest level of security are covered — enough food, safe housing, ability to handle ordinary expenses — extra income adds far less to day-to-day happiness than most people expect. Yet many of us live as if the next pay bump, the next upgrade, the next "win" in the market will finally make us feel safe and satisfied. Often, the chase does the opposite: more hours, less sleep, more pressure, less time with the people and habits that protect our health.

Comparison pours gasoline on this fire. The human brain wasn't built for constant exposure to everyone else's highlight reel. Your neighbor's car, your colleague's kitchen renovation, your friend's vacation posts — none of these tell you about their debt, their stress, or their trade-offs. You see the possession, not the price their nervous system pays.

Another modern trap is speculative investing — day trading, trying to "beat the market" minute by minute. For many people, this turns the stock market into a 24/7 casino: charts open, heart racing, mood tied to tick-by-tick changes they cannot control. The body can respond as if it's facing danger: stress hormones rise, sleep can fragment, and relationships get whatever is left over. Meanwhile, a slow, diversified, long-term approach — the financial equivalent of walking and eating your vegetables — tends to perform well over time with far less stress.

Money itself is not the enemy. Wealth can buy time, safety, and choices — all of which support health and purpose. The danger is in trying to get there too fast and in wanting more than you truly need. When financial goals pull you so hard that you chronically sacrifice sleep, movement, relationships, and sanity, the "wealth plan" becomes a health drain.

A healthier approach is simpler and kinder. Aim for "enough" rather than "as much as possible" — enough to cover basics, handle emergencies, and create some breathing room. Treat basic money skills as health interventions: a simple budget, a small weekly or monthly savings habit, gradually building a cash buffer. Clarity reduces the unknowns your nervous system spins on. Choose investments that let you sleep: long-term, boring, diversified, automatic. If your blood pressure spikes every time you check a price, the instrument you're trading is probably not worth the cost.

And remember: you don't need a new car every 2–3 years, a bigger house, or a backyard pool to support your health. Clean, safe, "good enough" often outperforms fancy-but-stressful in the long run. True wealth is basic needs met, a bit of margin, a body that works, and a mind that is not constantly on fire. Trying to find the fastest way to wealth is often the surest way to burn through the health that makes wealth worth having.

Real-life snapshot

Aris and Theo were brothers with similar incomes and very different strategies.

Aris wanted to "catch up" fast. He leased new cars, stretched for a bigger house in a "better" neighborhood, and spent nights glued to stock charts, trading individual stocks and making frequent, high-stakes trades. Every dip in the market hit him in the gut. He checked prices in the middle of the night, slept poorly, and drank more to wind down. By his mid-40s, he had a nice house, impressive stuff — and rising blood pressure, reflux, and chronic anxiety.

Theo lived more quietly. His car was older but paid off. He chose a smaller home that left room in the budget. He and his partner had a simple written budget, an emergency fund they slowly built, and automatic contributions to a broadly diversified index fund each month. He rarely checked the market. "I'm investing for 20–30 years," he said. "I don't need to watch it every day." Even when money was tight, he tried to protect sleep, home-cooked meals, and time with his kids.

Twenty years later, Aris had cycled through booms and busts. Some trades did well; others wiped out gains. The stress left its mark: he was on multiple medications for blood pressure and anxiety, and burnout forced him to cut back his work. Theo was not a millionaire on magazine covers, but he had steady savings, relatively low stress, and a body that still let him travel, play, and work on his own terms.

"I thought the fast lane was the smart lane," Aris admitted. "But the toll it took on my health was higher than I realized. Theo's lane wasn't flashy, but he got both — health and enough."

Quick science

- Financial stress is associated with anxiety, depression, poor sleep, high blood pressure, and increased risk of cardiovascular disease.
- Chronic debt and money worries can drive persistent sympathetic nervous system activation ("fight-or-flight"), raising cortisol and impairing immune and metabolic health.
- Research on income and wellbeing suggests that beyond covering basic needs and a reasonable level of security, additional income yields diminishing returns on daily happiness; how you live with what you have often matters more than the raw number.[48]

Inspiration note

A simple, sustainable plan that lets you sleep is healthier than a "brilliant" plan that keeps you in fight-or-flight.

Today's Invitation

One thing I will do for myself today:

- ☐ I lower money stress by handling one small money task in a 10-minute window, then closing the tab.
- ☐ I reduce money stress by cutting comparison today (unfollow one account or take a social break).
- ☐ I steady money stress at the root by calming my body first: one minute of slow breathing before decisions.

Action Step:
Choose the easiest one today. Do it now or set one reminder and do it when it best fits your schedule.

Reflection:
After I took the step today, I felt: ☐ calmer ☐ clearer ☐ steadier ☐ proud ☐ no change yet (effort still counts)

Bottom line

Wealth matters for freedom and health — but only if the way you pursue it doesn't break you. Aim for enough. Protect your pillars. Let your money plan support your life, not consume it.

Your lines

(write one thought, one insight, or rewrite one sentence that rang true)

_____

_____

_____

☐ Done for today

Why this matters
Writing just a few lines by hand locks the concept into memory and gently primes your subconscious mind to adopt and act on it, leading to better recall and follow-through.

DAY 49

"You cannot pour from an empty cup."
— Proverb

You are not here to abandon yourself in the name of helping others.
Your wellbeing is your service.
Your vitality is your offering.

Reflection

There is a quiet tragedy that unfolds in countless lives: people who give and give until the thread holding them together begins to fray. They are the reliable ones — the helpers, the late-night problem solvers, the ones who say, "It's fine, I've got it," even when they are barely standing. They show up for their family, their patients, their colleagues, their community — but slowly disappear from their own story.

    The teaching behind this quote is gentle and blunt at the same time: do not neglect your own good in the name of serving others. See your own welfare clearly and protect it. The point is not to make you self-centered. It is to remind you that collapse helps no one. A depleted person cannot offer strength. A burned-out person cannot offer clarity. An exhausted parent, partner, clinician, or friend may love deeply, but when they abandon the roots that keep them steady, their body and mind eventually give out.

    Your body usually warns you long before that point. It whispers in the tightening of your chest, the heaviness you feel getting out of bed, the short temper you don't recognize, the strange mix of fatigue and restlessness, the sense that life is happening just beyond your reach. These are not character flaws. They are early alarm bells — signals that the instrument you use to love and serve is being pushed past its limits.

    Self-neglect is not compassion; it is a slow walking away from the very vessel you were given to do good in this world. True compassion begins with stewardship: sleeping when your body asks, eating food that nourishes instead of just numbing, moving daily so energy can circulate again, setting boundaries so your soul has room to breathe, giving yourself pockets of stillness so your mind can come back to center. These practices are not indulgences reserved for people with easier lives. They are responsibilities for anyone who wants to keep showing up.

The deeper truth is simple: your wellbeing is the force that allows you to serve without shattering. Your vitality is your offering. Your steadiness is your gift. When you guard your health, you are not retreating from the world; you are preparing yourself to re-enter it with more clarity, more warmth, and far more power.

Real-life snapshot

Maria was the "strong one" in every room — the dependable one, the helper, the late-night problem solver. She covered extra shifts, took every call, answered every message. When her body whispered, she brushed it off. "Other people have it worse," she told herself. "They need me more."

Over time, the whispers turned into alarms: a racing heart, tightness in her chest, waking at 3 a.m. with panic, snapping at people she loved. She began to dread phone calls. One night, after pulling over on the side of the road to catch her breath during a near-panic attack, she finally heard the message underneath: she was breaking her own instrument.

With her doctor's encouragement, she made changes that felt almost selfish at first. She set a real bedtime and honored it. She protected one true day off each week. She ate actual meals at a table instead of crumbs between crises. She walked outside most days, even if only for 10 minutes. She drew one clear line: no work messages after a certain hour. And, hardest of all, she started saying gentle noes when she hit her limit.

Months later, she was still helping others — but from a different place. Her sleep had returned. Her panic had eased. Her laughter was back. She could listen without feeling drained and offer support without resenting it.

"I didn't stop serving," she said. "I just stopped sacrificing myself to do it. Taking care of me is how I make sure I can keep showing up for them."

Quick science

- Chronic over-giving without recovery can keep the stress response elevated, which can weaken sleep, mood, and immune resilience over time.
- Clear boundaries and periods of true rest reduce sympathetic overactivation and can improve heart rate variability (HRV), a marker of resilience and recovery capacity.
- Consistent self-care practices — sleep, movement, nourishing food, and healthy limits — improve emotional regulation and increase long-term caregiving capacity.[49]

Inspiration note

A candle cannot light another when its own flame is out.

Today's Invitation

One thing I will do for myself today:

- ☐ I refill my cup today with a 10-minute quiet reset (no screen): sit, breathe slowly, and let my shoulders drop.
- ☐ I set one clean boundary today (one 'not today,' one delayed yes, or one protected break).
- ☐ I protect recovery tonight with an earlier bedtime and a simple lights-down cue.

Action Step:
Choose the easiest one today. Do it now or set one reminder and do it when it best fits your schedule.

Reflection:
After I took the step today, I felt: ☐ calmer ☐ clearer ☐ steadier ☐ proud ☐ no change yet (effort still counts)

Bottom line

Caring for yourself is not selfish. It is how you make your love sustainable.

Your lines

(write one thought, one insight, or rewrite one sentence that rang true)

_____

_____

_____

☐ Done for today

Why this matters

Writing just a few lines by hand locks the concept into memory and gently primes your subconscious mind to adopt and act on it, leading to better recall and follow-through.

DAY 50

"The morning sun has gold in its mouth."
— Ben Franklin

Light is a powerful signal you take in through your eyes — use it wisely.
Morning light tells your body, It's time to be alive.
Darkness later tells your body, It's safe to let go.

Reflection

Your brain runs on light signals. Tiny cells in the eye send a powerful message to your master clock: Day has begun or Night is here. That clock sets the timing for almost everything — alertness, mood, hunger, body temperature, and the release of sleep hormones. The problem is not that we don't have enough light and dark. It's that we often use both backwards.

A few common patterns work against you: phone light before daylight, sunglasses too early, indoor-dim mornings paired with bright evenings, and screens or overhead LEDs late at night.

You don't need perfection, but you do need better patterns. Think of light as a powerful medicine:

Morning light: As soon as you reasonably can after waking, get light in your eyes outside — if it's comfortable, try a few minutes without dark sunglasses; never stare at the sun. Even on cloudy days, outdoor light is many times stronger than indoor bulbs. For many people, 5–10 minutes helps; more if it's heavily overcast, less if it's very bright.

If you work indoors, treat morning and lunchtime like light appointments. A few minutes by a window is okay, but stepping outside is best.

Gentle evenings: As the sun goes down, let your home copy the sky: lights lower and warmer, screens dimmer and earlier off. Your brain is watching.

Photoreceptors in your eyes — and, remarkably, light-sensing pathways even in some blind individuals — send timing signals to the brain's master clock. That clock helps schedule daily hormone rhythms, including cortisol and melatonin.

Morning light tells cortisol, Rise now — then ease off later.
Evening darkness tells melatonin, It's your turn.

When you protect that sequence, sleep often comes easier, energy feels smoother, cravings tend to quiet down, and mood steadies.

You cannot control every sunrise or every evening, but you can stop making light work against you and start letting it work for you.

Real-life snapshot

Karen dragged herself out of bed each morning, shuffled to the kitchen, and stared at her phone in the dark. Most days, the only "morning light" her brain got was from a screen. She hurried into a car, drove to work, and spent daylight hours under fluorescent bulbs. At night, she wound down with bright TV and a lit-up phone in bed. "I'm always tired but can't sleep," she told her friend.

After learning about light's power, she tried a new plan for one month:

- No phone for the first 15 minutes after waking.
- Within 30 minutes of getting up, she stepped outside — even just on the front step — and looked toward the sky (not at the sun) for about 5–10 minutes, without sunglasses unless the light truly bothered her eyes.
- At lunch, she walked outside for another 5–10 minutes instead of staying under office lights.
- After sunset, she turned off overhead lights, used lamps instead, and set a screens mostly off time an hour before bed.

Within a week, she felt more awake in the morning and naturally sleepier at night. Within a month, she was falling asleep faster, waking less often, and relying less on sugar and caffeine to prop her up.

"It felt like my days finally had a beginning and an end," she said. "Once I fixed the light, my body seemed to remember what to do."

Quick science

- Morning outdoor light activates specialized cells in the retina that signal the suprachiasmatic nucleus (SCN), the brain's master clock, anchoring circadian rhythm.
- Bright morning light boosts daytime alertness and helps set the timing for an evening rise in melatonin, improving sleep onset and sleep quality.
- Excessive bright light and blue-rich screens at night suppress melatonin and delay sleep, fragmenting deep rest and increasing next-day sleepiness and cravings.[50]

Inspiration note

The morning sun is free medicine — and most people walk past the pharmacy.

Today's Invitation

One thing I will do for myself today:

- ☐ I get outdoor light early today (even 5 minutes helps).
- ☐ I take one midday daylight break outside (quick walk or stand in light).
- ☐ I dim lights and screens 30–60 minutes before bed tonight.

Action Step:
Choose the easiest one today. Do it now or set one reminder and do it when it best fits your schedule.

Reflection:
After I took the step today, I felt: ☐ calmer ☐ clearer ☐ steadier ☐ proud ☐ no change yet (effort still counts)

Bottom line

Letting light lead your day is one of the simplest, strongest ways to steady your sleep, mood, and energy.

Your lines

(write one thought, one insight, or rewrite one sentence that rang true)

_____

_____

_____

☐ Done for today

Why this matters
Writing just a few lines by hand locks the concept into memory and gently primes your subconscious mind to adopt and act on it, leading to better recall and follow-through.

DAY 51

"Sedatives knock you out; they don't let you sleep."
— A. Smyrlis, MD

Asleep is not the same as restored.
Sedation mimics sleep on the outside but breaks it on the inside.
Don't trade depth for drowsiness.

Reflection

Sedation is not sleep — and your body knows the difference. When someone says, I slept, but I'm still exhausted, this is often part of the puzzle.

Alcohol and many sedating aids (including some prescription sleep medications) can make you drowsy or unconscious, but they don't always create the same restorative sleep architecture your brain and body need. They may help you fall asleep, yet still disrupt the stages you rely on: deep sleep for repair and REM for memory and emotional reset.

The cost often hides in the second half of the night. Sedation can splinter sleep into lighter fragments, increase awakenings, reduce REM, and keep the body more activated when your nervous system should be settling. What feels like helping me sleep can quietly borrow from tomorrow: groggy mornings, higher anxiety or irritability, stronger cravings for sugar or caffeine, and slower balance and reflexes — especially risky if you get up at night to use the bathroom.

For older adults in particular, this matters. Sedation can mean waking at 3 a.m. a little disoriented, with slower coordination. One misstep can become a fall, a fracture, and a hospital stay — all from something that was supposed to help.

True sleep is an orchestra of stages, temperature shifts, hormone pulses, and neural housekeeping. Sedation, by contrast, is like throwing a blanket over the conductor. Things get quieter, but not necessarily better.

Safety rail: If you're taking a prescription sleep medication, don't stop it suddenly or change your dose on your own. Any change should be guided by your clinician.

Real-life snapshot

Katerina used to pour her first glass while cleaning the kitchen, almost on autopilot. It felt like a soft landing after a long day. But by 3 a.m., she was often wide awake — heart thumping, mind racing, bargaining for more sleep. The next day had a pattern too: foggy morning, afternoon crash, and a restless, edgy feeling she didn't recognize as mild withdrawal.

Her clinician suggested a 30-day experiment. Weeknights: no alcohol. Weekends: if she chose to drink, always with food and finished at least three hours before bed. She added a simple lights-down hour: dim lights, no work email, no heavy news. A warm shower, a cup of chamomile or lemon-ginger tea, and ten pages of calming fiction. If appropriate for her and cleared by her clinician, gentle supports like magnesium glycinate in the evening or a drop of lavender on the pillow.

The first change wasn't dramatic. It was quieter: fewer 3 a.m. jolts. Then a smoother morning. Then a calmer afternoon. Two weeks in, she said, I forgot what real sleep feels like. I thought I needed something to knock me out. What I needed was to stop interrupting my body while it was trying to repair.

Quick science

- Alcohol may shorten the time it takes to fall asleep, but it fragments the night, suppresses REM, and worsens sleep quality — especially in the second half of the night.
- Many prescription sleep medications distort normal sleep stages and can cause next-day impairment; stopping them suddenly can trigger rebound insomnia, so any change must be guided by a clinician.
- Reducing sedatives or alcohol while improving sleep habits often improves sleep continuity and next-day alertness over time.[51]

Inspiration note

Your body isn't asking for sedation — it's begging for real sleep.

Today's Invitation

One thing I will do for myself today:

- ☐ I keep my nights clean by skipping alcohol and sedatives tonight (or keeping them earlier and rare).
- ☐ I build a true wind-down tonight: dim lights, no heavy news, and one low-input activity for 20 minutes.
- ☐ I keep changes safe by talking with my clinician before adjusting any sleep medication, while I improve habits I control now.

Action Step:
Choose the easiest one today. Do it now or set one reminder and do it when it best fits your schedule.

Reflection:
After I took the step today, I felt: ☐ calmer ☐ clearer ☐ steadier ☐ proud ☐ no change yet (effort still counts)

Bottom line

Don't sedate — restore. Real sleep heals what sedation only hides and helps keep you steadier, clearer, and safer — day and night.

Your lines

(write one thought, one insight, or rewrite one sentence that rang true)

_____
_____
_____

☐ Done for today

Why this matters
Writing just a few lines by hand locks the concept into memory and gently primes your subconscious mind to adopt and act on it, leading to better recall and follow-through.

DAY 52

"The best doctor gives the least medicine."
— Benjamin Franklin

The strongest medicine is often the simplest habit.
The best doctor doesn't just prescribe — they teach and inspire.
Real healing begins when the forces of nature are finally on your side.

Reflection

If this book has a heart, this is it. Pills and procedures save lives. As a doctor, I've seen them rescue people from the edge more times than I can count. But they were never meant to do the daily work of health. Foundations do that: sleep that tracks the sun, food that looks like ingredients, bodies that move, minds that have somewhere to lay their burdens down. When the roots are right, the branches need less constant pruning.

We don't have to guess. Long-term studies of real communities — the Blue Zones and other high-longevity pockets — show the same pattern over and over. People live longer and die later not because they had the most advanced pharmacies, but because their everyday lives lined up with nature: circadian rhythms, fresh food, walking built into the day, work with meaning, friendships that held them, relatively low toxic load. Modern medicine is a miracle on top of that foundation. Without the foundation, it spends most of its time bailing water out of a leaking boat.

The modern psyche loves quick fixes. We are wired to want numbers that change fast. Blood pressure down by tomorrow. Sugar normalized by next visit. Cholesterol cut in half on the next lab slip. Medications can often do that — and sometimes they must, for safety. But a balance created only by medication is like a scaffold around a damaged building. Essential? Yes. Stabilizing? Absolutely. But it isn't the structure. If you never rebuild what's underneath, you'll need support forever.

The best medicine uses support as a bridge, not a permanent way of living. It steadies the system while you do the slower, harder, truer work: changing mindsets and habits, and harnessing the forces that actually heal — circadian alignment, sleep that replenishes, movement that builds muscle and vascular health, nutrition that lowers inflammation and smooths glucose, detoxification that lightens the liver's load, connection that calms the nervous system. These forces can calm symptoms, improve risk factors, and in some cases help put early disease on a better course.

A good question to ask of every intervention is: What root is being addressed? If the answer is none, begin there. There is almost always at least one root you can touch: protect a sleep window, keep a daily walk, swap one ultra-processed habit for real food, and soften stress with breathing, boundaries, or support.

Often, the smallest root — consistency — matters most. One month of steady basics can shrink mystery symptoms more than three new prescriptions. As doctors, our deepest work is not just to adjust doses, but to ignite conviction: to help you see that your daily choices are not background noise but the main event. To remind you that nature still wants to heal you — and that you are allowed to work with it.

Use medicine as a bridge; let habits become the road.

Real-life snapshot

Caroline had seen almost everyone. Rheumatology for joint pain. Endocrinology for fatigue and weight gain. Neurology for brain fog. Each visit added a pill or a new supplement. Nothing truly changed. She was collecting labels and bottles, not her life back.

Finally, she landed with a clinician who asked a different set of questions: What time do you actually fall asleep? What do most of your meals look like? How much do you move in a normal week? Who helps you carry stress? At first she was annoyed. I came here for answers, she thought, not a lecture on sleep and vegetables.

But she was tired enough to try. They made a simple, unglamorous plan:

- A fixed sleep window most nights — in bed around the same time, up around the same time, with screens off at least 30 minutes before.
- A daily 15–20 minute walk after her largest meal, no phone.
- One real meal each day built from mostly whole foods: protein, vegetables, healthy fat, and calmer carbohydrates.
- A review of her meds with the explicit goal: Use them now, so we might use less later.

Over the next few months, her joint pain eased, her energy improved, and her lab markers began moving in a better direction. Over more time, with careful supervision, her medication list shrank.

Quick science

- Lifestyle interventions — nutrition, movement, sleep, and stress reduction — are associated with lower risk and better outcomes across many chronic conditions.
- Consistent routines that respect circadian rhythms help regulate hormones, appetite, and metabolism, improving blood pressure, glucose control, weight, and mood.
- Medications used without foundational changes often have diminishing returns over time or require more and more support drugs; medications combined with lifestyle change tend to produce better and more durable outcomes.[52]

Inspiration note

Strong roots do what no prescription can: they change the soil, not just the symptoms.

Today's Invitation

One thing I will do for myself today:

- ☐ I protect a real sleep window tonight (wind-down and lights-down on time).
- ☐ I take a 10-minute walk today, ideally after a meal.
- ☐ I eat one real-food meal today: protein + plants + healthy fat.

Action Step:
Choose the easiest one today. Do it now or set one reminder and do it when it best fits your schedule.

Reflection:
After I took the step today, I felt: ☐ calmer ☐ clearer ☐ steadier ☐ proud ☐ no change yet (effort still counts)

Bottom line

Let medicine support you — but let habits define you.

Your lines

(write one thought, one insight, or rewrite one sentence that rang true)

_____

_____

_____

☐ Done for today

Why this matters
Writing just a few lines by hand locks the concept into memory and gently primes your subconscious mind to adopt and act on it, leading to better recall and follow-through.

DAY 53

> "Let there be spaces in your togetherness…
> And stand together yet not too near together"
> — Kahlil Gibran

Love is not fusion — it's two whole lives standing side by side.
Closeness heals best when there is room to breathe.
Strong marriages learn to hold both togetherness and space.

Reflection

Health and marriage are braided together. When one shakes, the other feels it. Chronic fatigue, pain, insomnia, weight gain, brain fog — any of these can quietly strain a relationship. One partner feels guilty for not being who they used to be. The other feels helpless or resentful, carrying extra weight at home, at work, with the kids. Many couples love each other deeply and still find themselves drifting apart under the pressure.

Gibran's image is gentle and wise: pillars of a temple standing apart, trees growing near but not inside each other's shadow. A healthy marriage is not two people merged into one blurred identity. It is two whole beings, each with their own roots and light, choosing to lean together without swallowing each other.

When health is shaken, the temptation is to either cling too tightly — monitoring every bite, every pill, every step — or to pull away and shut down. Both responses come from fear. But neither brings real closeness. The art is to stay near enough to care, and spacious enough to breathe.

That looks like listening without interrupting or fixing. Saying, I see how hard this is for you, instead of, You just need to. Letting your partner have their pace with health changes while you keep your own healthy floor. And building both shared routines and protected personal space, so closeness doesn't become pressure.

You are not your partner's doctor. You are their companion. Your steadiness, kindness, and boundaries are medicine, too. You are allowed your own needs. You are allowed to say, I love you, and I'm tired — I need a rest as well.

A marriage that can talk honestly about health, fear, and limits — without shaming, lecturing, or abandoning — is a rare and powerful thing. It becomes a place where both people can heal, instead of one person always rescuing and the other always collapsing.

Real-life snapshot

When Andrew's autoimmune symptoms flared in his mid-40s, everything shifted. He went from the strong one to the one who needed help getting out of bed some mornings. His wife, Rachel, picked up more work at home and with the kids. At first, she tried to be endlessly strong: no complaint, no pause, just more doing.

Quietly, resentment started to grow. She felt alone in the burden. He felt like a problem to be managed. They argued more over small things — dishes, appointments, money — because neither could say the larger truth: I'm scared. I miss who we were. I don't know how to do this.

At counseling, the therapist used Gibran's image. You are not broken pillars, she said. You are two pillars that need space and alignment. Together they worked on two things:

- Shared togetherness: one short evening walk most nights, even when Andrew was slow; a weekly check-in where they asked, How is your body? How is your heart?
- Honoring space: each got one protected block of time weekly — Andrew for quiet and journaling, Rachel for exercise or seeing a friend — no guilt, no scorekeeping.

They also agreed on one boundary: health talk without problem-solving for a few minutes. Just, Tell me what it's like, and, Thank you for listening.

Their circumstances didn't magically fix. Some days were still hard. But the marriage felt less like one person dragging the other and more like two people carrying a shared load. We're still us, Rachel said later. We're just learning a different kind of togetherness.

Quick science

- The quality of a close relationship is associated with health outcomes: supportive, low-conflict relationships are linked with better longevity and cardiovascular markers, while chronic high-conflict relationships are linked with higher stress and worse health over time.
- Feeling emotionally seen and understood by a partner calms the nervous system, lowering blood pressure and improving heart-rate variability.
- Having both closeness and room for personal autonomy (time alone, own interests) is associated with better relationship satisfaction and individual wellbeing than fusion or chronic distance.[53]

Inspiration note

Healthy love holds hands without erasing fingerprints.

Today's Invitation

One thing I will do for myself today:

- ☐ I strengthen our health braid by giving my partner 5 minutes of listening (no fixing, no minimizing).
- ☐ I protect our closeness by doing one supportive thing together (a walk, a shared meal, or a gentle check-in).
- ☐ I keep love spacious and honest by naming one need kindly: I love you, and I need rest/help/space tonight.

Action Step:
Choose the easiest one today. Do it now or set one reminder and do it when it best fits your schedule.

Reflection:
After I took the step today, I felt: ☐ calmer ☐ clearer ☐ steadier ☐ proud ☐ no change yet (effort still counts)

Bottom line

You are not meant to disappear into someone else — nor to walk alone. The music of a strong relationship comes when two whole lives stand side by side, with just enough space for both to breathe and grow.

Your lines

(write one thought, one insight, or rewrite one sentence that rang true)

_____

_____

_____

☐ Done for today

Why this matters
Writing just a few lines by hand locks the concept into memory and gently primes your subconscious mind to adopt and act on it, leading to better recall and follow-through.

DAY 54

> "The fear and worry of suffering does more damage to our health than suffering itself."
> — A. Smyrlis, MD

A lot of suffering doesn't start in the body — it starts in our thoughts. Chronic worry quietly tears at your chemistry, your sleep, and your choices. When love and purpose move in, fear has less room to stay.

Reflection

Not every health problem begins with food, cigarettes, or a couch. Many begin with fear. Fear of getting sick. Fear of being left. Fear of losing your job, your money, your reputation. Fear of being hurt again. The event might happen once — the betrayal, the firing, the accident, the harsh words — but the fear and worry replay hundreds of times in your mind.

The body can respond to a remembered threat like it's happening now when you relive it with full intensity. Every replay can bring a stress surge — heart rate up, muscles tight, breath shallow, sleep lighter. Over months and years, that load can show up as higher blood pressure, digestive flares, pain sensitivity, headaches, insomnia, fatigue, and mood instability.

This is not about blame. Most of this happens without you choosing it. The mind is trying to protect you. If I worry enough, it thinks, maybe I won't be blindsided again. But the cost is high. You get hurt in multiples: once by what happened, and again and again by the constant replay.

So how do you keep fear and worry from running your life and wrecking your health? There is no single magic trick, but there are two powerful routes: rest and love.

Rest: Good sleep helps your brain process emotional memories. During certain stages of sleep, your brain replays the day's events with the body mostly quiet. It can uncouple some of the raw emotion from the memory. When sleep is broken, that processing is weaker. Yesterday's fear keeps feeling like today's emergency. Protecting sleep is one of the most underrated nervous-system reset tools we have.

Love and service: Fear curls you inward. Love turns you outward. When you are fully engaged in caring for something beyond yourself — your family, your customers, your community, your craft — your attention leaves the fear loop, even if only for a few minutes. You remember, I can still do some good. I am more than what was done to me.

This doesn't mean ignoring your pain. It means balancing it. You can acknowledge and work through your hurt with safe people (therapist, trusted friend, support group). You can gently care for your body with sleep, food, movement, and light so the nervous system can calm. And at the same time, even in the middle of your own storms, you can choose small acts of love: helping, listening, creating, serving.

You can't stop every wave of fear from rising. But you can teach your body that fear is not the only reality. Gratitude, kindness, and service are not sentimental ideas. They change what your brain focuses on and how your chemistry flows. When love, service, and gratitude have regular space in your life, fear still knocks — but it no longer gets to run the house.

Real-life snapshot

After a betrayal and a job loss in the same year, Karen lived in constant fear. She woke at 3 a.m. replaying conversations. Any email from her new boss made her chest tighten. She stopped exercising, ate irregularly, and withdrew from friends. Her sleep thinned, and her stomach stayed in knots.

Her doctor treated the reflux and the blood pressure, but also asked gently, Who's helping you carry all this? She realized the answer was no one.

Over time, with a therapist, she named the hurt and grief. She worked on sleep — no doom-scrolling in bed, a simple wind-down routine, a regular bedtime. As her nights softened, her mind had a little more room.

Then she did something surprising even to herself: she started volunteering two Saturdays a month at a local community center, helping kids with homework. At first it felt strange — Why am I helping anyone when my life is a mess? — but she kept going. Those hours became the only time she wasn't circling her own story.

Months later, the fear hadn't vanished, but it no longer filled the whole sky. Her body felt steadier, and she laughed more often.

Helping those kids didn't erase what happened to me, she said. But it reminded me that I'm still capable of love and good work.

Quick science

- Chronic fear and worry keep the body's stress response activated, which can contribute to high blood pressure, blood sugar problems, digestive issues, and immune changes.

- Sleep plays a key role in processing emotional memories, helping separate the feeling from the fact over time. Poor sleep keeps emotional charge higher.
- Acts of kindness, connection, and gratitude are associated with lower perceived stress and a stronger sense of safety, which supports healing.[54]

Inspiration note

Fear may visit your heart — but love, service, and gratitude decide whether it gets to stay.

Today's Invitation

One thing I will do for myself today:

- ☐ I protect sleep tonight with a gentle wind-down to give my mind fewer loops.
- ☐ I do one small act of love or service today to turn my attention outward.
- ☐ I write three gratitudes today to remind my nervous system there is still good here.

Action Step:
Choose the easiest one today. Do it now or set one reminder and do it when it best fits your schedule.

Reflection:
After I took the step today, I felt: ☐ calmer ☐ clearer ☐ steadier ☐ proud ☐ no change yet (effort still counts)

Bottom line

Not every illness begins with bad habits in the usual sense. Many begin with long years of fear and worry.

Your lines

(write one thought, one insight, or rewrite one sentence that rang true)

☐ Done for today

Why this matters
Writing just a few lines by hand locks the concept into memory and gently primes your subconscious mind to adopt and act on it, leading to better recall and follow-through.

DAY 55

"Anger is not cooled by anger; only by calm."
— Dhammapada

Anger is powerful — but only calm can steer it.
Heat uncontrolled burns; heat contained becomes light.
Your work is not to suppress anger, but to aim it.

Reflection

Anger is like fire — the same force that can warm a home or burn it down. In a power plant, heat is contained and directed into something useful. In an explosion, it is dumped all at once and harms everything nearby. The difference isn't the energy. It's the container.

Your job is to build the plant. Anger itself is not the enemy. It's fast, bodily, primal — a signal that something feels wrong, unsafe, unfair, or out of alignment. Used wisely, anger clarifies boundaries, fuels needed change, and protects what matters. Used impulsively, it burns sleep, relationships, trust, and even health. What matters is whether you catch anger early enough to guide it, rather than be swallowed by it.

Start by learning your earliest signals: heat rising in the face, tight jaw or clenched fists, a surge in the chest, fast, sharp thoughts, shallow, choppy breath. These are not failures. They are invitations. When you pause and name the emotion — I feel angry — your thinking brain comes back online. That simple act brings your thinking brain back online and turns down the fight-or-flight alarm, like a hand gently turning the valve.

Then comes containment. Calm isn't weakness; it's control. Six long exhales. Two minutes of walking away to breathe and reset. A simple grounding phrase like, "I can respond, not explode." Containment is what keeps a moment of anger from becoming a night of regret. It gives you enough space to decide what you want to do with the energy instead of letting the energy decide for you.

Once steady, you can channel anger. Ask: What am I really trying to protect? What needs to change? What is one constructive step I can take — today — toward fixing this? Anger becomes useful when it becomes movement: a boundary drawn, a conversation prepared, a plan made, a truth honored.

Real-life snapshot

Simone's anger ignited in an instant — a reckless driver cut her off and her pulse shot up. She used to chase such drivers, swearing the whole way, arriving wired and shaken.

One day she tried something different. She said quietly, I'm angry and startled, took six long exhales, loosened her grip on the wheel, and asked, What keeps me safe right now? She let the car go. She arrived calm, not explosive. Same trigger. Different handling.

Dev's anger was different — slow, simmering, chronic. A demeaning manager eroded his nights and shortened his temper at home. At first, he snapped at his family, replayed arguments in his head, and slept badly.

With help, he learned to contain his anger first — breathwork at night instead of replaying the day, dumping thoughts into a journal, singing along to his favorite song on the drive back home, taking short walks after work. Then he channeled it: documenting incidents, scheduling a boundary meeting with HR present, and quietly applying for roles that matched his values. A few weeks later, he transferred. His shoulders dropped. His sleep improved. Same anger — newly directed.

Quick science

- Naming emotions (I feel angry, I feel hurt) reduces reactivity in the brain's alarm centers and increases activity in regions involved in control and decision-making.
- Longer exhales activate the parasympathetic brake, slowing heart rate and lowering arousal.
- Rumination fuels anger; brief physical movement and cognitive reframing reduce its intensity and shorten how long it lasts.[55]

Inspiration note

Heat becomes harm without direction — but becomes strength when guided by calm.

Today's Invitation

One thing I will do for myself today:

- ☐ I grow my anger into wisdom by naming the feeling out loud: I feel angry.
- ☐ I use my brake first by taking 6 slow exhales before I respond.
- ☐ I channel the energy well by turning it into one wise action (a boundary, a hard conversation, or a brisk walk).

Action Step:
Choose the easiest one today. Do it now or set one reminder and do it when it best fits your schedule.

Reflection:
After I took the step today, I felt: ☐ calmer ☐ clearer ☐ steadier ☐ proud ☐ no change yet (effort still counts)

Bottom line

The goal isn't to suppress anger. It's to recognize it early, cool it with calm, and aim it toward repair instead of damage.

Your lines

(write one thought, one insight, or rewrite one sentence that rang true)

☐ Done for today

Why this matters
Writing just a few lines by hand locks the concept into memory and gently primes your subconscious mind to adopt and act on it, leading to better recall and follow-through.

DAY 56

> "Everything happens twice — first in
> the mind, then in the world."
> — A. Smyrlis, MD

Your mind is where reality begins.
When you rehearse the scene, your body recognizes it when it arrives.
Clear inner pictures make outer action easier.

Reflection

If you want a different life, you can't skip the inner rehearsal. Every meaningful change begins as an inner picture. Before your body ever moves, your mind runs a quiet preview — a rehearsal that tells your nervous system what to expect and how to respond. Visualization isn't magic or wishful thinking. It is neurological priming. It is mental training. It is practice without sweat.

Your brain can respond to vividly imagined action in ways that resemble real practice. When you vividly picture lacing your shoes, stepping outside, feeling the ground, breathing in rhythm, your motor networks light up as if you were actually doing it. You're not pretending — you're installing a blueprint.

Most people aim visualization too far away: one day when I'm healthy, one day when I'm fit. The real power lies in near-term scenes: tomorrow's walk, tonight's wind-down routine, your next no when you usually say yes, your next workout, the moment you choose a home-prepped meal instead of default takeout.

Keep the scene small, clear, and embodied. Where are you? What time is it? What do you see, hear, feel in your body? What is the exact last step of the scene? Then link it to a cue so your body follows the script at the right moment: After coffee, I run my scene. Before bed, I run my scene.

Visualization also softens fear. When you internally experience something before it happens, your nervous system stops seeing it as pure threat. The unknown becomes familiar. The effort becomes possible. This is why athletes, musicians, surgeons, pilots, and performers use visualization: it makes unfamiliar actions feel less foreign and more natural.

For your health journey, visualization is a quiet advantage most people underestimate. It is one of the tools that can turn I hope I can into my body recognizes this; we've been here before.

Real-life snapshot

Sara was rehabbing a knee injury and felt afraid to push herself. Every time she thought about longer walks, she saw herself stumbling, re-tearing something, ending up back on the couch. Her body tightened before she even moved.

Her physical therapist suggested a two-minute mental script. Twice a day, she closed her eyes and pictured: standing up with confidence; stepping onto a curb smoothly; walking fifteen minutes with easy breath and steady steps; finishing proud, not panicked. Her cue was simple: After coffee, I run my script.

At first, it felt silly. But after a week, she noticed something strange: when it was time to walk, her body didn't freeze in the same way. The path felt less scary because her mind had walked it first. Over time, her distance grew, her fear eased, and her confidence returned.

Sitting still and imagining didn't fix my knee, she said. But it let my body believe I could move again. That changed everything.

Quick science

- Motor imagery (mentally rehearsing a movement) activates many of the same brain regions as physical practice and can improve learning and performance.
- Visualizing a specific, near-term action and then linking it to a cue (when–then planning) increases the likelihood that you'll follow through.
- Repeated mental rehearsal strengthens self-efficacy — the belief that I can do this — which is strongly linked to long-term habit success.[56]

Inspiration note

A rehearsed mind makes the body braver.

Today's Invitation

One thing I will do for myself today:

- ☐ I rehearse my next right action by visualizing it for 60 seconds (where, when, and how it starts).
- ☐ I make the action easier by linking it to a reliable cue (after breakfast, after lunch, or when I get home).
- ☐ I set myself up to follow through by preparing the stage now (shoes out, food prepped, lights dimmed).

Action Step:
Choose the easiest one today. Do it now or set one reminder and do it when it best fits your schedule.

Reflection:
After I took the step today, I felt: ☐ calmer ☐ clearer ☐ steadier ☐ proud ☐ no change yet (effort still counts)

Bottom line

Rehearsal makes real life easier. Train the brain; the body follows.

Your lines

(write one thought, one insight, or rewrite one sentence that rang true)

_____
_____
_____

☐ Done for today

Why this matters
Writing just a few lines by hand locks the concept into memory and gently primes your subconscious mind to adopt and act on it, leading to better recall and follow-through.

DAY 57

> "We are what we repeatedly do. Excellence, then, is not an act, but a habit."
> — attributed to Aristotle

Excellence isn't about peaks — it's about what you do on ordinary days.
Your identity is shaped more by your floor than your ceiling.
Tiny, repeatable habits quietly build a powerful life.

Reflection

Excellence isn't a lightning strike; it's a floor you build, brick by brick. The body and brain adapt to whatever you repeat. A single early night helps, but a month of early nights rewires your sleep drive. One post-meal walk lowers glucose; a hundred walks train your metabolism. A protein-anchored breakfast quiets cravings in a day; consistency reshapes appetite over time.

We spend most of our lives chasing ceilings — big goals, perfect plans, best shape of my life bursts. Ceilings feel exciting, but they're unstable. They depend on motivation, willpower, the stars lining up. Floors are different. Floors hold you when motivation disappears. They are the small, non-negotiable acts that keep you aligned on your worst days: a 10-minute walk, a fixed wake time, a glass of water upon waking. Floors keep you steady when ceilings collapse.

Here's the secret most people miss: set the floor so low you can trip over it on your worst day. Not 10,000 steps and a perfect workout, but I walk for 10 minutes after my largest meal, no matter what. Not I will never eat sugar again, but I always start dinner with something green. When the floor is simple and repeatable, you stop failing. You just keep showing up.

Over time, something profound happens. The habit stops feeling like effort and starts feeling like who I am. Stress chemistry cools. Self-trust grows. Identity shifts from I'm someone who always falls off to I'm someone who does this, even when life is messy.

Real-life snapshot

For years, Jenna lived on the weight-loss roller coaster. January meant an all-in diet: no sugar, no carbs, daily intense workouts. By March she was exhausted, sore, and back to old habits. The scale yo-yo'd. Each regain felt heavier than the last — not just in pounds, but in shame. I can't stick to anything, she told herself.

One day, her clinician asked her to forget about goal weight for a moment. Let's build your floor, not your perfect week, she said. Together they wrote down a short habit menu — walk after her largest meal, protein-plus-fiber breakfast, a simple overnight eating window, vegetables at lunch and dinner, more water, two weekly strength sessions, and a basic wind-down for sleep.

Then came the key question: Which of these can you keep doing even on your worst day? That became her floor. She picked just two to start: a 10-minute walk and a protein-plus-fiber breakfast. Everything else was optional. For 21 days, she did only those. No heroics. No perfection. Just the floor — again and again. Then she added a fixed wake time. Weeks later, she layered in a simple dinner window.

The scale began trending down — slowly, but steadily. More importantly, the wild swings quieted.

Quick science

- Habits automate behavior by shifting control from effortful decision-making to more automatic brain circuits; this reduces reliance on willpower and makes healthy actions easier to repeat.
- Repeated small actions strengthen specific neural pathways (I'm someone who walks after dinner), which reinforces identity and makes future choices in that direction more likely.
- Consistent, moderate behaviors — like daily walking, steady eating patterns, and regular sleep — are more effective for long-term health and weight stability than intense-but-short bursts of extreme effort.[57]

Inspiration note

A strong floor lets you reach higher without fear of crashing.

Today's Invitation

One thing I will do for myself today:

☐ I choose one minimum habit today so easy I can do it even on a bad day.
☐ I tie it to a cue: After _____, I will _____ (no debate, just do).
☐ I mark the streak with one simple check mark on paper.

Action Step:
Choose the easiest one today. Do it now or set one reminder and do it when it best fits your schedule.

Reflection:
After I took the step today, I felt: ☐ calmer ☐ clearer ☐ steadier ☐ proud ☐ no change yet (effort still counts)

Bottom line

Excellence is built from the floor up — one small habit at a time, repeated until it becomes who you are.

Your lines

(write one thought, one insight, or rewrite one sentence that rang true)

_____
_____
_____

☐ Done for today

Why this matters
Writing just a few lines by hand locks the concept into memory and gently primes your subconscious mind to adopt and act on it, leading to better recall and follow-through.

DAY 58

> **"Anything that lasts is well-insulated —
> your health is no different."**
> — A. Smyrlis, MD

Your health depends less on willpower and more on what you protect. When your essentials are insulated, life's noise stops knocking them over. Insulation isn't isolation — it's protection for what matters most.

Reflection

Think of your life like a house in a place with wild weather. You don't control the wind, the heat, the storms — or the neighbors with leaf blowers at 7 a.m. What you can control is how well your house is insulated.

Insulation isn't hiding. It's smart engineering. You decide which doors stay open, which windows get sealed, and what temperature you keep inside — no matter what's happening out there. Your health works the same way. If every door is open to noise, bright light, breaking news, and other people's crises, the inside climate swings all over the place. Sleep frays. Eating gets reactive. Movement feels like too much work.

Nature already understands this. Everything truly precious is insulated. Your brain sits inside a hard skull. Your heart and lungs rest behind your rib cage and chest wall. A baby grows inside the womb. What matters is almost always wrapped, padded, or sealed — so it can last.

Your health needs the same kind of protection. You don't need more toughness; you need better weatherproofing. Instead of trying to be endlessly strong in a chaotic environment, change the environment so strength isn't required every second. A few small seals can make a big difference: dim lights before bed, protect sleep from screens, tame the noise and digital input around meals and mornings, keep real food easy to reach and junk food harder to grab, carve out a protected focus window and one device-free moment of connection.

These are not moral rules. They're practical seals so that what matters — rest, real food, movement, presence — doesn't get washed away by the daily storm.

Insulation is love in practical form. It's you telling your brain, I won't flood you with junk light, junk noise, and junk information, then blame you for being anxious and tired.

Real-life snapshot

Mara's palpitations always showed up the same way: at night, in a quiet house. She would finally lie down, and her heart would thud once, then race. Her mind would sprint right behind it: "What if something's wrong with my heart? What if I don't wake up?" She'd sit up, check her watch, take a few frantic breaths, and reach for her phone "to distract herself." Ten minutes of news and texts later, she was wide awake — shaky, wired, and scared.

She did get checked (because new or changing palpitations deserve that). The tests were reassuring. But the pattern kept repeating. That's when she tried insulation instead of willpower. Her phone started charging in the kitchen. Lights went down 30 minutes before bed. Mornings began with a protein-plus-fiber breakfast so she wasn't riding a blood-sugar roller coaster. And when the first flutter hit at night, she had one practiced move: feet on the floor, hand on chest, and a slow exhale longer than the inhale.

Two weeks later, the world hadn't gotten calmer. But the episodes were shorter, rarer, and less terrifying. As she put it, "My heart stopped feeling like an alarm. It started feeling like a signal I could respond to."

Quick science

- Boundary-setting around light, noise, and digital input is associated with better sleep and lower perceived stress and anxiety.
- Environment design — staging healthy choices to be easier and unhealthy ones to be less convenient — significantly increases the odds of following through on habits.
- Stable anchors in your day (regular sleep time, protected meals, consistent movement) help regulate hormones and mood without relying on constant willpower.[58]

Inspiration note

Insulation isn't about hiding — it's about making space for what keeps you alive and well.

Today's Invitation

One thing I will do for myself today:

- ☐ I create one protected pocket today (phone parked, quiet corner, or a real break).
- ☐ I anchor one rhythm today (consistent wake time, meal time, or lights-down time).
- ☐ I set up one cue in my space that makes the healthy choice easier (shoes visible, healthy food ready, or screens dim at night).

Action Step:
Choose the easiest one today. Do it now or set one reminder and do it when it best fits your schedule.

Reflection:
After I took the step today, I felt: ☐ calmer ☐ clearer ☐ steadier ☐ proud ☐ no change yet (effort still counts)

Bottom line

You don't need to be tougher. You need better weatherproofing. When you insulate what matters, you can face storms without losing your center.

Your lines

(write one thought, one insight, or rewrite one sentence that rang true)

_____

_____

_____

☐ Done for today

Why this matters
Writing just a few lines by hand locks the concept into memory and gently primes your subconscious mind to adopt and act on it, leading to better recall and follow-through.

DAY 59

"Motion feeds life as much as food and breathing."
— A. Smyrlis, MD

Motion feeds life.
Workouts build fitness; daily movement keeps it.
Break sitting; bank health.

Reflection

Walking is not just exercise. For your body, moving is as fundamental as eating and breathing. Long stretches of stillness send a quiet signal of decline. Movement says, I'm alive and I intend to stay that way.

When you take even a few steps, the internal machinery wakes up. The heart beats a little faster, pushing fresh, oxygen-rich blood to every organ. The lungs expand more fully, bringing in oxygen and clearing carbon dioxide. Blood stops pooling; the calf muscles act as pumps, helping prevent clots. The brain gets a rise in circulation, bringing fuel and oxygen that support focus, creativity, and mood.

This is why long stretches of sitting can be risky: stagnation adds strain. Short movement breaks push things back toward normal. After surgery or illness, physical therapists push early walking because movement supports recovery. Fresh blood brings nutrients to tissues; circulation helps clear byproducts. Immobility, on the other hand, raises the risk for clots, pneumonia, loss of muscle, and faster decline.

And then there's the brain. Walking increases cerebral blood flow and boosts growth factors that protect neurons and support learning and mood. Problems that feel stuck at a desk often start to untangle on a sidewalk. Over and over, solutions arrive once the feet move.

So how much is enough? A helpful anchor is to aim for about 7,000–9,000 steps most days. Many studies suggest the biggest gains happen as you move from low steps to moderate steps, with benefits tending to plateau around 6,000–8,000 steps/day in older adults and around 8,000–10,000 steps/day in younger adults. If you're far below that, don't jump to a big number — add 500–1,000 steps/day and let it compound.

This isn't about obsessing over a number. It's about understanding that regular, sprinkled movement is one of the most powerful, underrated medicines you have: better circulation, steadier mood, smoother glucose, and a calmer nervous system — wrapped into one simple act.

Real-life snapshot

Daniel sat for a living. Eight hours at a desk, a commute, then a couch. By 2 p.m. he felt like his brain was wrapped in cotton. His hips were stiff when he stood up. His cravings hit hard at night, and caffeine became his "solution" for everything.

He told himself the same line every week: I don't have time to work out. His clinician didn't argue. She gave him a smaller target: Don't train. Just interrupt sitting.

So Daniel made movement "automatic." Every time he refilled his water, he took a two-minute loop. Every time he finished a meeting, he stood and did ten slow sit-to-stands. After dinner, he walked for ten minutes — no earbuds, no phone, just air and steps.

Nothing felt dramatic. But the pattern changed. His afternoons stopped crashing as often. His body felt less stuck. The night cravings softened because he wasn't running on stress and stagnation all day.

Same job. Same hours. Same stress. Different signals.

He didn't change his whole life. He changed the defaults — and his body started paying him back.

Quick science

- Walking improves circulation, oxygenation, and lymph flow, lowering clot risk and supporting recovery. Movement increases cerebral blood flow and boosts brain growth factors tied to mood, memory, and learning.
- Higher sedentary time is associated with higher cardiometabolic risk, even in people who work out; frequent short breaks are associated with better markers and lower risk.
- A 10-minute post-meal walk can smooth glucose spikes and support metabolic health for hours.[59]

Inspiration note

Rivers stay clear because they move. Stagnant water grows trouble.
Your body is the same.

Today's Invitation

One thing I will do for myself today:

- ☐ I walk like it's essential by taking a 20-minute walk today (or two 10-minute walks).
- ☐ I make walking effortless by turning one call into a walking call.
- ☐ I use a post-meal walk as medicine by walking 10 minutes after one meal to steady blood sugar and mood.

Action Step:
Choose the easiest one today. Do it now or set one reminder and do it when it best fits your schedule.

Reflection:
After I took the step today, I felt: ☐ calmer ☐ clearer ☐ steadier ☐ proud ☐ no change yet (effort still counts)

Bottom line

Your body runs best on small doses of movement all day.

Your lines

(write one thought, one insight, or rewrite one sentence that rang true)

_____

_____

☐ Done for today

Why this matters
Writing just a few lines by hand locks the concept into memory and gently primes your subconscious mind to adopt and act on it, leading to better recall and follow-through.

DAY 60

"Sometimes enemy and friend can look alike."
— A. Smyrlis, MD

Food that looks the same on the plate can act very differently in the body.
How your food was raised matters as much as what it's called.
Don't be fooled by appearance — choose what truly supports your biology.

Reflection

Two steaks, two stories. Two glasses of milk, two outcomes. Two cartons of berries, two very different long-term effects. Food that looks identical on the surface can behave very differently once it's inside you.

Take beef. A 100% grass-fed, pasture-raised cow eats what its biology recognizes — grass — while moving, grazing, and living outdoors. A confinement, grain-fed cow is pushed on corn and soy, kept mostly indoors, and grown for speed. Those upstream differences ripple downstream: on average, grass-fed beef contains more omega-3 fats and some antioxidants (including vitamin E) and CLA, while grain-finished beef tends to be higher in omega-6 fats and lower in some of those compounds. The two cuts may look the same in the pan — but they don't act the same in your system.

Dairy follows a similar pattern. Milk, yogurt, cheese, and butter from grass-fed or pasture-raised herds often contain more of certain beneficial fats and fat-soluble vitamins. Two cartons in your fridge may look identical — but the chemistry your cells receive is not.

Then there's produce — the quiet highway through which you ingest tiny traces of the world your food grew in. Non-organic berries, spinach, apples, kale, peppers, potatoes, and lettuce consistently sit high on residue lists. These aren't doses that cause obvious poisoning. They're low-level exposures that can add to your body's overall load over time — often invisible day to day, but worth taking seriously across years. A blueberry isn't just a blueberry; it's a carrier for whatever touched it on its way to your bowl.

Organic isn't perfection. It's simply less burden — fewer residues, fewer synthetic chemicals, fewer quiet irritants for your body to work around. Over years, those small differences can add up — especially for people who are sensitive, inflamed, or already overloaded.

And then there are ultra-processed foods — the boxed, bagged, flavored, engineered products that dominate modern diets. These combinations of refined starches, industrial oils, and additives can disrupt satiety, shift gut microbes, and raise inflammation markers — and diets high in ultra-processed foods are consistently associated with higher cardiometabolic risk and earlier mortality. This isn't fringe; it's one of the clearest signals in nutrition research.

Here's the truth: your body becomes what your food once was. If you want different outcomes — better energy, better mood, less inflammation, deeper sleep — you must choose different inputs. Food is chemistry. Food is instruction. Food is information. Select information that supports your biology rather than sabotages it.

Real-life snapshot

Larry, 55, lived with unpredictable low-back pain. Weeks of relief, then sudden flares. He blamed aging, posture, and stress — but never food.

His clinician noticed a deeply inflammatory pattern: cheap meats, non-organic high-residue produce, seed-oil-based dressings, and lots of ultra-processed snacks. Larry didn't want to become a health nut, but he agreed to upgrade a few staples: grass-fed ground beef instead of bargain grain-fed; pasture-raised eggs; organic berries and leafy greens; organic whole-milk yogurt; extra-virgin olive oil instead of generic seed oils for most cooking; fewer boxes and bottles, more single-ingredient foods.

He didn't change jobs, mattresses, or routines. He changed inputs.

By six months, the flares were far less frequent and less intense. Same spine. Same workload. Same life. Different signals to his cells.

Quick science

- Grass-fed and pasture-raised beef and dairy generally contain more beneficial fats (like omega-3s and CLA) and antioxidants, while grain-fed and confinement products tend to lean toward more omega-6 and fewer of some protective nutrients.
- Organic versions of high-residue produce (such as berries and leafy greens) lower pesticide exposure and can reduce overall exposure burden over time.
- Diets high in ultra-processed foods are associated with higher inflammation markers and higher risk of cardiometabolic disease and early mortality; links to other outcomes are still being studied.[60]

Inspiration note

Your body becomes what your food once was — choose ingredients raised in ways that respect life.

Today's Invitation

One thing I will do for myself today:

- ☐ I choose cleaner inputs by swapping one ultra-processed item for a simpler version today.
- ☐ I improve my inputs by making one high-impact produce choice today (organic berries/leafy greens, or wash well).
- ☐ I choose with clarity by reading one label today: fewer ingredients, more recognizable foods.

Action Step:
Choose the easiest one today. Do it now or set one reminder and do it when it best fits your schedule.

Reflection:
After I took the step today, I felt: ☐ calmer ☐ clearer ☐ steadier ☐ proud ☐ no change yet (effort still counts)

Bottom line

If you want a different outcome, choose different inputs — foods raised and grown in ways that support your biology, not fight it.

Your lines

(write one thought, one insight, or rewrite one sentence that rang true)

_____

_____

_____

☐ Done for today

Why this matters
Writing just a few lines by hand locks the concept into memory and gently primes your subconscious mind to adopt and act on it, leading to better recall and follow-through.

DAY 61

> **"Snoring isn't just noise — it's your airway asking for help."**
> — A. Smyrlis, MD

If you're tired no matter how long you sleep, don't blame your character.
If the chain is frayed, you don't need more willpower.
Sometimes the culprit is breathing.

Reflection

You can do "everything right" and still wake up exhausted if your airway is collapsing all night.

Sleep-disordered breathing is a hidden saboteur of brain fog. It can look like snoring, mouth breathing, dry mouth on waking, morning headaches, waking to pee, or a bed partner noticing pauses and gasps. Some people don't snore much at all — they just grind, toss, and wake unrefreshed.

Here's why it matters: your brain can't do deep repair if it keeps being yanked toward the surface. When breathing gets blocked, your oxygen can dip and your body hits an emergency switch. Stress hormones surge. Your heart rate spikes. Your nervous system jolts you just enough to reopen the airway — sometimes dozens or even hundreds of times a night. You may never fully "wake up," so you don't remember it. But your body does.

Instead of resting, your system is on night watch. Not repairing. Not restoring. Fighting — again and again — to keep you alive and breathing.

This is not about fear. It's about accuracy. If you suspect this, don't blame your character. Don't double down on caffeine. Get curious. A simple conversation, a sleep test, or a dental/ENT evaluation can change your whole trajectory.

Real-life snapshot

Maira thought she had "insomnia." She fell asleep fine, but woke up tired and wired. Her Fitbit said she slept seven hours, yet she felt like she ran a marathon.

Her husband finally said, gently, "You stop breathing sometimes. Then you snort and roll over."

Maira resisted the idea. She was fit. She wasn't "the sleep apnea type." But she did a home sleep test. The result wasn't dramatic — just enough breathing disruption to keep her nervous system on alert.

She started with simple changes: side sleeping, no alcohol late, nasal breathing support, and follow-up care. Within weeks, the morning dread softened. By month two, her brain fog began to lift.

Quick science

- Repeated micro-arousals fragment deep sleep even when total hours look "normal."
- Intermittent drops in airflow can trigger stress hormones that raise heart rate and blood pressure overnight.
- Treating sleep-disordered breathing often improves daytime energy, mood, and focus because sleep becomes truly restorative. [61]

Inspiration note

You don't need more time in bed. You need better air.

Today's Invitation

One thing I will do for myself today:

- ☐ I run a simple airway check by noticing two signs: snoring/mouth-dryness, and morning headache or fog.
- ☐ I support nasal breathing tonight by trying one low-risk step (saline rinse, nasal strip, or humidifier) and sleeping on my side.
- ☐ I protect my future energy by messaging my clinician about a sleep test if I have loud snoring, witnessed pauses, or persistent unrefreshing sleep.

Action Step:
Choose the easiest one today. Do it now or set one reminder and do it when it best fits your schedule.

Reflection:
After I took the step today, I felt: ☐ calmer ☐ clearer ☐ steadier ☐ proud ☐ no change yet (effort still counts)

Bottom line

If your sleep isn't restoring you, check the airway before you blame the person.

Your lines

(write one thought, one insight, or rewrite one sentence that rang true)

_____
_____
_____

☐ Done for today

Why this matters
Writing just a few lines by hand locks the concept into memory and gently primes your subconscious mind to adopt and act on it, leading to better recall and follow-through.

DAY 62

> **"Gratitude is not only the greatest of virtues, but the parent of all the others."**
> — Cicero

Gratitude doesn't change your circumstances — it can change your inner state. When you practice noticing what's good, your whole system shifts toward safety. Thankfulness is not denial; it's a recalibration of your inner world.

Reflection

Gratitude is more than being positive. It's a full-body act. To feel grateful, you have to pause, notice, and name something good. That tiny sequence does a lot of work: your attention moves away from threat for a moment, your breathing often slows, your muscles soften a bit, and the body gets a brief break from what's wrong to see what's here.

Your brain and body are always talking. When you dwell only on what's broken, your nervous system hears unsafe and responds with tension, stress hormones, blood pressure spikes, shallow sleep, and frantic thoughts. When you deliberately practice gratitude, you send a different message: There are problems, yes — but also supports. I am not completely alone. There is something good, right now.

Practice that message enough, and it leaves fingerprints on your physiology. Studies of gratitude journaling and exercises show benefits that aren't just emotional: better sleep quality, improved mood, and, in some studies, modest improvements in blood pressure and other health markers.

What's happening under the hood? Gratitude is associated with a calmer stress response and better emotional regulation — a shift toward steadier, safer physiology.

Over time, this isn't just feeling nicer. A calmer, more balanced system sleeps deeper, repairs better, digests more smoothly, and is more capable of making good choices. Chronic disease risk is shaped heavily by stress, sleep, immunity, and behavior. Gratitude touches all of these: it lightens the mental load, steadies emotions, improves sleep, and encourages you to care for yourself and others.

None of this means you must be grateful for every event. Some things are not okay. Gratitude is not about lying to yourself or erasing pain. It is about refusing to let pain be the only story. Even in hard seasons, you can thank a warm bowl of soup, a nurse's kindness, a text from a friend, sunlight through the window. These are medicines too.

Gratitude practiced daily is like cleaning a window. The world outside doesn't instantly change — but you can finally see more of it: the help that is present, the love that still exists, the strength you do have. From that clearer place, your thoughts get cleaner — and the actions that follow tend to be wiser and kinder.

Real-life snapshot

After a brutal stretch at work and a string of medical tests, Luis felt like his life had collapsed into problems. Bills, lab results, arguments, worries about the future — his mind replayed them on a loop. Sleep was thin. His appetite swung between no interest and comfort food.

A counselor suggested a tiny experiment: each night, before touching his phone, write down three very specific things he was grateful for. Not generalities — concrete details.

One night he wrote: Sun on the stoop while I drank coffee. Maria's voice note that made me laugh. The nurse who joked about my shoes during blood draws. Then he sent one text: Thank you for the voice note today — it really helped.

The next morning, nothing magical had changed. The tests were still pending. The bills were still there. But he felt a fraction lighter. After a week, his sleep was a bit deeper. He wasn't as quick to snap.

Quick science

- Randomized gratitude interventions (like writing down blessings) are associated with improved sleep quality, optimism, and overall well-being, and in some studies reduced diastolic blood pressure.
- Regular gratitude is associated with fewer physical symptoms, less pain, better sleep quality, and even more consistent exercise in some participants.
- Meta-analytic data show gratitude is linked with lower depression and better mood; gratitude-based practices may also support cardiovascular health and long-term well-being.[62]

Inspiration note

Gratitude doesn't change your life overnight. It changes your lens.

Today's Invitation

One thing I will do for myself today:

- ☐ I practice gratitude by writing three lines: something I saw, someone I appreciate, something I did right.
- ☐ I strengthen gratitude by thanking one person today (a text counts).
- ☐ I let gratitude land by savoring one ordinary moment for 10 seconds.

Action Step:
Choose the easiest one today. Do it now or set one reminder and do it when it best fits your schedule.

Reflection:
After I took the step today, I felt: ☐ calmer ☐ clearer ☐ steadier ☐ proud ☐ no change yet (effort still counts)

Bottom line

Gratitude is not pretending everything is fine. It's practicing the skill of seeing what is still good — and letting that steady your brain, your body, and your next choice.

Your lines

(write one thought, one insight, or rewrite one sentence that rang true)

_____

_____

_____

☐ Done for today

Why this matters
Writing just a few lines by hand locks the concept into memory and gently primes your subconscious mind to adopt and act on it, leading to better recall and follow-through.

DAY 63

> "Just as a rock cannot be shaken by the wind,
> a mindful person is not shaken by praise,
> blame, pleasure, or pain."
> — Modern rendering, Dhammapada

Steadiness is the quiet crown of a conscious life.
When you walk in truth, the weather of the world cannot move you.
What once pulled you off-center becomes small beside the law of love.

Reflection

Health and happiness are not just physical achievements. They are also a spiritual path.

When you begin walking consciously — seeing health for what it truly is — something shifts. Praise and criticism. Pleasure and pain. Gain and loss. You start to recognize them as winds. They blow, but they don't have to steer you. You were never meant to live like a leaf.

As awareness grows, you begin to sense a deeper order beneath life — call it God's way, truth, or the law of love. It's the same quiet rhythm woven into giving and receiving, sowing and reaping, light and dark, inhale and exhale.

When we live out of rhythm — expending without replenishing, consuming without gratitude, taking without contribution — we feel it. Not as punishment, but as feedback. A gentle signal that we've drifted and can return.

Health, at its deepest level, is alignment. It's living from truth instead of fear. It's choosing steadiness over reaction. It's letting love guide your decisions more than ego or urgency.

Anchor your inner life in what does not change — God, truth, love, or the highest good you trust. The winds still blow. But when you walk in that alignment, they no longer own you.

Real-life snapshot

Ava spent years chasing approval — perfecting every detail at work, tracking every comment online, bending herself to avoid criticism. She looked successful, but inside she felt hollow and on edge.

During a personal crisis, she began practicing stillness each morning: five quiet minutes of breathing, turning her attention to God — whom she understood as a spirit of love — and asking one question: "What is the loving thing to do now?"

At first, nothing outside changed. The job was the same. The inbox kept coming. But over months, the winds that once controlled her lost their force. Praise felt pleasant, but no longer addictive. Criticism still stung, but it didn't pierce. She began eating, moving, resting, and choosing from alignment instead of anxiety.

"I finally understand," she said. "Health is not just habits. It's my spirit remembering where home is."

Quick science

- Meditation and contemplative prayer can reduce reactivity to daily stressors and support steadier emotional regulation.
- Living with purpose and aligned values is associated with better stress recovery and overall wellbeing, and in some studies with healthier inflammatory markers.
- Practices of compassion and loving-kindness are associated with better emotional regulation and resilience.[63]

Inspiration note

Stillness is not the absence of movement — it is the presence of truth.

Today's Invitation

One thing I will do for myself today:

☐ I take 2 minutes today for prayer, stillness, or quiet reflection.
☐ In one hard moment, I ask: What would love choose here?
☐ I make love practical today with one small act of compassion or service.

Action Step:
Choose the easiest one today. Do it now or set one reminder and do it when it best fits your schedule.

Reflection:
After I took the step today, I felt: ☐ calmer ☐ clearer ☐ steadier ☐ proud ☐ no change yet (effort still counts)

Bottom line

Health is alignment with the law of love. When you walk in that law — one honest step at a time — the winds still blow, but they cannot shake your center.

Your lines

(write one thought, one insight, or rewrite one sentence that rang true)

_____

_____

_____

☐ Done for today

Why this matters
Writing just a few lines by hand locks the concept into memory and gently primes your subconscious mind to adopt and act on it, leading to better recall and follow-through.

DAY 64

"Well done is better than well said."
— Benjamin Franklin

Your life is shaped by what you do, not what you intend.
A tiny action has more power than a perfect plan on paper.
Starting small is how big things quietly begin.

Reflection

Talk fades. Tiny action stays.

We love to live in the realm of ideas — thinking about getting healthy, reading about it, talking about it. The mind feels busy and satisfied: "I know what I should do." But knowing is not enough. Knowing without doing becomes a kind of fog. You feel worse, not better, because the gap between what you understand and how you live keeps widening.

Action cuts through that fog. It slices past excuses, overthinking, and performance and shows you what you're actually willing to live. Even the smallest step tells the truth: ten squats, one glass of water, a two-minute walk, a single "no" to something that drains you. These aren't symbolic gestures. They're real votes for the person you are becoming.

If you want a simple way to start, use the two-minute rule. Lower the bar to doable. Put on shoes. Fill the water bottle. Chop the veggies. Once momentum starts, add a little more. Tie actions to cues: "After coffee, I stretch." "After lunch, I walk five minutes." And record your streaks — the checkmark is a tiny spark that keeps the fire.

Doing also asks something deeper from you: alignment. When your mind, body, and spirit are pointed in the same direction, even small actions feel different. You're not just following a tip; you're giving a piece of your day to health — and to the purpose behind it: to be present for the people you love, to serve well, to walk your path with strength. When the act matches the truth you hold inside, many people feel their nervous system settle, and the habit starts to feel natural.

Small done beats big promised. Speed favors starters.

Real-life snapshot

Omar and Lena made the same promise: "I'm getting in shape."

Omar made a beautiful plan — new shoes, a spreadsheet, a Monday start date. But his days stayed the same: late calls, skipped lunch, tired evenings. When it was time to act, he'd think, "I'll do it right when life calms down."

Lena chose a different game. She picked one tiny move she could do on her worst day: ten pushups before her shower. Then she added one more anchor she could repeat: a five-minute walk after lunch, even if it was just around the building. No heroics. Just a start that could survive real life.

Four weeks later, Lena had a quiet streak and better energy. Omar still had a perfect plan — and no momentum.

Quick science

- Action creates internal feedback and a small sense of reward that reinforces new behaviors.
- The "two-minute rule" can reduce procrastination by lowering overwhelm and making the start easy.
- Repeated small actions often grow into larger efforts as confidence and identity ("I'm someone who does this") build.[64]

Inspiration note

The difference between "someday" and "today" is often just a two-minute action.

Today's Invitation

One thing I will do for myself today:

- ☐ I let action speak by doing a 2-minute starter step right now (shoes on, water poured, or veggies washed).
- ☐ I make action likely by scheduling the next tiny step with a specific time.
- ☐ I keep the chain alive by marking it when it's done (one check mark counts).

Action Step:
Choose the easiest one today. Do it now or set one reminder and do it when it best fits your schedule.

Reflection:
After I took the step today, I felt: ☐ calmer ☐ clearer ☐ steadier ☐ proud ☐ no change yet (effort still counts)

Bottom line

Well done beats well said — every time, and in every domain of health.

Your lines

(write one thought, one insight, or rewrite one sentence that rang true)

_____

_____

_____

☐ Done for today

Why this matters
Writing just a few lines by hand locks the concept into memory and gently primes your subconscious mind to adopt and act on it, leading to better recall and follow-through.

DAY 65

> "Life is now — not later. Retirement is not a life plan."
> — A. Smyrlis, MD

This is not a rehearsal — this is the run.
"Later" is where most health plans quietly die.
If you don't build a life you can live now, retirement becomes a repair shop, not a reward.

Reflection

You grind. Early trains, late emails. Deals closed. Metrics up. You tell yourself, "Push now, rest later." Retirement becomes the magic box where you'll finally sleep, cook, move, travel, be present.

But every day, you are shaping the body and brain you'll retire with.

Imagine you're building a house you'll have to live in for the rest of your life. Every late night, every skipped meal, every week without movement is one more corner cut in the foundation. The walls may stand — for a while. Then small cracks appear: foggy mornings, rising blood pressure, stubborn weight, a mood that frays too easily. Eventually, a bigger crack may arrive as chest pain, a strange scan, a diagnosis that rearranges your plans. It can feel sudden, but it usually isn't random.

Most people don't ignore health on purpose. They're trying to make it through the week. So we bargain: "I'll fix this when things calm down. When the kids are older. When I hit 65." But the body doesn't live in "someday." It responds to today's inputs: sleep, food, movement, stress, connection.

This doesn't mean you need a perfect life. It means you need a sustainable one — a way of living that doesn't quietly grind down your joints, your arteries, and your nervous system while you're saving for a future you may be too tired to enjoy.

You don't have to quit your job or move to the mountains. You do have to stop making deals your body can't afford. If the promotion costs your sleep, steps, and sanity, the price is wrong. If you're always "too busy" for real food, you're borrowing energy from tomorrow to feed today. Drive-thru and cafeteria meals can plug a hole, but they're not reliable building material. A simple lunch from home beats a hundred "whatever's available" meals. And if every ping gets an instant reply, your nervous system never clocks out.

Be firm with the world, kind to your body. Put the essentials on the calendar first: a sleep window, a little movement, at least one home-prepared meal, and a sliver of quiet or connection. Let work fit around that, not the other way around.

Retirement should not be the first time you meet your own life. Start building a livable future inside your present — one small choice at a time.

Real-life snapshot

Peter had a plan: grind hard, retire at 65, then "finally get healthy." He worked long hours, slept short nights, grabbed cafeteria food, and told himself it was temporary — just a season.

At 57, chest pain sent him to the ER. The cardiologist's face gave him the message before the words did: his body hadn't been waiting for his retirement date. It had been keeping score.

In cardiac rehab, surrounded by people his age and younger, he noticed the same sentence floating through the room: "I'll deal with this later." Later didn't arrive as a quiet reset. It arrived as treadmills with wires, monitors, and nurses watching.

Peter decided "later" was over. He started small: a daily walk, even if it was just around the block. An earlier bedtime — no more midnight emails. A few basic meals he could repeat, and lunch from home instead of whatever the cafeteria offered. One clear "no" to an extra project so he could make rehab and follow-ups without scrambling.

"I almost gambled my whole future on 'later,'" he admitted.

Quick science

- Midlife patterns — sleep, movement, diet, smoking, stress — are linked to later risk for heart disease, stroke, cognitive decline, and disability.
- Chronic, unmanaged stress can add to "allostatic load" — the body's long-term wear and tear — which is associated with earlier and more severe illness.
- Early, sustained changes (even modest ones) can improve daily function and may lower the odds of needing intensive care later.[65]

Inspiration note

Retirement is not a life plan — the way you live today is.

Today's Invitation

One thing I will do for myself today:

- ☐ Tonight I protect a real sleep window — the kind my future self will thank me for.
- ☐ Today I put 10 minutes of movement on the calendar (walk, stairs, or simple strength).
- ☐ I choose one real-food meal today instead of defaulting to convenience.

Action Step:
Choose the easiest one today. Do it now or set one reminder and do it when it best fits your schedule.

Reflection:
After I took the step today, I felt: ☐ calmer ☐ clearer ☐ steadier ☐ proud ☐ no change yet (effort still counts)

Bottom line

Life is now. If you want a livable future, start building a life your body can survive and enjoy — today.

Your lines

(write one thought, one insight, or rewrite one sentence that rang true)

☐ Done for today

Why this matters
Writing just a few lines by hand locks the concept into memory and gently primes your subconscious mind to adopt and act on it, leading to better recall and follow-through.

DAY 66

> **"Luck is what happens when preparation meets opportunity."**
> — attributed to Seneca

What looks like "luck" is often preparation becoming visible.
Your future health depends less on willpower and more on setup.
A well-prepared environment makes the right choice feel automatic.

Reflection

Luck doesn't just wander in — you set a place for it. Health works the same way. You don't wake up one day "suddenly disciplined." You quietly rig the game in your favor: you lay out the tools, remove the speed bumps, and make the next good step obvious.

What looks like "luck" is often preparation becoming visible. When your environment is staged, the right choice feels automatic. When it isn't, every good choice has to fight a dozen tiny frictions: Where are my shoes? What should I eat? Do I have time? That constant deciding is exhausting — and exhaustion pushes you toward whatever is easiest.

Success hides in the setup. A packed gym bag by the door. A lights-down alarm that actually lands you in bed. Water at eye level. Real food visible and ready. When your space points you forward, you don't have to push as hard; your environment quietly pulls.

Three simple levers do most of the work. Put it in your path (shoes by the door, journal on the pillow). Remove friction (fewer steps between you and the habit; phone charging outside the bedroom). Pair it with a cue (After I brush my teeth, I stretch two minutes. After dinner, we walk the block. After I sit down, I start with my priority project). Tie habits together like cars on a train.

Preparation isn't rigidity — it's kindness in advance. It's the night-before you leaving gifts for the morning-you who will be tired and distracted. Set the runway so the plane can land.

Real-life snapshot

Nina and Omar both felt too tired after work. Nina meant to exercise, but the couch kept winning. Omar bought gear and made plans, but nothing was staged — so decision time always turned into delay.

On a friend's suggestion, Nina tried something simple: a "movement kit." Each night, before bed, she set the scene — workout clothes and shoes by the door, a filled water bottle on the counter, and a mat already rolled out in the corner.

The next day, when she walked in, the choice was still hers — but the path of least resistance now pointed toward movement. She slipped on the sneakers and hit play on a short routine.

"By the time I debated it," she said, "I was already dressed." Within a few weeks, "too tired" turned into "this is just what I do when I get home."

Quick science

- Designing your environment ("choice architecture") can shape behavior more consistently than motivation alone.
- Reducing friction — fewer steps between you and the action — often boosts follow-through on healthy habits.
- Implementation intentions ("If X, then Y") can prime the brain to respond when a specific cue appears, turning decisions into simpler responses.[66]

Inspiration note

Kindness to your future self is one of the most powerful forms of preparation.

Today's Invitation

One thing I will do for myself today:

- ☐ Tonight, I set the runway by laying out one thing in advance (shoes, clothes, or a water bottle).
- ☐ Today, I reduce friction so the right choice is easier (add a helper, remove a temptation).
- ☐ When stress hits, I use one if–then rule: I pause, then choose a better next step.

Action Step:
Choose the easiest one today. Do it now or set one reminder and do it when it best fits your schedule.

Reflection:
After I took the step today, I felt: ☐ calmer ☐ clearer ☐ steadier ☐ proud ☐ no change yet (effort still counts)

Bottom line

You don't need more luck — you need better staging. Preparation opens the door so opportunity can walk through.

Your lines

(write one thought, one insight, or rewrite one sentence that rang true)

_____

_____

_____

☐ Done for today

Why this matters
Writing just a few lines by hand locks the concept into memory and gently primes your subconscious mind to adopt and act on it, leading to better recall and follow-through.

DAY 67

"No man is free who is not master of himself."
— Epictetus

Health is the foundation of all freedom.
Discipline isn't chains; it's rails that keep you out of the ditch.
Self-mastery is a kindness to your future self.

Reflection

We often picture freedom as no rules, no limits. But that world doesn't exist. There will always be clocks, bills, people who need you, and laws of biology that don't care about your calendar.

Real freedom isn't the absence of obligations; it's choosing commitments that serve what you believe. Epictetus had it right: if you're not master of yourself — your attention, your impulses, your defaults — you're not really free. You get pulled around by cravings, pings, and pressure.

Discipline gets a bad name because we confuse it with punishment or perfectionism. In reality, healthy discipline is gentle structure that protects what matters most. It sounds like: "Lights down by 10 p.m. most nights, because my brain deserves tomorrow." "Phone stays off the table at meals, because these people matter." "One meaningful task gets my best focus before the day splinters into fragments." These are not punishments. They're guardrails. When you choose your guardrails, your guardrails start choosing your day.

Think of discipline in four domains: body, mind, spirit, and people. For the body, it's a steady sleep window, mostly real food, some movement, morning light. For the mind, it's less noise, one daily focus block, a simple plan for your attention. For the spirit, it's a remembered why that you touch in small ways — service, prayer, reflection, learning. For people, it's daily connection — a shared meal, a check-in text, a hug that lasts more than a second.

Discipline gets easier when you design for it. Put **distance** in front of what drains you and remove distance from what feeds you. Charge your phone in another room at night. Keep the TV remote out of reach during your wind-down hour. Put your book or journal on the pillow. Keep a filled water bottle on your desk. Set tomorrow's lunch in the front of the fridge. Good design makes good choices feel like the default, not a heroic act.

Strong doesn't mean rigid. Emergencies happen, weeks go sideways. Mastery isn't "I never slip." Mastery is "When I slip, I know how to come back." Direction beats perfection. If you drift off plan, your next cue is your chance to return: lights down tonight, walk before screens tomorrow, one meal at the table instead of the couch.

You can't control everything around you. But you can craft how you move through it. That's self-mastery. That's freedom.

Real-life snapshot

Karim felt trapped by his schedule: constant messages, endless meetings, kids' activities, family obligations. Yet he said yes to every new request and let his phone interrupt him dozens of times an hour. By night, he felt wrung out and oddly unaccomplished — like he ran all day and still didn't arrive anywhere.

His doctor asked him to try a simple experiment: not a huge overhaul, just three self-chosen rules for a month. Phone charges outside the bedroom. Two 45-minute deep-work blocks daily — no email, no chat, just one important task. And one device-free meal with his family — no TV, no phones at the table.

The first week felt strange, like he was missing something. By week three, something else was missing: the feeling of being constantly yanked around. His sleep improved. His work felt more focused. Dinner felt like a human moment again instead of content with food attached.

I'm more free now with more structure, he said, because I'm finally choosing my constraints instead of letting everyone else choose them for me.

Quick science

- Self-chosen structure reduces decision fatigue and preserves willpower for meaningful choices.
- Boundaries around attention and rest can support better sleep and steadier stress and mood over time.
- Discipline that comes from autonomy ("rules I choose for myself") is more sustainable and less stressful than control imposed entirely from outside.[67]

Inspiration note

You can't control everything around you, but you can craft how you move through it.

Today's Invitation

One thing I will do for myself today:

- ☐ Today I pick one rule I choose and keep (lights down, walk after lunch, or a real breakfast).
- ☐ I add one speed bump to what drains me (move the charger, log out, or delete the app).
- ☐ Tonight I stage one small setup that makes tomorrow easier (shoes out, lunch packed, or water ready).

Action Step:
Choose the easiest one today. Do it now or set one reminder and do it when it best fits your schedule.

Reflection:
After I took the step today, I felt: ☐ calmer ☐ clearer ☐ steadier ☐ proud ☐ no change yet (effort still counts)

Bottom line

Freedom grows as you master your choices — not as you escape them.

Your lines

(write one thought, one insight, or rewrite one sentence that rang true)

_____

_____

_____

☐ Done for today

Why this matters
Writing just a few lines by hand locks the concept into memory and gently primes your subconscious mind to adopt and act on it, leading to better recall and follow-through.

DAY 68

> **"The part can never be well unless the whole is well."**
> — Plato

Your body doesn't operate in departments — everything is connected. A symptom in one place often starts with imbalance somewhere else. When the whole system is tuned, each part can finally rest.

Reflection

Your body is not a set of separate offices. It's one living system. A fast heartbeat might look like a heart problem — until you discover thyroid hormones are running high, sleep is depleted, or stimulants are overdoing it. High blood pressure and weight gain can look like "bad willpower"—until you see blood sugar and insulin have been running high for years, quietly driving cravings and fat storage.

Specialists are valuable. But if you only ever zoom in, you can miss the pattern that lives in the wide view. A thyroid issue, a gut issue, a sleep issue, a stress issue — each can echo through many organs at once. That's why a whole-person approach matters: it looks for shared roots instead of trimming branches one by one.

Think of your body as a choir. When one voice is off, you can scold the soloist (another pill, another test), or you can tune the whole group — sleep, food, movement, gut health, stress, relationships, purpose. The second approach is slower, but it holds. It doesn't just quiet a symptom; it changes the conditions that made the symptom necessary. Support the whole, and the parts often follow.

Real-life snapshot

For years, Maya bounced between specialists for fatigue, palpitations, weight gain, and high blood pressure. Cardiology checked her heart. Neurology scanned her brain. Each doctor focused on their part. No one was "wrong," but nothing made her feel right. She left most visits with another prescription and the same quiet line: "We'll keep watching."

Finally, one clinician stepped back and asked different questions: "How is your sleep? What's your caffeine like — coffee, tea, energy drinks? What supplements are you taking, and when?" Maya paused. She hadn't thought of those as "medical." They were just her routine.

It turned out she was drinking licorice and ginseng tea in the evening to "support energy," and taking B-vitamins at night because that's when she remembered. On rough weeks, she added a pre-workout in the afternoon and chased fatigue with a second coffee. None of it sounded dramatic. But together, it added up to a steady stream of activation at the exact hours her body was trying to downshift.

They ran a simple experiment — not a new diagnosis, just cleaner signals. Licorice and ginseng were replaced with a gentler morning tea, earlier in the day. B-vitamins moved to the morning, with food. Caffeine got a clear cutoff. Evenings got quieter: dimmer light, a calmer wind-down, and a consistent sleep window. Meals got simpler and more repeatable, and she added gentle walking — especially after dinner.

Over the next months, her palpitations became much less frequent and less scary. Her energy steadied. Her cravings softened. Her blood pressure began moving in a better direction. Nothing magical happened. Her system just stopped getting mixed messages — and as the noise dropped, the "mystery" symptoms began to shrink. The problem wasn't mysterious. It was a system getting contradictory cues.

Quick science

- Body systems (hormones, gut, nerves, immune signals, and the heart) constantly talk to each other; a shift in one area can show up somewhere else.
- Many symptoms are "system signals" — sleep loss, chronic stress, inflammation, and nutrient gaps can amplify multiple complaints at once.
- Foundational levers (sleep, movement, real food, stress relief) can improve several issues together because they support the body's shared control systems.[68]

Inspiration note

You're not a collection of parts — you're a living symphony.

Today's Invitation

One thing I will do for myself today:

- ☐ Today I support the whole by doing one small foundation step (sleep, real food, or movement).
- ☐ I remove one drain that throws my system off (late screens, ultra-processed snack, or no daylight).
- ☐ I add one root support that helps me stabilize (morning light, water, a short walk, or a real meal).

Action Step:
Choose the easiest one today. Do it now or set one reminder and do it when it best fits your schedule.

Reflection:
After I took the step today, I felt: ☐ calmer ☐ clearer ☐ steadier ☐ proud ☐ no change yet (effort still counts)

Bottom line

Lasting healing comes from tuning the whole, not just adjusting one note.

Your lines

(write one thought, one insight, or rewrite one sentence that rang true)

_____

_____

_____

☐ Done for today

Why this matters
Writing just a few lines by hand locks the concept into memory and gently primes your subconscious mind to adopt and act on it, leading to better recall and follow-through.

DAY 69

> "Balance isn't found at the extremes;
> it's protected between them."
> — A. Smyrlis, MD

Too much effort can break what apathy never could.
You can drown chasing breath and starve chasing leanness.
True health lives in rhythm, not rigidity.

Reflection

Your body tends to do best in waves, not straight lines.

It's designed for cycles: push, then recover; work, then rest; nourishment, then pause. Live only at the extremes — overtraining, over-restricting, overworking — and you flatten the very rhythms that keep you alive.

At first, extreme effort looks like progress. You feel productive, disciplined, even virtuous. But slowly, quietly, joy thins out. Your sleep lightens. Your strength plateaus. The spark that made the work possible begins to dim.

Balance is not the absence of striving. It is intelligent pacing.

When you stop measuring your life only by how much — how many reps, hours, calories, tasks — you start noticing subtler signals: steadier mornings, a natural desire to move, deeper sleep, more patience, more laughter at breakfast. These are your lane markers. They tell you when your training and routines are tuned, not tearing.

Balance isn't laziness; it is precision. It's the space where your physiology can adapt instead of defend, grow instead of brace. The middle is where health lives — not in the heroic extremes, but in the rhythmic tension between effort and ease.

Real-life snapshot

Alex trained six days a week and lived on low-carb meals. For a while he felt unstoppable — until his pull-ups dropped, his sleep thinned, and mornings went dull. He assumed the answer was to tighten up even more.

His coach stopped him with one line: "You don't need more grind. You need recovery." They tried an experiment: one true rest day each week, one lighter deload week each month, and slightly more food — especially around training.

Within days, his strength began to return. Soreness softened. Sleep deepened. He found himself joking again at the breakfast table instead of staring into space.

Quick science

- Healthy systems rely on oscillation — stress followed by true recovery.
- Chronic stress and persistently elevated cortisol can blunt normal rhythms and is often linked with lower HRV (one proxy of recovery/resilience).
- Wave-based training and flexible fueling often support better adaptation and long-term performance than constant maximal effort.[69]

Inspiration note

A violin string plays only when it is tuned.
    Too loose, and it whispers. Too tight, and it snaps.
    Your body is the same.

Today's Invitation

One thing I will do for myself today:

☐ Today I plan one push and one recovery on purpose (effort, then ease).
☐ Tonight I protect sleep as my main recovery tool — lights down earlier.
☐ I choose the sustainable dose: enough to help, not so much that it breaks me.

Action Step:
Choose the easiest one today. Do it now or set one reminder and do it when it best fits your schedule.

Reflection:
After I took the step today, I felt: ☐ calmer ☐ clearer ☐ steadier ☐ proud ☐ no change yet (effort still counts)

Bottom line

Listen to the lane markers before you hit the ditch. Balance isn't found at the extremes — it's protected in the space between effort and ease.

Your lines

(write one thought, one insight, or rewrite one sentence that rang true)

_____
_____
_____

☐ Done for today

Why this matters
Writing just a few lines by hand locks the concept into memory and gently primes your subconscious mind to adopt and act on it, leading to better recall and follow-through.

DAY 70

> **"Choose clinicians who remember you are a person, not just a chart."**
> — A. Smyrlis, MD

You are the expert on your life; your clinician is the expert on medicine.
Good care is not a solo act — it's a careful dance where both partners listen and lead in turn.
You deserve a partner in your health, not just a prescription.

Reflection

Not all clinicians practice the same way. Some are brilliant technicians but poor listeners. Some are kind but rushed. Some are thoughtful partners who see you as a whole person and are willing to think upstream — about sleep, food, movement, stress, and purpose — not just pills and procedures.

You deserve a clinician who helps you thrive, not just survive.

Start by noticing how they show up: do they seem present in the room or half-turned toward the computer the whole time? Do they ask open questions, or do they jump straight to prescriptions and orders? When you describe your symptoms, do they reflect back what they heard to make sure they understand, or do they move on as if it were obvious?

Pay attention to how you feel during and after the visit. Do you feel seen, respected, and calmer, even if the news is serious? Or do you feel dismissed, confused, or scolded? Your nervous system is a good sensor. A good clinician usually helps your nervous system settle, not spike.

A helpful clinician invites questions. You can test this gently: Can you explain what you think is going on in a simple way? What are my options? What would you recommend to a close family member in my shoes? Watch their reaction. If they get defensive, impatient, or annoyed, that's important information.

It's also reasonable to ask where lifestyle fits: How do sleep, food, movement, and stress play into this condition? Are there changes I can make that might help over time and, in some cases, reduce reliance on medication? A clinician who is willing to engage those questions — even if they're not an integrative or functional specialist — is telling you they see you as more than a body to be fixed.

Sometimes you will need a team: a primary care clinician to coordinate and screen; a specialist for a specific diagnosis or procedure; a therapist, nutritionist, or health coach for day-to-day habit change. Think of them as different instruments in an orchestra. What matters is that they are at least roughly playing the same piece of music and that you feel safe enough to speak.

If a clinician's style is not a fit, you are allowed to change. If you're unsure, consider a second opinion before making big changes.

When you find a clinician who is curious, honest, humble, and thorough — keep them. Show up prepared. Follow through on agreed plans. Bring them questions instead of silent resentment. Good clinicians are under pressure too; when they recognize a patient who wants to work as a partner, they often go the extra mile.

At its best, the relationship between you and your clinician is one of the strongest medicines available. It can calm fear, clarify priorities, and help you make decisions that honor both your biology and your values.

You are not just a chart or a collection of lab values. You are a person with a story, a family, and a future you care about. Choose clinicians who remember that — and let them help you write the next chapter of your health with wisdom, courage, and hope.

Real-life snapshot

Elena had seen the same primary care doctor for years. He was smart and efficient, but every visit felt rushed. He rarely looked up from the screen. When she tried to mention sleep and stress, he waved it off and added another prescription. She left each time more anxious than when she arrived.

Her coworker Daniel had a different doctor and kept saying, It shouldn't feel like this — you're allowed to find a better fit.

After a particularly confusing visit, she asked a friend for a recommendation and booked a new appointment. The new clinician greeted her, closed the laptop for the first few minutes, and asked, "What's the most important thing you want me to understand today?"

He listened, summarized what he'd heard, explained his thinking in plain language, and said, "Here's how medications help — and here's where sleep, food, and movement play in. Let's build a plan that fits your life."

The treatment plan wasn't magic. But Elena felt less scared and more engaged, and over the next weeks her sleep steadied and her blood pressure readings began trending in a better direction. "The biggest change," she said, "was realizing I was allowed to choose a doctor who actually sees me."

Quick science
- A strong therapeutic alliance (good relationship between clinician and patient) is associated with better adherence, satisfaction, and in some cases better health outcomes.
- Feeling heard and respected can lower anxiety and may improve blood pressure and heart-rate measures during and after visits.
- Patients who feel safe asking questions tend to understand their conditions better and are more likely to follow through with agreed plans.[70]

Inspiration note

You are not difficult for wanting to be heard — you are doing the sacred work of caring for the one body you'll ever live in.

Today's Invitation

One thing I will do for myself today:

- ☐ Today I write what I need from care in one line (listening, curiosity, whole-person thinking).
- ☐ I ask one clarifying question at my next visit: Can you explain what you think is going on in plain terms?
- ☐ If something doesn't fit, I protect my health by seeking a second opinion or a better partnership.

Action Step:
Choose the easiest one today. Do it now or set one reminder and do it when it best fits your schedule.

Reflection:
After I took the step today, I felt: ☐ calmer ☐ clearer ☐ steadier ☐ proud ☐ no change yet (effort still counts)

Bottom line

You are not just a chart. Choose clinicians who see your whole story — and let them help you build health that fits the life you actually want to live.

Your lines

(write one thought, one insight, or rewrite one sentence that rang true)

_____
_____
_____

☐ Done for today

Why this matters
Writing just a few lines by hand locks the concept into memory and gently primes your subconscious mind to adopt and act on it, leading to better recall and follow-through.

DAY 71

"Have no fear of perfection — you'll never reach it."
— Salvador Dalí

Perfectionism feels like safety, but it quietly makes you alone.
If you can't delegate, you can't rest — your nervous system never clocks out.
Trust is a health skill: let good enough hold, and let other hands help.

Reflection

Perfectionism rarely feels like vanity. It usually feels like responsibility.
 "If I don't hold it, it will drop."
 "If I don't do it, it won't be done right."
 So you become the manager of everything. Parenting without backup. A business that can't move unless you approve every detail. A household where you carry the invisible list: birthdays, prescriptions, appointments, groceries, repairs, forms, emails, plans. You don't just do the work — you also do the worrying.
 From the outside, it can look admirable. On the inside, it's expensive. Your nervous system stays slightly braced, like a computer with too many programs running at once. Sleep gets lighter. Patience gets thinner. Small mistakes feel dangerous because you're already running at the edge.
 Here's the pitfall: perfectionism turns you into a one-person system. And one-person systems don't have redundancy. They can't truly recover because they're always on-call.
 Delegation is not dumping your life on others. It's building a structure your body can survive. It's letting help in before you collapse. It's practicing a new belief: "Good enough can hold. I don't have to carry this alone."
 Yes, support costs something — time, money, ego, discomfort. But so does doing everything yourself. And over years, the cost of "I've got it, always" is often worse: burnout, resentment, health symptoms, and a life that feels like it's happening just out of reach.
 You are not weak for needing other people. You are human.

Real-life snapshot

Noah owned a small but growing business. On paper he was successful. In real life, he was exhausted. He answered every email, approved every purchase, scheduled every shift, and rewrote half of what his team produced. If anyone made a mistake, he told himself, "It's easier if I just do it myself."

A friend ran a similar business and had one simple rule: if you delegate it, you let it stay delegated. Noah laughed at that — and then felt the truth of it in his chest.

At home, the pattern continued. Two young kids, and Noah insisted on doing bedtime himself "so it's done right." He handled most errands. He refused help because it felt faster to push through than to explain.

Headaches grew. Sleep shrank. His blood pressure crept up. At a visit, his doctor asked gently, "What would it look like to let this be a team — at work and at home?"

Noah started small. One employee took scheduling, with clear rules. A bookkeeper handled monthly accounting. And he said yes when his parents offered to take the kids every other Saturday morning. The hardest part wasn't the logistics — it was the trust. He still hovered at first. He still wanted to check everything. But he practiced letting "good enough" stand.

Within a few months, his evenings felt less frantic. He walked more. He ate a real meal a couple of nights a week. He had actual conversations with his partner again. His headaches eased. His blood pressure readings began trending in a better direction.

"I didn't get weaker when I asked for help," he said. "I got healthier. The business ran better — and so did my body."

Quick science

- Higher perceived social support is linked with lower stress markers and better health outcomes, and some studies associate it with lower cardiovascular risk and longer life.
- Chronic role overload and perfectionism are linked with higher risk of burnout, anxiety, and stress-related physical symptoms.
- Sharing tasks and receiving emotional support can improve mood and sleep and may reduce physiologic stress over time. [71]

Inspiration note

"Good enough" is not giving up — it's letting your body come down.

Today's Invitation

One thing I will do for myself today:

- ☐ Ask one person for a small, specific help today (a call, a pickup, or a 10-minute cover).
- ☐ Delegate one task and let it be good enough so your nervous system can come down.
- ☐ Put one point of connection on the calendar (walk, call, or shared meal).

Action Step:
Choose the easiest one today. Do it now or set one reminder and do it when it best fits your schedule.

Reflection:
After I took the step today, I felt: ☐ calmer ☐ clearer ☐ steadier ☐ proud ☐ no change yet (effort still counts)

Bottom line

Perfectionism is a lonely load. Delegation is medicine.

Your lines

(write one thought, one insight, or rewrite one sentence that rang true)

☐ Done for today

Why this matters
Writing just a few lines by hand locks the concept into memory and gently primes your subconscious mind to adopt and act on it, leading to better recall and follow-through.

DAY 72

> "Lay the brick in your hand as honestly as you can; the wall will always take care of itself."
> — A. Smyrlis, MD

You shape the present — the future shapes itself.
One honest action steadies the whole day.
Peace often returns when you give your best to this moment, not the next.

Reflection

Most of us spend our lives anywhere but here. We live in the future — worrying about where we're headed. Or in the past — replaying what we should have done differently. The body is in the chair, but the mind and soul are somewhere else.

Health is built in the present. In the one brick you're laying right now.

Picture a builder with a long wall to construct. One type of builder keeps staring at the empty stretch still ahead and feels overwhelmed. Another keeps staring at the beautiful section already done and worries they'll never match it. The master builder looks at the brick in their hand. They feel its weight. They check the line. They remember why this wall needs to stand — who it will protect, what it will hold. Then they lay that one brick as straight and true as they can. And only then do they reach for the next.

That's what it means to align body, mind, and soul in the present moment. The body is fully engaged in the physical act — chopping vegetables, walking, stretching, studying, breathing. The mind is placed gently on just this task — no scoreboard, no "what if," no "I'm so far behind," just attention. The soul remembers the why behind it — "I'm doing this to be there for my kids," "to serve well," "to walk my years with clarity and strength."

When those three line up, the moment becomes a kind of consecration. Ordinary acts turn into honest offerings. One well-cooked meal. One sincere walk. One focused study block. One real conversation.

Here's the paradox: the more you obsess about the entire wall — perfect labs, perfect weight, perfect life — the more your nervous system tightens. Stress tends to rise. Sleep can fracture. Your thinking can get noisy. The wall wobbles. When you bring your attention back to the single brick in front of you — this breath, this bite, this step, this page — the system calms. You're no longer trying to live your whole life at once. You're just laying one true brick.

You don't have to know exactly what the finished wall will look like. You just have to keep placing today's brick flat and aligned with what you know to be right. Walls built that way tend to become masterpieces without anyone forcing the ending.

Real-life snapshot

Jasmine was studying for her boards with her stomach in a knot. Every session started with "What if I fail?" and ended with avoidance: checking her phone, doing random chores, opening the book and closing it again. In her head, she was trying to pass the entire exam every time she sat down.

Her classmate Marco wasn't calmer by personality — he just did one timed block a day and stopped, even when he wanted to do more.

Her mentor listened and said, "Right now, your mind is staring at the whole wall. Let's just lay bricks."

They agreed on a simple pattern: one 45-minute focused study block — no phone, one topic; five minutes of handwritten recall, writing what she remembered without looking; and a short walk to reset.

Her only job was to lay that brick honestly each day — show up, focus on the page in front of her, and remember why she was doing this: to be the kind of doctor her patients could trust. She stopped judging days by how "ready" she felt and started counting bricks laid.

Two weeks later, the fear wasn't gone, but the panic had softened. Her practice scores began to rise. More importantly, she felt less like she was drowning and more like she was building.

Quick science

- Focusing fully on a single task (present-moment attention) can reduce mental noise and stress, freeing up cognitive resources for accuracy, learning, and recall.
- Mindful, single-task actions — like deliberate breathing, eating with awareness, or focused work — are associated with lower perceived stress, steadier emotional regulation, and better performance.
- Bringing attention back to the present moment can interrupt worry about the future and rumination about the past — common drivers of anxiety and burnout.[72]

Inspiration note

You don't control the whole journey — just the way you take the next step.

Today's Invitation

One thing I will do for myself today:

- ☐ Today, I'll do one 5-4-3-2-1 grounding reset by naming 5 things I see, 4 I feel, 3 I hear, 2 I smell, and 1 I taste.
- ☐ For one ordinary task, I single-task for 2 minutes (no multitasking).
- ☐ On a 10-minute walk, I notice three things I see and two sounds I hear.

Action Step:
Choose the easiest one today. Do it now or set one reminder and do it when it best fits your schedule.

Reflection:
After I took the step today, I felt: ☐ calmer ☐ clearer ☐ steadier ☐ proud ☐ no change yet (effort still counts)

Bottom line

Aim your effort at what you can actually touch — the brick in your hand. Lay it true. The wall will take care of itself.

Your lines

(write one thought, one insight, or rewrite one sentence that rang true)

_____
_____
_____

☐ Done for today

Why this matters

Writing just a few lines by hand locks the concept into memory and gently primes your subconscious mind to adopt and act on it, leading to better recall and follow-through.

DAY 73

> "We cannot solve our problems with the same thinking we used when we created them."
> — attributed to Albert Einstein

Real change never starts on the outside.
When your thinking shifts, your choices — and health — slowly follow.
One small, honest insight can rewrite the way you live.

Reflection

Most of the problems we face today weren't created by bad intentions. They were created by old patterns — ways of thinking and living that made sense at the time, or that we never really examined. Late nights for "productivity," fast food for "convenience," stress as "normal," ignoring pain as "toughness."

Einstein's line is a hard but hopeful truth: you can't solve new problems with the same level of thinking that quietly helped create them. That doesn't mean you caused your illness on purpose. It means that at least part of the solution will involve looking inward, with compassion, and asking, "What in my life is quietly feeding this?"

Modern medicine often caters (understandably) to our natural desire for quick fixes: a pill to mute the symptom, a procedure to patch the visible damage, a scan to reassure us nothing catastrophic is happening. These can all be important and life-saving. There is no blame in needing them. But if we stop there, we're operating at the same level of thinking: "The problem is out there. I just need something done to me."

Durable change often asks a harder question: "What needs to change in me — in my schedule, my beliefs about rest, my relationship with food, my boundaries, my way of handling stress — for this problem to truly improve?"

This is not about self-blame. Most patterns were built unconsciously: family habits, cultural norms, survival strategies. You did the best you could with what you knew. Now you know more.

New thinking might sound like: "My blood pressure isn't just bad luck. Where am I constantly rushing, saying yes, eating on the run?" "My reflux isn't just a broken valve. What am I putting in my body late at night? How am I eating?" "My fatigue isn't just 'getting older.' How have I been treating sleep, movement, light, and my own limits?"

From that new level of thinking, you start to see root causes: chronic sleep debt, ultra-processed food, unrelenting stress, no real recovery, loneliness, lack of meaning. Many of these won't show up neatly on a single lab test, but they can influence every system.

Real change is slow and humbling. It asks for small experiments: one boundary where you used to say "yes" from fear; one simple home meal where you used to default to takeout; one honest conversation instead of swallowing frustration; one protected sleep window instead of another late-night scroll. Each small act says, "I'm willing to live differently now." Over time, your body often responds. Symptoms may not vanish overnight, but the trajectory can shift. When the roots are tended, the leaves can green again.

Real-life snapshot

Rita wanted relief fast. She cycled through antacids, stronger reflux meds, sleep aids, energy drinks, and extra supplements. She'd feel better for a short stretch, then slide back. "My body is broken," she thought.

One clinician gently asked, "If your body weren't the enemy, what might it be trying to show you?"

She took that question home. At first, it stung. Then she got curious. She wrote down a few patterns she'd been avoiding: late heavy takeout after 9 p.m., working into the night with no wind-down, drinking more on stressful evenings, saying yes to everyone and resting only when she crashed.

None of this made her a bad person. It made her human. But she could see, for the first time, how her days were quietly feeding the very problems she wanted to escape.

She didn't fix everything at once. She started with two changes: no big meals after 7 p.m. and fewer drinks in the evening, plus a simple lights-down routine and an in-bed time she tried to honor most nights.

Over months, with careful help from her doctor, she simplified some of her medications and felt less chained to her symptoms.

Quick science

- Reframing can change how stress feels in the body. Interpreting stress as a challenge rather than a threat can shift nervous-system response and influence recovery over time.
- Implementation intentions often outperform willpower alone. Simple if–then plans reduce decision fatigue and make the next step more automatic.
- Identity-based habits can stick longer. When actions tie to identity (I'm someone who protects sleep), small wins tend to reinforce the loop.[73]

Inspiration note

You didn't choose every pattern that shaped you — but you can choose new ones to shape who you become.

Today's Invitation

One thing I will do for myself today:

- ☐ Today I ask one root question and write one honest answer: What might be feeding this in my daily life?
- ☐ I use one if–then plan today (when X happens, I do Y).
- ☐ I finish one identity line and act once: I'm someone who _____.

Action Step:
Choose the easiest one today. Do it now or set one reminder and do it when it best fits your schedule.

Reflection:
After I took the step today, I felt: ☐ calmer ☐ clearer ☐ steadier ☐ proud ☐ no change yet (effort still counts)

Bottom line

Most health problems can't be solved at the same level of thinking that quietly helped create them. Look inward with kindness.

Your lines

(write one thought, one insight, or rewrite one sentence that rang true)

☐ Done for today

Why this matters
Writing just a few lines by hand locks the concept into memory and gently primes your subconscious mind to adopt and act on it, leading to better recall and follow-through.

DAY 74

"Set your heart upon your work, but never on its reward."
— Modern rendering, Bhagavad Gita

Chasing applause burns you out.
Doing the right thing builds you up.
Detach from outcome; attach to excellence.

Reflection

Most of us are trained to live by the scoreboard. We watch numbers — salary, title, likes, weight, ratings, rankings — and measure our worth against things we can't fully control. When the numbers rise, we feel briefly safe. When they falter, the ground shakes. The nervous system reads this as constant threat: Am I enough? Am I winning? Am I behind? It's exhausting.

Outcome-attachment is a stress loop. You cannot control the market, the scale, other people's approval, or the timing of recognition. You can only own the next right action. When you hitch your peace to results, your biology stays braced. Sleep suffers. Anxiety rises. Work becomes a tight, breathless performance instead of an honest offering.

The invitation is different: set your heart on the work itself.

When you pour yourself into the craft — the quality of the call, the care in the chart, the honesty of the conversation, the attention to the patient, the love in the meal — something shifts. Your nervous system can shift from threat toward flow. You act from purpose rather than fear. Paradoxically, results may improve when you stop clutching at them.

Honor the craft and your body can relax. The work becomes a form of prayer — something you offer because it's who you are, not because of what it buys. Care about why and how you work. Let outcomes arrive on their own schedule.

Real-life snapshot

Richard wanted the promotion. He spent months refreshing email, replaying conversations, and wondering how he was perceived. He slept poorly and lived on caffeine. Every day felt like a referendum on whether the promotion would come.

At his mother's suggestion, he changed his approach. He decided to set his heart on the work itself. He stopped chasing the outcome and started loving the craft. Each day, he mentored one junior colleague, fixed one broken process, and left one area better than he found it. He made excellence the point, not the promotion.

Three months later, his sleep began to stabilize, his caffeine use dropped, and his work got cleaner and calmer. Team performance improved — and the promotion arrived. But it no longer felt like his oxygen.

Quick science

- Focusing on process rather than outcome reduces performance anxiety and improves consistency.
- Flow states — supported by clear goals plus full presence — can reduce mental "noise" and deepen learning.
- Autonomy, mastery, and purpose are linked with stronger intrinsic motivation and can support long-term follow-through more than external rewards.[74]

Inspiration note

Honor the craft. Excellence, done quietly, is a form of prayer.

Today's Invitation

One thing I will do for myself today:

☐ Today I choose one process goal I can control (walk, meal, or sleep cue).
☐ For 25 minutes, I do focused work with full presence (no multitasking).
☐ One check mark today is for showing up — not for the outcome.

Action Step:
Choose the easiest one today. Do it now or set one reminder and do it when it best fits your schedule.

Reflection:
After I took the step today, I felt: ☐ calmer ☐ clearer ☐ steadier ☐ proud ☐ no change yet (effort still counts)

Bottom line

Care about why and how you work — outcomes will follow in their own time.

Your lines

(write one thought, one insight, or rewrite one sentence that rang true)

_____

_____

_____

☐ Done for today

Why this matters
Writing just a few lines by hand locks the concept into memory and gently primes your subconscious mind to adopt and act on it, leading to better recall and follow-through.

DAY 75

> **"Grow a garden, and you'll rediscover the rules your body lives by."**
> — A. Smyrlis, MD

Tending life outside teaches you how life works inside.
Roots, seasons, soil, light — your body is built on the same laws.
Gardeners don't just eat better; they understand what health needs to flourish.

Reflection

If you want to understand health, grow something. It might be a full garden, a raised bed, or just three pots on a sunny windowsill. The size doesn't matter. What matters is the relationship. Gardening quietly teaches the same rules your body lives by: feed the roots first, protect the soil, respect seasons, water regularly, pull weeds early, and work with the light instead of fighting it.

As a doctor, I see the same patterns in people that I see in plants.

Neglect the roots (sleep, food, movement, connection), and the leaves eventually show it. Overwater or overfertilize (excess, extremes), and things rot. Ignore the seasons, and you burn out trying to force summer in winter.

When you plant, you think a season ahead. When you harvest, you remember that patience and small daily actions turned seeds into food. When you tend soil, you see that life below the surface is what makes growth possible above it. All of this mirrors metabolic health, emotional health, and spiritual health.

People who garden often walk more, bend and lift more, spend more time outside, and eat more plants. But even beyond those obvious benefits, they live inside a story of care, continuity, and growth. Each day has something to check on, something to nurture, something to anticipate. That can be powerful support for sleep, mood, metabolism, and meaning.

Real-life snapshot

After retiring, Carla felt unmoored. She slept late, watched more TV than she wanted to admit, and felt her energy and mood decline. Her daughter suggested starting a small garden on the balcony — just herbs and a few cherry tomato plants.

At first, it felt trivial. But tending those few pots pulled her outside every morning: check the soil, water a little, pinch off a dead leaf, notice a new flower. She began walking around the block to stretch her legs before checking the plants.

By midsummer, she was walking most days without forcing herself, sleeping more soundly with extra daylight and gentle movement, adding fresh herbs and tomatoes to meals, and feeling a quiet joy each time she saw new growth.

"The garden gave me a reason to step outside," she said. "And it keeps reminding me that growth takes time, care, and good roots. That's true for my body too."

Quick science

- Gardening can increase daily physical activity (walking, bending, lifting) in an enjoyable, low-pressure way.
- Time in green spaces is associated with better mood and lower stress, and may support cardiovascular and metabolic health over time.
- Caring for something living can reduce loneliness and add structure and meaning to the day, supporting resilience.[75]

Inspiration note

The garden is a kaleidoscope of truth: tend the roots, respect the season, and life will often meet you halfway.

Today's Invitation

One thing I will do for myself today:

☐ Today I water or tend one living thing (plant, herb, or garden).
☐ At one meal, I add one plant (greens, beans, berries, or a vegetable).
☐ I step outside for 10–20 minutes and let daylight do its work.

Action Step:
Choose the easiest one today. Do it now or set one reminder and do it when it best fits your schedule.

Reflection:
After I took the step today, I felt: ☐ calmer ☐ clearer ☐ steadier ☐ proud ☐ no change yet (effort still counts)

Bottom line

Gardening is not just a hobby. It's a teacher and a mirror. When you care for living things — soil, plants, even a single pot — you learn, day by day, how your own health and life really work.

Your lines

(write one thought, one insight, or rewrite one sentence that rang true)

___

___

___

☐ Done for today

Why this matters
Writing just a few lines by hand locks the concept into memory and gently primes your subconscious mind to adopt and act on it, leading to better recall and follow-through.

DAY 76

"Growth begins at the edge of comfort."
— A. Smyrlis, MD

Growth doesn't live in comfort — it lives just past it.
The edge is where your body and mind learn they can do more.
Stretch, don't snap — that's the art of productive strain.

Reflection

Very little in the body changes without a signal. Muscles strengthen when they meet resistance. Minds sharpen when they wrestle with challenge. Character deepens when patience is tested. The secret isn't brute force — it's calibration: enough strain to spark adaptation, enough recovery to let it take root.

Too little challenge and capacity quietly shrinks. "Use it or lose it" is one of nature's laws. Sit all winter, drive everywhere, rarely raise your heart rate, and by early spring stairs feel harder than they should. Nothing "broke." The system simply wasn't asked to stay strong.

Too much strain and the system buckles. The sweet spot is the middle — the narrow band where steady discomfort tells your biology, Build more capacity. That's where growth lives.

Think of a fruit-bearing branch. In the early years it can hold only a little. Season by season it carries more weight, then rests. Over time, the wood thickens and becomes reliable. But overload it too quickly — or hit it with a storm when it's already maxed out — and it cracks.

Your tissues learn the same way. Small increases, followed by real recovery, teach the body where to reinforce. You become sturdier not from punishment, but from repeated, honest nudges at the edge.

The mind follows the same rule. Tasks that are slightly above your current ability — hard enough to stretch you, not so hard you drown — create "desirable difficulty." That's where learning, memory, and focus improve most.

Your biology is trainable. It wants the edge, not the cliff. Move the line a little, let rest cement the gain, and capacity grows. Ignore the signal and it fades. Respect it — and it builds.

Real-life snapshot

Emily and Jordan both wanted to get fit. Emily had been mostly sedentary for years, but every time she jumped into intense workouts, her knees flared and she quit. Jordan kept starting big too — then disappearing for weeks after the soreness hit.

This time, Emily chose the tree-branch approach: small load, repeated, then rest. She started with a 10-minute walk, three times a week. When that felt routine, she nudged the edge: 12 minutes, then 15. Some weeks she didn't increase time at all; she just chose a slightly hillier route one day. Every fourth week she kept the load the same and focused on sleep and stretching.

After a few months, she was walking 30 minutes most days, with fewer aches and more confidence than any previous attempt.

Quick science

- After a stressor (exercise or deep learning), the body can rebound above baseline — often described as super-compensation — especially when recovery is real.
- Long periods of underuse can lead to losses in fitness and strength over time — deconditioning isn't neutral.
- Slightly challenging work ("desirable difficulty") can improve learning and retention, while sharp pain, collapsing sleep, or persistent irritability can signal overreach.[76]

Inspiration note

Pressure refines when it is measured, paced, and paired with rest.

Today's Invitation

One thing I will do for myself today:

- ☐ Today I do one moderate-effort strength set and stop before I grind.
- ☐ I pair effort with recovery by choosing one easy reset (walk, stretch, or earlier bedtime).
- ☐ For 25 minutes, I do one slightly challenging task with no multitasking.

Action Step:
Choose the easiest one today. Do it now or set one reminder and do it when it best fits your schedule.

Reflection:
After I took the step today, I felt: ☐ calmer ☐ clearer ☐ steadier ☐ proud ☐ no change yet (effort still counts)

Bottom line

Growth begins just past comfort — not miles beyond it. Too little and you can lose capacity; too much and you can break down. The art is in the edge.

Your lines

(write one thought, one insight, or rewrite one sentence that rang true)

_____
_____
_____

☐ Done for today

Why this matters

Writing just a few lines by hand locks the concept into memory and gently primes your subconscious mind to adopt and act on it, leading to better recall and follow-through.

DAY 77

"Be kind, for everyone you meet is fighting a hard battle."
— attributed to Plato

Everyone is carrying something.
A private weight, an unseen wound, a story with nowhere easy to rest.
Kindness is how you move through that battlefield without adding more wounds.

Reflection

If we could see what people are carrying, we would rarely be as harsh as we are. Everyone has a private struggle — grief, fear, shame, pressure, loneliness, pain — sometimes all at once. But most of it is hidden. That blind spot makes us quicker to judge, and it makes others feel alone.

Kindness isn't weakness. It's wisdom. It's moving through the day without adding weight to someone else's burden — and often without adding more weight to your own.

The driver who cuts you off might be racing to a hospital. The nurse who snaps at you might be on her fourth shift. The student who fails might have spent the night in an ER waiting room with his sick mother. The barista who gets the order wrong might be barely holding it together.

All we see is the surface: the sharp tone, the missed deadline, the dropped ball. Our reflex is to judge the outcome: How could they do that? What's wrong with them? But underneath is usually a tired body, a braced nervous system, and a mind trying to survive something you can't see.

Kindness doesn't mean pretending the problem isn't real. It means seeing the person before the problem.

When you answer harshness with harshness, your body joins the fight — heart rate up, jaw tight, thoughts fast. When you answer with gentleness — a slower exhale, a softer voice, a brief pause to wonder, What might they be facing?—your system shifts first. Threat lowers. Breath deepens. The room changes, even if only inside you.

We treat kindness like a moral extra, something nice to add when life calms down. In truth, it's stabilizing. It's nervous-system regulation in human form. When you aim to leave people more peaceful than you found them, you tend to leave yourself that way too.

You're never wrong to be kind. You may still need boundaries, firm words, and clear decisions — but you can lay them down without poison if you remember one simple line: everyone is fighting a hard battle, just like me.

Real-life snapshot

A man boarded the plane with two little kids and one carry-on that looked like it had been packed in a hurry. Ten minutes after takeoff, the kids started melting down — crying, kicking the seat, asking for their mom. The father just stared forward, frozen, barely moving. The cabin tightened. You could feel the shared irritation rising.

Across the aisle, a passenger finally snapped. He leaned in, swore at the dad, and said something like, "Do your job and control your kids." The kids cried harder. The father didn't fight back. He looked like someone underwater.

A few rows up, the passenger next to him asked quietly, "Hey…are you okay?" The father's voice broke. "My wife died yesterday," he said. "We were on vacation. I'm flying home with them. I don't even know how to be a person right now."

Nothing about the noise changed instantly. But the meaning did. The cabin softened. Someone offered to walk one child up the aisle. Another handed him water and tissues. The angry passenger went silent.

Quick science

- Compassion and loving-kindness practices can reduce sympathetic arousal and may support steadier blood pressure over time.
- Non-verbal warmth — soft eyes, relaxed jaw, gentle posture — can signal safety and support cooperation and trust.
- Brief compassion or loving-kindness practices are linked with improved mood and emotion regulation, even in high-stress settings.[77]

Inspiration note

Aim to leave people more peaceful than you found them — and notice how your own peace grows.

Today's Invitation

One thing I will do for myself today:

☐ Before I speak once today, I pause and soften my tone.

- ☐ I do one small act of compassion (hold a door, send a kind text, or be patient).
- ☐ I offer kindness inward: one kind sentence to myself instead of self-attack.

Action Step:
Choose the easiest one today. Do it now or set one reminder and do it when it best fits your schedule.

Reflection:
After I took the step today, I felt: ☐ calmer ☐ clearer ☐ steadier ☐ proud ☐ no change yet (effort still counts)

Bottom line

Kindness doesn't just help others. It calms you first.

Your lines

(write one thought, one insight, or rewrite one sentence that rang true)

☐ Done for today

Why this matters
Writing just a few lines by hand locks the concept into memory and gently primes your subconscious mind to adopt and act on it, leading to better recall and follow-through.

DAY 78

> "He who knows that enough is enough
> will always have enough."
> — Lao Tzu

Fullness comes from boundaries, not excess.
"Enough" is a doorway to peace your body can feel.
When you honor your limits, life becomes gentler.

Reflection

In places that practice "enough," life feels different. In the World Happiness Report, Finland has ranked near the top for years; the United States tends to rank lower. This isn't about who is better — it's about the thermostat we set on everyday life. A culture that prizes "good enough" turns the heat down before the room overheats. A culture that glorifies "more" leaves the dial stuck on high — later nights, bigger carts, longer hours — until circuits trip.

Think of desire as a cup. In the "never enough" life, the cup has no rim. You keep pouring in — work, upgrades, attention — and it never feels full. In "enough," the cup has an edge. You pour, you notice, you taste. Satisfaction is possible because there is a place to stop. That rim — those limits around sleep, food, spending, screens, and status — does not shrink your life; it shapes it so you can finally feel full.

"Enough" is not giving up; it's getting back the parts of life that make you glad to be alive. When you know where to stop, you recover presence. Your home is good enough. Your car is good enough. Your job is good enough for this season. Mornings start without panic. You have time left for family dinners, a walk in the park, or your morning workout. You become easier to live with, and people around you soften in response. Contentment is not just an idea; it's a nervous system that finally stops bracing.

Real-life snapshot

Helena spent decades in New York City living in "more mode" — more hours, more projects, more purchases, more plans. Her calendar was packed, her inbox overflowing, and her mind always half a step ahead of the present moment. Meals blurred into meetings. Online shopping became her evening "treat." Sleep was something she squeezed into the cracks.

Then her company asked her to spend six months in Copenhagen to help set up a branch office. She expected the same rush in a different language. What she found instead startled her. People took lunch away from their desks. Cafés were full of conversation, not just laptops. Shops closed earlier. Weeknights were quiet. Colleagues left the office on time — not because they lacked ambition, but because their lives outside work mattered just as much.

Work still got done — very well — but it moved at a steadier pace. Projects were planned with human limits in mind. Evenings were for family, friends, and simple pleasures: cooking at home, bike rides, walks by the water. Helena noticed something unsettling: people seemed content. Not flashy, not chasing — just present. Their faces looked less strained. Their eyes seemed less tired.

At first she felt restless, like there was "not enough" happening. But slowly, the quieter rhythm began to feel like a relief. When she returned to New York, she knew she couldn't go back to the old thermostat setting. She began practicing daily "enough moments": a hard stop on work most nights, a real wind-down and steadier bedtime, stopping when she felt satisfied at dessert, and putting her phone down after one scroll instead of falling into a long hole.

Within months, her sleep felt deeper, her eating felt steadier, and she felt less keyed up. She still worked hard and cared about her career — but she no longer treated her body and time as bottomless. "Enough gave me back my life," she said. "Nothing huge changed on the outside, but inside, I stopped living like a cup with no rim."

Quick science

- Chasing constant "more" — more alerts, more purchases, more stimulation — can keep the reward system revved up, which may leave you feeling restless and empty instead of satisfied.
- Reducing sensory overload (fewer notifications, less multitasking, quieter evenings) can help lower stress signaling and help your body relax.
- Practicing mindful stopping — at meals, with work, with screens — can support digestion, steadier mood, and easier sleep.[78]

Inspiration note

Enoughness is the art of choosing presence over pressure.

Today's Invitation

One thing I will do for myself today:

- ☐ Choose a stop: Set a hard end to work tonight, then do one restoring thing for 20 minutes (walk, shower, stretch, or reading).
- ☐ Practice enough at one meal: Eat to satisfied and stop when your body says enough, even if food is left.
- ☐ Lower the noise: Silence non-urgent notifications for 30 minutes and do one thing at a time.

Action Step:
Choose the easiest one today. Do it now or set one reminder and do it when it best fits your schedule.

Reflection:
After I took the step today, I felt: ☐ calmer ☐ clearer ☐ steadier ☐ proud ☐ no change yet (effort still counts)

Bottom line

Enoughness restores what excess erodes.

Your lines

(write one thought, one insight, or rewrite one sentence that rang true)

_____

_____

_____

☐ Done for today

Why this matters
Writing just a few lines by hand locks the concept into memory and gently primes your subconscious mind to adopt and act on it, leading to better recall and follow-through.

DAY 79

"No one has ever become poor by giving."
— attributed to Anne Frank

Giving doesn't drain you when it's done wisely — it fills you. Generosity shifts your body from scarcity into a sense of safety. Small, honest acts of giving can rebalance a stressful day.

Reflection

Give what you can keep giving. Deep down, many traditions and teachers agree on one thing: true success begins with meaningful giving. Not showy charity, but real contribution — time, presence, skill, care. Life runs on cause and effect. When you offer something genuinely helpful into the world, that action doesn't vanish. It ripples. It shapes the lives around you — and it also shapes you.

Generosity is not subtraction; it multiplies. When you help someone — listening fully for ten minutes, sharing a skill, cooking a simple meal, offering a ride, writing a warm note — your chemistry shifts. The body can release bonding and reward chemicals like oxytocin and dopamine, and stress can feel less sharp. Perspective returns. Problems stop feeling like a private prison and become something you face as part of a human family.

Healthy giving is sustainable giving. It doesn't mean bleeding yourself dry or saying yes to everything. It means offering what you can continue to offer without collapsing — a steady trickle, not a one-time flood. That might look like one hour a week of tutoring, one neighbor you check on, one community you serve, one skill you donate. When giving is sized to your reality, it doesn't crush you; it strengthens you.

Over time, giving rewires how you see the world. You stop living only in What do I still lack? and start tasting What do I have that I can share? That shift from scarcity to contribution is powerful for health. It lightens the chest, steadies the mind, and can become the soil where new opportunities quietly grow. Many people discover that meaningful work — and sometimes new directions — can begin with something they first did for free, simply because it mattered.

Real-life snapshot

After losing his job, Miguel felt useless and ashamed. His days blurred into worry and scrolling job boards. The more he stared at what he'd lost, the smaller his world became.

One afternoon, a neighbor knocked and asked a simple favor: "Could you help my son with math? He's really struggling." Miguel had always been good with numbers. Unlike his friend Daniel, also job searching, who stayed isolated and spiraled most nights, Miguel said yes to one hour a week.

Something shifted. For that hour, he wasn't unemployed. He was useful. He was steady. He was a teacher. The boy improved. Word spread. Another neighbor asked. Then a cousin. Within a few months, Miguel was tutoring three evenings a week. His income wasn't fully back, but his posture was. His mood lifted, his purpose returned, and his anxiety eased. He slept better and ate more regularly.

Over the next year, those few hours of giving became the seed of a new direction. Miguel expanded tutoring, added a few online sessions, and built a steadier path forward. "The business came later," he said. "The real change started the day I stopped staring at what I'd lost and started giving what I still had."

Quick science

- Generous acts can activate reward circuits in the brain and may increase chemicals linked with bonding and meaning (like dopamine and oxytocin).
- Helping others is associated with lower perceived stress and better mood; many people describe a helper's high.
- Prosocial behavior — small, regular acts of service — is linked with better psychological health and resilience, and some studies associate it with longer life.[79]

Inspiration note

You are never so empty that you have nothing to give; often what you give is what starts to heal you.

Today's Invitation

One thing I will do for myself today:

- ☐ Today I do one small act of service (2–10 minutes).
- ☐ I set one clear limit so my giving stays clean and sustainable.

☐ I choose one recurring way to help (weekly check-in, meal, ride, or support).

Action Step:
Choose the easiest one today. Do it now or set one reminder and do it when it best fits your schedule.

Reflection:
After I took the step today, I felt: ☐ calmer ☐ clearer ☐ steadier ☐ proud ☐ no change yet (effort still counts)

Bottom line

Thoughtful, sustainable giving enriches the giver first — in chemistry, in meaning, and in health.

Your lines

(write one thought, one insight, or rewrite one sentence that rang true)

_____

_____

_____

☐ Done for today

Why this matters
Writing just a few lines by hand locks the concept into memory and gently primes your subconscious mind to adopt and act on it, leading to better recall and follow-through.

DAY 80

> "Your time is limited, so don't waste it living someone else's life."
> — Steve Jobs

A life that looks right but feels wrong will quietly drain you.
Your body knows when you're off your true path — it calls it stress.
Health thrives when your days match your deepest convictions.

Reflection

Answer your own call. A genuine life isn't a script you memorize; it's a voice you learn to trust. When you spend years living by other people's priorities — parents, bosses, culture, what someone like me is supposed to do — you can look successful and still feel starved. The cost shows up quietly: restless sleep, a short fuse, cravings that won't quit, a fog that hangs. Misalignment can feel like friction in the nervous system; it can leak energy all day.

Living your own life doesn't mean walking away from responsibility. It means letting your deepest beliefs set the order of your day. What do you love? What would you keep doing even if no one clapped? What do you care about enough to practice when no one is watching? Following that thread is not indulgence; it is integrity. Integrity can calm the body. When you stop performing and start aligning, stress can feel less sharp, breathing can soften, and steadiness becomes easier to access.

Clarity rarely arrives as a thunderclap. It begins as a whisper — a curiosity, a pull, a small yes. You move toward it by taking one honest step, then another. Expect some fear. Fear often means you're near the edge of something true. Give yourself permission to choose one thing because you love it — not because it checks a box, not because it will impress anyone, but because it rings like a bell inside you.

To live your own life, you'll need boundaries. Every real yes needs space. That space appears when you gently put down borrowed priorities: one weekly commitment that isn't yours, one task you do only to avoid disappointing someone, one role that no longer fits. Make room for the thing that does.

Health isn't only food and steps; it's alignment. A day lived in alignment is lighter on the heart, quieter on the nerves, clearer in the mind. Your time is limited. Spend it on what you were made to make.

Real-life snapshot

Arman followed the expected path — the career his family encouraged, the schedule his workplace demanded, the image his culture praised. Outwardly, he was successful. Inwardly, he was exhausted and numb. His lab work began to show it: rising blood pressure, creeping A1c, stubborn weight despite doing the right things. He was doing everything for everyone — except himself.

On a particularly hard night, he wrote one line in his journal: If my life were truly mine, I would spend more time _____. The blank filled itself: writing, mentoring, and solving complex problems in a way that lit him up. Those were the moments he felt most alive — and they barely existed in his week.

With his clinician's encouragement, he carved out just 15 minutes a day for his work — early morning writing, mentoring a younger colleague, reading in his field out of curiosity rather than obligation. He also set a few gentle boundaries: no more late-night emails, one evening a week reserved for what mattered to him, not just to others.

Over the next months, something shifted. His energy improved. His anxiety eased. And as he sustained the basics more consistently, his numbers began trending in a better direction.

Quick science
- Living in alignment with your core values is associated with lower stress, better psychological wellbeing, and greater life satisfaction.
- Chronic misalignment — saying yes while your whole body says no — increases anxiety, burnout risk, and perceived stress load.
- Autonomy and a sense of purpose are linked with resilience, and some studies associate them with better health and longer life; people who feel their life is theirs often cope better during hard seasons.[80]

Inspiration note

Alignment is less about grand gestures and more about daily, honest steps toward what matters.

Today's Invitation

One thing I will do for myself today:

- ☐ Today I write one honest sentence about what I need most right now.
- ☐ I say one small, clean no to protect sleep, energy, or values.
- ☐ I do one action that matches my values — even if no one applauds.

Action Step:
Choose the easiest one today. Do it now or set one reminder and do it when it best fits your schedule.

Reflection:
After I took the step today, I felt: ☐ calmer ☐ clearer ☐ steadier ☐ proud ☐ no change yet (effort still counts)

Bottom line

You can't be fully well living someone else's script — your health depends on answering your own call.

Your lines

(write one thought, one insight, or rewrite one sentence that rang true)

_____

_____

_____

☐ Done for today

Why this matters
Writing just a few lines by hand locks the concept into memory and gently primes your subconscious mind to adopt and act on it, leading to better recall and follow-through.

DAY 81

> "All of humanity's problems stem from man's inability to sit quietly in a room alone."
> — Blaise Pascal

Noise is not only sound.
It is pressure.
And your nervous system keeps score.

Reflection

We talk about food toxins and air toxins, but we ignore a loud one: chronic noise.

Noise isn't only volume. It's constant input. A brain that never gets a quiet minute stays slightly braced, like it's waiting for the next demand — traffic rumble, TV as background "comfort," podcasts in every gap, notifications flicking attention like a light switch. The body reads that as pressure.

And when the body feels pressure, it guards itself. Shoulders stay a little high. Jaw stays a little tight. Breathing stays a little shallow. Even if you "get through the day," you do it on a low simmer of alertness.

At night, noise steals sleep in sneaky ways. You might not fully wake up, but your brain gets pulled toward lighter sleep — again and again. It's like trying to recharge a phone while someone keeps tapping the screen. The next morning you wake with fog and a shorter fuse, and the instinct is to add more stimulation to cope: more news, more caffeine, more sound. The loop tightens.

Silence is not emptiness. It is medicine for a nervous system that has been on edge.

You don't need a silent monastery. You need small pockets of quiet that tell your body: nothing is chasing you right now.

If nighttime noise is part of your story, make a simple "sound plan":
Start with masking (fastest wins):

- Earplugs — cheap, easy, and they can help on night one.
- A steady, "boring" sound (fan / white noise) — masks sudden spikes.
- After lights-down, remove voices (TV, podcasts, talk radio) — speech keeps the brain listening.

Then reduce noise at the source:

- Seal leaks: door sweep, weather stripping, draft stopper.
- Add softness: thicker curtains, a rug, or other fabric to cut echo.
- If traffic is intense, consider upgrading the bedroom windows — even one room can be a game changer.

Train quiet in daylight, too:

- One 5-minute "no-input" pocket each day.
- One block a day with no background noise (during a drive, cooking, or work).

Quiet is a boundary your nervous system has been begging for. Protect it, and sleep can get deeper — and mornings can get clearer.

Real-life snapshot

Jorge fell asleep to the TV every night. He told himself it helped him "turn his brain off." But he woke up tired most mornings, with a low-level buzz of anxiety that followed him into the day. He didn't remember waking much — he just never felt fully restored.

One night he tried a different experiment: no voices after lights-down. No TV. No podcasts. He kept the room dark and used a steady, boring sound instead — a fan — so his brain didn't have to track a story.

The first night felt strange, almost too quiet. By the fourth night, he noticed he was falling asleep faster. By day ten, his mornings felt less jagged. The anxiety edge softened.

"It's like my brain finally got a clean rinse," he said. "I didn't realize how loud my nights were."

Quick science

- Chronic noise exposure is associated with higher stress hormones and higher cardiovascular strain over time.
- Sound can fragment sleep even without full awakening, reducing deep restorative stages.
- Quiet time downshifts the nervous system and supports attention, mood, and emotional control. [81]

Inspiration note

Quiet is a boundary your brain has been begging for.

Today's Invitation

One thing I will do for myself today:

- ☐ I give my nervous system a break by taking five minutes of no-input quiet (no music, no podcast, no scrolling).
- ☐ I protect tonight's sleep by creating a lights-down sound plan (earplugs, fan, or steady white noise) and removing voices after bedtime.
- ☐ I lower my daily noise load by turning off one background sound for one block of time (drive, cooking, or work) and letting my mind settle.

Action Step:
Choose the easiest one today. Do it now or set one reminder and do it when it best fits your schedule.

Reflection:
After I took the step today, I felt: ☐ calmer ☐ clearer ☐ steadier ☐ proud ☐ no change yet (effort still counts)

Bottom line

Protect quiet the way you protect sleep — it's the same kind of repair.

Your lines

(write one thought, one insight, or rewrite one sentence that rang true)

_____

_____

_____

☐ Done for today

Why this matters
Writing just a few lines by hand locks the concept into memory and gently primes your subconscious mind to adopt and act on it, leading to better recall and follow-through.

DAY 82

"When hurt, heal first."
— A. Smyrlis, MD

If you're bleeding, stop sprinting.
Protect the injury, then rebuild.
Rest now so you can return stronger later.

Reflection

The body runs on a steady rule: healing tends to come before progress. When something hurts — an ankle, a tendon, your back, your sleep, your mind — the instinct is often to prove you're still strong. "I'll push through." "Let me test it again." "Maybe it's fine now."

But pushing through real pain is like pouring gasoline on a fire you're trying to put out. You don't speed up the result you want — you delay it and risk burning down the whole house.

Injuries are not rare accidents reserved for the unlucky. They are built into the price of real effort. Most serious athletes get hurt at some point. Every demanding career brushes up against burnout or overload. Every intense season of study strains the mind. Sometimes the "injury" is spiritual — the ache when your work no longer lines up with your values, or when you've said "yes" to something that quietly violates what you believe.

Pros and masters in every field don't avoid injury; they expect it and learn how to respond. What separates them from quitters is not that they never get hurt — it's that they know how to pause, repair, and then continue, wiser.

Real healing follows a timeless sequence: Protect → Repair → Rebuild. Skip a phase and your body may circle back, louder the next time.

When you're hurt, think like a captain at sea. First, stop the leak — protect the irritated tissue, reduce the load, avoid the motions that keep tearing it open. Then, pump the water out — bring inflammation down, support repair with real protein, plenty of deep sleep, gentle pain-free movement. Only when the foundation is ready do you sail forward again — gradually reloading: lightly, slowly, and thoughtfully.

Rest is not the same as doing nothing. Smart rest is active healing: the right things, in the right order, at the right time.

Some people see rest as weakness. In reality, strategic rest is strength. Climbers reach the summit because base camps exist — push, then repair, then rise. Recovery is not avoidance. It is intelligent progression.

Real-life snapshot

Jess rolled her ankle on a run. She "tested" it again three days later, then again the next week. Three re-sprains later, she could barely walk without pain.

Finally, she rewrote the plan: no more testing runs; brace and elevate when needed; gentle range-of-motion work; earlier bedtimes; protein at each meal; and a progression ladder — pool walking → bike → short flat walks → light jogs.

Six weeks later, she was back to short runs with little to no pain. She didn't heal by pretending nothing happened. She healed by doing the right things in the right order: protect, ease, then rebuild.

Quick science

- Tissue repair follows phases (inflammation → repair → remodeling); loading too hard or too early can disrupt healing and cause re-injury.
- Adequate protein and good sleep support collagen building, tissue remodeling, and immune function.
- Pain-free, low-load movement preserves function, reduces stiffness, and may help recovery compared with complete immobilization in some cases.[82]

Inspiration note

Even the best progress has pit stops — the pause is part of the climb.

Today's Invitation

One thing I will do for myself today:

- ☐ Move: Choose pain-free movement today (easy walk, gentle mobility, or light strength).
- ☐ Fuel: Add protein to one meal today to support repair.
- ☐ Sleep: Set a lights-down alarm tonight and protect bedtime (a lot of repair happens during sleep).

Action Step:
Choose the easiest one today. Do it now or set one reminder and do it when it best fits your schedule.

Reflection:
After I took the step today, I felt: ☐ calmer ☐ clearer ☐ steadier ☐ proud ☐ no change yet (effort still counts)

Bottom line

Heal first; perform later. That's how you come back more reliably — and stronger.

Your lines

(write one thought, one insight, or rewrite one sentence that rang true)

_____
_____
_____

☐ Done for today

Why this matters
Writing just a few lines by hand locks the concept into memory and gently primes your subconscious mind to adopt and act on it, leading to better recall and follow-through.

DAY 83

> "All things come to him who will but wait."
> — Henry Wadsworth Longfellow

Slow change is real change.
Time is the partner your health has been waiting for.
Good things grow quietly before they grow obviously.

Reflection

Health tends to obey slow laws. Anyone who tells you, "You can flip everything in a week," is either confused or trying to sell you a shiny shortcut. Your body is not a vending machine; it's more like a kiln (a slow, hot oven for pottery), a vineyard, or a jar of cold brew on the counter. You set the right conditions, and time does quiet chemistry. Rush the heat and the pottery cracks. Pick the grapes early and the wine is thin. Cut the steep short and the coffee is weak. Patience isn't doing nothing; it's tending what matters and letting time multiply the gain.

This is why so many people quit too soon. Pounds don't vanish overnight. High sugar or cholesterol won't normalize in a week. Brain fog rarely lifts after one early bedtime. The work is happening — just out of sight. Nerves downshift after many steady nights. Muscles rebuild from small, repeated efforts. The gut lining renews when meals have a beginning and an end. Mitochondria grow from consistent movement, not one heroic workout. If you stop because fireworks don't appear, you miss the sunrise that was already forming.

Impatience pushes us toward shortcuts — more caffeine, stronger stimulants, GLP-1 shots with no lifestyle behind them, harsher diets, last-minute "resets." They feel powerful for a day and taxing for a week. Quick fixes always borrow from tomorrow: wired now, weary later. A good question to ask yourself is, "What's the catch?" There is usually one. Real change tends to choose roots over glitter. It keeps the oven low and steady. It waits for flavor to deepen.

The way forward is simple, not easy: plant what you can keep planting. Choose one habit you can repeat on your worst day, not just your best — dim lights an hour before bed, take a 10-minute walk after dinner, eat protein with breakfast, step into morning light, pause to breathe between tasks. Hold the line for a few weeks and watch for quiet signs — clearer mornings, steadier mood, fewer cravings. That's the steep. That's time paying interest.

Real-life snapshot

Olivia and Grace were close friends who did almost everything together — until their 60s, when a routine bone density scan gave them both the same unwelcome news: osteoporosis. Same age, same diagnosis, similar family history. The scan printouts looked nearly identical.

At her appointment, Olivia's doctor took a few extra minutes. "Yes, we can use medicine to lower your fracture risk," she said. "But your bones also listen to what you do every day. If we give them the right signals, there's a lot we can improve over time." She suggested a gradual plan: review her long-term acid-suppressing medication with her clinician (some can affect mineral absorption), and build a safer reflux plan if changes are made. She also suggested gentle resistance training three times a week (bands, light weights, simple movements), more calcium and vitamin D from food (and supplements if needed), plus daily walking and a little more safe sun exposure. "It will take years, not weeks," she added. "Think of this as planting a new tree." Olivia sighed, but agreed.

Grace saw a different clinician. Her visit was shorter. "You have osteoporosis," he said. "We'll start an osteoporosis medication (often given as an injection on a set schedule) to help lower fracture risk." When she asked about exercise and food, he waved a hand. "Those are fine if you can fit them in, but this shot is the main thing." Grace was relieved. "I don't have time for a whole lifestyle overhaul," she thought. The injection felt like a strong, simple answer.

Five years later, their paths had diverged. Olivia's follow-up scan showed modest improvement — trending closer to the osteopenia range. She still lifted light weights, walked most days, and treated her bones like a long project. She hadn't been perfect, but she had been patient.

Grace's story was rougher. After a few years, she had side effects and stopped the medication. Her bones, never supported by movement or nutrition changes, remained fragile. A minor fall in her kitchen was followed by a compression fracture. Weeks of pain and bed rest followed, and each week in bed weakened her further.

Quick science

- Habits tend to become more automatic after repetition: practicing the same small action in the same context (same time, same cue) makes it easier to repeat.
- Mitochondrial biogenesis (building more "energy factories" in cells) typically responds to consistent movement over weeks and months, not a few intense days.

- The gut lining turns over in days, and the gut microbiome can shift over weeks to months with consistent food patterns — steady inputs matter more than occasional "perfect" days.[83]

Inspiration note

Trust the rise you can't see yet.

Today's Invitation

One thing I will do for myself today:

- ☐ Sleep: Set a lights-down time tonight — and end work when it arrives.
- ☐ Move: Take a 10–15 minute walk after dinner, even at an easy pace.
- ☐ Fuel: Make one simple real-food plate today (protein + vegetables + healthy fat).

Action Step:
Choose the easiest one today. Do it now or set one reminder and do it when it best fits your schedule.

Reflection:
After I took the step today, I felt: ☐ calmer ☐ clearer ☐ steadier ☐ proud ☐ no change yet (effort still counts)

Bottom line

Slow is sustainable — and sustainable is unbeatable.

Your lines

(write one thought, one insight, or rewrite one sentence that rang true)

_____

_____

_____

☐ Done for today

Why this matters
Writing just a few lines by hand locks the concept into memory and gently primes your subconscious mind to adopt and act on it, leading to better recall and follow-through.

DAY 84

> "Be faithful in small things because it is in them that your strength lies."
> — Mother Teresa

Tiny is not failure — tiny is how real change begins.
On exhausted days, tiny efforts still count as deposits.
Small, repeatable habits quietly re-engineer your life.

Reflection

On exhausted days, big plans can feel like a mountain. This is where most people quit — not because they don't care, but because the plan demands a version of them that isn't available today.

So here's a different way to think about it: your health is a seam. When life gets rough, the seam starts to pull. You don't need to sew the whole garment tonight. You just need one stitch — one small act that keeps the seam from tearing further.

Small signals still count. A body doesn't only respond to intensity. It responds to consistency. One earlier lights-down. One protein-forward breakfast. One three-minute walk while the coffee brews. One glass of water before anything else. One minute of slow breathing in the bathroom before you walk back into the noise. These are not "nothing." They are proof. They tell your nervous system, "I'm still here. I'm still caring for you."

The goal in hard seasons is not to be impressive. It's to stay in relationship with your body. Choose the smallest version you can keep, repeat it without drama, and let it be enough. Over time, those stitches become strength. Not because you pushed harder, but because you stopped disappearing from your own care.

Real-life snapshot

Keisha was in a brutal season — two kids, a demanding job, and a parent who needed help. She kept telling herself she'd "get serious" when life calmed down. She'd download a new plan, buy groceries for a perfect week, and then crash by day three. The failure wasn't willpower. The plan required a rested person.

One night, after skipping dinner and snapping at her family, she decided to stop aiming for a full reset and start aiming for one stitch. She picked a tiny "faithful" practice she could do even when depleted: lights down at the same time most nights. No perfect bedtime — just a clear shut-down cue. If she could manage one more thing, she added a second stitch: a protein-first breakfast she didn't have to think about.

The first week looked almost too small to matter. But it changed her mood at night. She stopped falling into the late-scroll spiral as often. Her mornings felt less jagged. Two weeks later, she had enough steadiness to add a short walk after dinner — sometimes five minutes, sometimes ten.

Three months in, her life was still busy. But she wasn't free-falling anymore. "I didn't fix everything," she said. "I just stopped tearing the seam."

Quick science

- Tiny, consistent behaviors are often easier for the brain to accept, which can help habits form with less internal resistance.
- Repeating small actions in the same context (same time, same cue) can shift behavior toward more automatic patterns, reducing reliance on willpower.
- Completing small, realistic goals builds self-efficacy (I can do this), which is linked with better follow-through over time.[84]

Inspiration note

Strength isn't built in one heroic day — it's built in a thousand quiet, almost invisible moments.

Today's Invitation

One thing I will do for myself today:

- ☐ Today I choose one tiny habit I can do even on a terrible day (2 minutes counts).
- ☐ I attach it to a cue I already have (after breakfast, after lunch, or when I get home).
- ☐ When it's done, I mark one visible check so the win is real.

Action Step:
Choose the easiest one today. Do it now or set one reminder and do it when it best fits your schedule.

Reflection:
After I took the step today, I felt: ☐ calmer ☐ clearer ☐ steadier ☐ proud ☐ no change yet (effort still counts)

Bottom line

Be faithful in the small things — they are the bricks that build your future health. Tiny is enough to begin.

Your lines

(write one thought, one insight, or rewrite one sentence that rang true)

_____
_____
_____

☐ Done for today

Why this matters
Writing just a few lines by hand locks the concept into memory and gently primes your subconscious mind to adopt and act on it, leading to better recall and follow-through.

DAY 85

> "Rest is not laziness, but the pause that gives strength to all work."
> — John Lubbock

Your strength is not in nonstop motion; it's in the pauses that restore you.
Rest is not the absence of effort; it's the refueling stop that lets you keep going without breaking down.
When you learn to pause on purpose, you gain more control over your energy, mood, and clarity.

Reflection

Rest is powerful medicine. We live in a culture that treats exhaustion like a badge of honor and calls it drive. We stack tasks until the body groans or breaks, and then we wonder why mood, focus, and health fall apart. Rest isn't a prize you earn at the end — it's the ingredient that lets you keep going.

Think of a traditional archer's bow. You string it to shoot, then you unstring it to protect its power. Leave it strung and the wood warps, the string frays, and the bow becomes useless. Your body works the same way. You were made to draw and release — to work with focus, then let your system come down so it stays strong for tomorrow.

Not everything that looks like a break is real rest — that's the trap. Scrolling, "just checking" email, online shopping, or chasing one more notification keeps your mind revved up. Quick hits like sugar, nicotine, or extra caffeine can numb you for a moment, then rebound you into more tension. Real rest is screen-free, simple, and short: a few minutes outside, a cup of tea without your phone, three long breaths with eyes closed, a gentle stretch or slow walk, a brief lie-down. Use this test: if you return clearer, looser, and more present, it was rest. If you return scattered or craving another hit, it wasn't.

You don't need a week off to begin. You need permission to pause on purpose — briefly and often. Practice these tiny, honest rests, and your body relearns how to downshift. True rest doesn't take you away from your life. It gives you back the strength to live it.

Real-life snapshot

Maria, a 39-year-old nurse practitioner, pushed herself through every shift — double coffees, skipped lunches, late-night charting. She believed rest was weakness until the day she almost fainted while walking a patient back to their room. Her doctor looked at her labs, then at her schedule, and said gently, "Your body isn't failing you. It's exhausted."

Maria agreed to two five-minute rest breaks per shift — no phone, just breathing and stretching — and a simple nightly wind-down routine: dimmed lights, a warm shower, and three slow breaths before bed. And whenever she felt tension rising, she gave herself a 60-second "reset" in the bathroom: door closed, eyes shut, a few long exhales — just enough to turn the volume down before she walked back out.

Within a few weeks her irritability eased, she made fewer mistakes, and her energy felt steady instead of spiky.

Quick science

- Short rest breaks can improve decision-making and reduce errors.
- Longer exhales activate the vagus nerve, shifting the body into parasympathetic calm.
- Recovery boosts immune repair, memory consolidation, and emotional regulation across the day.[85]

Inspiration note

A bow that stays strung eventually breaks; a bow unstrung keeps its power ready.

Today's Invitation

One thing I will do for myself today:

- ☐ I treat rest like medicine by taking one 10-minute real break today (no phone, no input).
- ☐ I downshift on purpose by doing 5 slow breaths the moment I notice I'm rushing (longer exhale).
- ☐ I protect recovery tonight by choosing one restoring activity for 20 minutes (walk, stretch, shower/bath, or quiet reading).

Action Step:
Choose the easiest one today. Do it now or set one reminder and do it when it best fits your schedule.

Reflection:
After I took the step today, I felt: ☐ calmer ☐ clearer ☐ steadier ☐ proud ☐ no change yet (effort still counts)

Bottom line

Rest is not retreat — it is repair, and it's non-negotiable for long-term health.

Your lines

(write one thought, one insight, or rewrite one sentence that rang true)

_____

_____

_____

☐ Done for today

Why this matters
Writing just a few lines by hand locks the concept into memory and gently primes your subconscious mind to adopt and act on it, leading to better recall and follow-through.

DAY 86

> "Spirit, mind, and body are like an old radio
> — only when they're tuned together does the
> music of your life come through."
> — A. Smyrlis, MD

At first, all you hear is static.
As you tune, bits of the song begin to appear.
Keep tuning, and the whole melody finally comes through.

Reflection

If you've ever used an old analog radio, you know the feeling. At first there's only static — noise, crackle, and faint hints of something underneath. As you slowly turn the dial, you catch pieces of the music: a drum beat here, a voice there. Then, if you're patient and keep tuning, the signal locks in. Suddenly the song is clear, rich, and whole.

Your health works the same way. At the beginning, there's a lot of static: poor sleep, irregular meals, rushed mornings, late nights, constant screens, stress about money, status, and what other people think. You decide to "get healthy," so you turn the first dials — earlier bedtime, more movement, simpler food. The static doesn't vanish overnight, but you notice small changes: a little less fog, slightly better mornings, one notch more patience. That's the first glimpse of the song.

But there is a deeper level of tuning. You can fix sleep, improve diet, and stick to workouts, and still feel off if your mind and spirit are tuned to a different station — comparison, hurry, fear, people-pleasing, "never enough." The glitter and pressure of the world pull you back into overwork, overthinking, and overcommitting. You can have a perfect workout plan and still feel like you're drowning in static if your deepest priorities and your daily choices are pointing in opposite directions.

Health tends to improve most when you tune the whole station. Spirit, mind, and body have to be turning the same way. When you begin to ask, "What truly matters to me?" and let the answers shape your schedule, a different signal comes in. Gratitude practice, honest boundaries, a few minutes of quiet reflection, choosing service over status — these are dials too. As you slowly align how you sleep, eat, move, think, and choose, the noise drops. Anxiety and resentment soften. You begin to hear more of the underlying "music" — a sense of meaning, connection, and rightness that no lab test can fully capture.

You don't tune an old radio with one violent twist; you tune it with many small, careful adjustments. Your life is the same. You don't need to be perfect. You just need to keep turning the dial, bit by bit, toward what feels truer and kinder — for your body, your mind, and your soul.

Real-life snapshot

Elias thought health was just "numbers and macros." He tracked every calorie, hit his protein, and never missed a workout. His labs looked good on paper. But inside, he felt empty, irritable, and wired at night. "I'm doing everything right," he told a friend, "so why do I feel so wrong?"

Together they looked at his life like a radio dial. Sleep was decent. Food was cleaned up. Workouts were strong. But the rest of the station was static: days packed with work he didn't care about, late-night online shopping as the default reward, little real time with family, and zero space for anything that felt meaningful.

So he decided to tune more than just his macros. He made three small changes: one phone-free family dinner every Sunday, one nightly "three gratitudes" line before bed, and one hour a week using his skills to help someone else.

Within a month, his workouts felt easier. Sleep deepened. The constant sense that something was missing softened. Nothing dramatic changed on the outside — same job, same gym, same body — but life started to feel more worth living inside.

Quick science

- A strong sense of purpose is associated with lower risk of heart disease, depression, and earlier death in observational studies.
- Gratitude practices are associated with better sleep quality, improved mood, and healthier inflammation-related markers in some studies.
- Living in line with your values can reduce stress signaling and may improve heart-rate variability (HRV), a sign of a more flexible, resilient nervous system.[86]

Inspiration note

Your dials aren't just sleep, food, and steps — they're also what you love, what you serve, and what you say yes or no to.

Today's Invitation

One thing I will do for myself today:

- ☐ Gratitude: Write one quick line about what went right today.
- ☐ Boundary: Set one honest stop time (or one clean no) and keep it.
- ☐ Values: Take one small action that matches the person I want to be today.

Action Step:
Choose the easiest one today. Do it now or set one reminder and do it when it best fits your schedule.

Reflection:
After I took the step today, I felt: ☐ calmer ☐ clearer ☐ steadier ☐ proud ☐ no change yet (effort still counts)

Bottom line

Fixing the parts helps, but only tuning your whole life lets the music come through.

Your lines

(write one thought, one insight, or rewrite one sentence that rang true)

_____

_____

_____

☐ Done for today

Why this matters
Writing just a few lines by hand locks the concept into memory and gently primes your subconscious mind to adopt and act on it, leading to better recall and follow-through.

DAY 87

> "The impediment to action advances action.
> What stands in the way becomes the way."
> — Marcus Aurelius

What you call "in the way" may be exactly what you need.
Resistance isn't just friction — it's feedback.
The obstacle, handled wisely, becomes the training ground.

Reflection

Obstacles aren't detours from life — they are part of the path. When something blocks you — an injury, a setback, a bad lab result, a hard conversation — you didn't choose the terrain, but you can choose how you move on it. With the right response, resistance becomes training, and training becomes strength.

In health, obstacles show up as the exact thing you wish weren't there: fatigue that forces rest, pain that changes how you move, a diagnosis that demands attention. The first reflex is usually, Why me? Why now? If you stay there, it's just a wall. But if you ask, "What's the next wise move here?" the wall often turns into a doorway.

Maybe the flare in your back is inviting you to strengthen your core, change how you sit, or finally ask for help. Maybe the burnout is forcing you to put boundaries where there have been none. Maybe the relapse is asking you to simplify your plan instead of making it more extreme. None of this romanticizes suffering. It simply admits that, since obstacles are part of every life, the most powerful stance is to use them.

When you stop fighting the existence of the obstacle and start learning from it, something quiet shifts. You don't have to like it. You just have to let it shape you into someone wiser and steadier. The stone is still real — but handled well, it becomes your next step.

Real-life snapshot

Running was Victor's therapy. Long miles, fast miles, any miles — as long as he could run, he felt like himself. Then a knee injury stopped him cold. One sharp pain on a downhill, and suddenly he couldn't run without limping.

At first, he was furious and depressed. "If I can't run, what's the point?" he thought. His doctor cleared him for swimming and strength training while his knee healed. Victor resisted. It didn't feel the same. But after a few weeks of sulking, he decided to treat the injury as an experiment instead of a verdict.

He started with short swims and light strength work: gentle laps, band exercises, careful squats under supervision. He hated it at first — awkward, slow, nothing like the high of running. But he stayed with it. Months later, something surprised him. His knee was stronger. His upper body and core were more developed than ever. His posture improved. He felt more balanced overall, and his mood was steadier than when he ran every day. When he finally returned to running, he was more resilient, not less.

"The injury felt like a wall," he said. "It turned out to be a door into a better version of me. If I hadn't been forced to change, I never would have built the strength that's protecting me now."

Quick science

- Reframing stress as a challenge (instead of a threat) can improve performance and reduce physiological stress reactivity.
- Facing and adapting to obstacles — instead of avoiding them or quitting — builds resilience over time; your nervous system learns that you can survive difficulty and recover.
- Skillful modification of effort (such as cross-training during injury instead of stopping all movement) maintains capacity, protects mental health, and reduces risk of re-injury when you return to your original activity.[87]

Inspiration note

The stone in your path can become the step under your foot.

Today's Invitation

One thing I will do for myself today:

- ☐ I turn the obstacle into training by writing one honest line: "What is this asking me to learn or practice right now?"
- ☐ I keep moving through the obstacle by doing a "Plan B" version of my habit today (smaller still counts).
- ☐ I build resilience from the obstacle by making one protective adjustment today (move differently, rest on purpose, or ask for support) instead of quitting.

Action Step:
Choose the easiest one today. Do it now or set one reminder and do it when it best fits your schedule.

Reflection:
After I took the step today, I felt: ☐ calmer ☐ clearer ☐ steadier ☐ proud ☐ no change yet (effort still counts)

Bottom line

You don't grow around obstacles — you grow through them.

Your lines

(write one thought, one insight, or rewrite one sentence that rang true)

_____

_____

_____

☐ Done for today

Why this matters

Writing just a few lines by hand locks the concept into memory and gently primes your subconscious mind to adopt and act on it, leading to better recall and follow-through.

DAY 88

> "You are the expert on your life; your doctor is the expert on disease. Good care happens when both voices are heard."
> — A. Smyrlis, MD

You can't control the system, but you can speak for yourself.
Being your own advocate isn't being difficult — it's being awake.
Your body, your life, your voice at the center of your care.

Reflection

Modern healthcare moves fast. Visits are short. Screens are loud. Systems reward speed and checkboxes. None of that is your fault — but you feel it when you leave with more confusion than clarity.

Advocacy isn't aggression. It's remembering one simple truth: this is your body and your life. You're allowed to slow the moment down long enough to understand what's happening and why.

Start before you walk in. Write your top one or two concerns in plain language. If you bring ten problems, the system will choose what gets addressed. If you bring one or two, you choose.

When a test or procedure is proposed, use four calm questions:

1. What are we trying to learn?
2. How would the result change the plan?
3. Is there a simpler or safer first step?
4. If we wait, what would make it unsafe — and for how long is it reasonable?

If the language gets too technical, ask for translation: "Can you give me the big picture in two sentences?" or "Can you explain it like you would to a family member?"

Bring a second set of ears if you can. If you're alone, take 60 seconds right after the visit — before you leave the building — to jot three things: what they think is going on, what the plan is, and when follow-up happens.

Also speak your values. If a treatment could help but at a cost you don't want to pay, say so: "My priority is staying independent," or "I care most about being clear-minded and present with my family." Plans change when values are clear.

And if something doesn't fit — if a recommendation feels extreme, or you feel brushed off — consider a second opinion. That isn't disloyalty. It's stewardship.

You can't fix the whole system. But you can claim your small circle of control: clear priorities, honest questions, written notes, and decisions that match your values. That is advocacy. Not a fight — a partnership where your voice belongs at the center.

Real-life snapshot

Carla often left appointments feeling small and confused. Her doctors were smart and busy, but the visits were fast. She nodded, went home, and realized she couldn't explain what had just been said.

After one particularly rushed visit, she tried a different approach. For her next appointment, she wrote down two main concerns on a card, brought her sister as a second set of ears, and kept four questions in her pocket.

The visit felt different. The pace slowed. Her doctor, instead of seeming annoyed, actually relaxed. He realized he didn't need to order two of the tests he'd clicked out of habit. They agreed on a clear plan and follow-up.

Quick science

- Patients who prepare questions and express their priorities tend to have better understanding of their conditions and are more likely to follow through with agreed plans.
- Shared decision-making — where clinician and patient decide together — is associated with better satisfaction, less regret, and sometimes fewer unnecessary tests and procedures.
- Feeling heard and respected in healthcare settings can lower anxiety and make it easier to implement lifestyle and medication changes.[88]

Inspiration note

You're not "difficult" for wanting to understand. You're doing the sacred work of caring for the one body you'll ever live in.

Today's Invitation

One thing I will do for myself today:

- ☐ Before my next visit, I'll write my top 1–2 concerns in plain language.

- ☐ I'll bring four questions: what are we looking for, how would it change the plan, is there a simpler first step, what if we wait?
- ☐ I'll bring one clear data point (med list, symptom notes, or a simple log) instead of relying on memory.

Action Step:
Choose the easiest one today. Do it now or set one reminder and do it when it best fits your schedule.

Reflection:
After I took the step today, I felt: ☐ calmer ☐ clearer ☐ steadier ☐ proud ☐ no change yet (effort still counts)

Bottom line

The system is busy, loud, and often hurried. You can't fix all of that. But you can bring clear priorities, honest questions, and your own values into the conversation. That's advocacy. That's partnership. That's how care becomes truly yours.

Your lines

(write one thought, one insight, or rewrite one sentence that rang true)

_____

_____

_____

☐ Done for today

Why this matters
Writing just a few lines by hand locks the concept into memory and gently primes your subconscious mind to adopt and act on it, leading to better recall and follow-through.

DAY 89

> **"Health is the best wealth; contentment, greater still."**
> — Dhammapada (Verse 204, paraphrase)

Health is wealth — and contentment is how you enjoy it.
"Enough" is the line between thriving and constant chasing.
Right-sizing your life creates room for your body and soul to breathe.

Reflection

We're trained to believe that "more" is the answer. More income, more upgrades, more trips, more everything. But "more" isn't a strategy — it's an appetite.

Every new thing you bring into your life — car, phone, subscription, project — comes with a hidden cost: the attention to maintain it, the hours to pay for it, the stress of thinking about it. Over time, those costs often land in your body: shorter sleep, rushed meals, skipped movement, a nervous system that never fully unwinds.

Contentment isn't about giving up. It's about right-sizing — choosing a dose of life that your health, relationships, and nervous system can actually support. Too little leaves you deprived. Too much leaves you overstimulated and exhausted. The right amount gives you margin: time to rest, to cook something simple, to walk, to be present with people you love.

Sufficiency means you fund your real wealth first — your health, your closest relationships, your inner life — and let everything else fit around that. It's not "settling." It's choosing the version of life that you can live without slowly burning yourself down.

When you stop chasing every upgrade, your nervous system softens. Breathing deepens. Small pleasures start to register again: warm food, a quiet morning, a conversation without rushing, a simple walk that actually feels good instead of like another to-do. You begin to see that you already have more than you realized.

Contentment is not passivity. It's wisdom in motion. It says:
"I will live fully — but not at the cost of my sleep, my peace, or my soul."

Real-life snapshot

The Parkers weren't reckless. They were just "keeping up."

They upgraded to a new SUV lease, swapped phones every launch day, packed holidays with gadgets and tickets, and said yes to every activity that made their kids look "involved." To finance the life, they worked later hours, took clients they didn't align with, and cut back on rest.

Evenings turned rushed. Most meals were takeout or eaten in the car. Their sleep drifted later and later. Both gained weight. Patience at home wore thin. No crisis, just a constant sense of being squeezed.

After a particularly tense month, they decided to try an "enoughness reset" for one season: keep the car two more years; skip the phone upgrades; focus on simpler local weekends instead of constant travel; set a lights-down alarm most nights; bring back a Sunday dinner with friends — home-cooked, nothing fancy.

Three months later, the facts were simple: they were sleeping more, spending less, arguing less, and laughing more. The house felt less pressured. Their health markers nudged in the right direction.

"We thought we needed more money to feel this way," Mr. Parker said. "What we actually needed was less pressure to chase what we didn't truly need."

Quick science

- The "high" from new possessions often fades quickly as your brain adapts, while stable relationships, meaningful work, and simple pleasures contribute more to long-term wellbeing.
- Chronic sleep loss and stress from overcommitted, overstretched lives can increase cravings, impulsive choices, blood pressure, and inflammation over time.
- Gratitude and sufficiency practices can lower perceived material strain and improve life satisfaction, making it easier to choose health-supportive behaviors.[89]

Inspiration note

A simple life, well-lived, is often the most luxurious of all.

Today's Invitation

One thing I will do for myself today:

- ☐ Choose enough: Say no to one extra thing today (an upgrade, a commitment, or an impulse buy).
- ☐ Savor one thing: Take a simple pleasure without multitasking (a walk, tea, music, or sunset).
- ☐ Name today's sufficiency: Write one line — What I have is enough for today because _____.

Action Step:
Choose the easiest one today. Do it now or set one reminder and do it when it best fits your schedule.

Reflection:
After I took the step today, I felt: ☐ calmer ☐ clearer ☐ steadier ☐ proud ☐ no change yet (effort still counts)

Bottom line

Fund your health and peace first. When life is right-sized, everything else gets cheaper — especially stress.

Your lines

(write one thought, one insight, or rewrite one sentence that rang true)

_____

_____

_____

☐ Done for today

Why this matters
Writing just a few lines by hand locks the concept into memory and gently primes your subconscious mind to adopt and act on it, leading to better recall and follow-through.

DAY 90

> **"If the joy fades, the signal's red."**
> — A. Smyrlis, MD

When movement becomes punishment, health turns hostile.
When food feels like math, appetite for life fades too.
Joy is the body's yes-signal.

Reflection

Discipline can start a habit, but joy often helps it last. That's why, when you're starting a new routine, it matters to personalize it to your taste, your season, your capacity, and your real life. The "best" plan on paper is useless if you secretly hate it. A good plan is one you can do without bracing.

When every workout becomes a penance and every meal feels like a test, your nervous system shifts from openness to defense. You may still check the boxes for a while — but dread grows, the body tightens, and eventually you drift away because something inside you knows: this isn't living.

Joy is not a bonus — it's guidance. It tells you your relationship with any health habit is still connected to life, not just numbers. When you protect even a sliver of delight — music in your ears during a walk, a sport you genuinely enjoy, a meal you savor slowly — you send a quieter message to your body: safe, steady, allowed. Health is supposed to expand your life, not shrink it.

Joy doesn't mean "easy" or "undisciplined." It means the work you're doing still feels tethered to something meaningful. It means the path still feels like yours.

Real-life snapshot

Janelle used to love running — the sunsets, the breath, the rhythm. Then training logs and pace charts took over. She stopped noticing the sky. She hit every pace but smiled at none.

Her performance dropped. Her coach finally told her, "Leave your watch at home. Run like a kid for one week."

She came back lighter, faster, and laughing.

Quick science

- Positive emotion is associated with better adherence to health behaviors and can support resilience over time.
- Enjoyment and reward signals (involving dopamine and related pathways) can make habits easier to repeat than relying on willpower alone.
- Flow states — being absorbed in an activity — are linked with better performance and lower perceived effort, especially when the activity feels meaningful.[90]

Inspiration note

Think of children running — no stopwatch, no metrics, just wonder. That's your calibration point.

Today's Invitation

One thing I will do for myself today:

- ☐ Choose joy-movement: Pick a form of movement I actually enjoy today.
- ☐ Add one brightener: Pair it with something pleasant (music, sunlight, a friend, or a favorite tea).
- ☐ Notice the win: Write one word after — done — and let it count.

Action Step:
Choose the easiest one today. Do it now or set one reminder and do it when it best fits your schedule.

Reflection:
After I took the step today, I felt: ☐ calmer ☐ clearer ☐ steadier ☐ proud ☐ no change yet (effort still counts)

Bottom line

When joy disappears, it's a useful signal you may have drifted. Steer gently back.

Your lines

(write one thought, one insight, or rewrite one sentence that rang true)

_____

_____

_____

☐ Done for today

Why this matters
Writing just a few lines by hand locks the concept into memory and gently primes your subconscious mind to adopt and act on it, leading to better recall and follow-through.

DAY 91

"Hatred does not cease by hatred; by love alone does it cease."
— Dhammapada

Harm multiplies unless someone chooses to stop the cycle.
You can be that someone.
Your body and soul are the first to benefit.

Reflection

When someone wounds you, the first instinct is to tighten. You brace. You defend. You reach for the sharpest reply. It feels powerful in the moment — a way to reclaim control, a way to prove you won't be walked over.

But inside the body, something very different unfolds. Hatred can send stress signals surging through your body. Your heart beats harder. Your blood pressure rises. Your breathing becomes thin and fast. Your attention narrows into a tunnel — the same cramped place where fear lives. Your body can stay tense as if preparing for a fight that may never end.

The original wound may have come from someone else,
but the damage now lives in you.
This is the health truth almost no one teaches:
Retaliation can keep the body stuck in stress.
Love — the calm, steady, principled kind — can help the body settle and recover.

Love is not weakness. Love is not letting people walk over you. Love is choosing not to become the thing that hurt you. It is speaking clearly, without cruelty. It is setting boundaries without bitterness. It is walking away without hate. It is remembering that your nervous system, your heart, and your long-term health cannot afford to carry poison.

You choose the healing response not because the other person deserves it — but because your body does.

Real-life snapshot

Omar drafted an email in the heat of anger — the kind that could scorch a room and end relationships. His whole body buzzed: tight chest, clenched jaw, racing thoughts.

Then he remembered what his grandmother used to tell him: "Hatred burns the hand that holds it. Love protects the one who chooses it."

Instead of sending it, he closed the laptop, went to bed, and let the storm settle.

In the morning, he rewrote the message: firm boundary, calm tone, clear next steps. The project improved. His sleep improved. His stomach unwound.

He avoided a feud — and likely avoided weeks of inflammation and regret. He didn't "win" the argument. He won back his health.

Quick science

- Hostility carried over months and years is associated with higher rates of cardiovascular disease and shorter lifespan.
- Reframing a hurt — even slightly — can soften amygdala activation and calm the threat response.
- Sleeping before reacting strengthens emotional regulation and restores access to wise choices.[91]

Inspiration note

Strength and kindness are not opposites. The strongest people are often those who refuse to pass their pain forward.

Today's Invitation

One thing I will do for myself today:

- ☐ Sleep on it: If I'm hurt, I'll wait until tomorrow before I respond.
- ☐ Create a pause: Take 6 slow exhales when I feel the urge to strike back.
- ☐ Choose clean love: Set one boundary without bitterness (distance, clarity, or a calm no).

Action Step:
Choose the easiest one today. Do it now or set one reminder and do it when it best fits your schedule.

Reflection:
After I took the step today, I felt: ☐ calmer ☐ clearer ☐ steadier ☐ proud ☐ no change yet (effort still counts)

Bottom line

Choosing love over hatred isn't naïve. It's medicine — nervous-system medicine, cardiovascular medicine, and spiritual medicine. You end the cycle inside yourself first. The rest follows.

Your lines

(write one thought, one insight, or rewrite one sentence that rang true)

_____
_____
_____

☐ Done for today

Why this matters
Writing just a few lines by hand locks the concept into memory and gently primes your subconscious mind to adopt and act on it, leading to better recall and follow-through.

DAY 92

> "Remembering that I'll be dead soon is the most important tool I've ever encountered to help me make the big choices in life."
> — Steve Jobs, Stanford Commencement Address, 2005

Life feels different when you remember it is finite.
Time becomes sharper, priorities clearer, and noise quieter.
Wisdom grows when you live as if each day actually counts.

Reflection

Thinking about the end isn't morbid — it's a clear mirror. When you remember that your days are numbered, the unimportant parts of life fall away. Petty comparisons, other people's expectations, fear of looking foolish — none of it survives very long in the light of, "My time here is limited." Mortality doesn't just bring sadness; it brings clarity.

When you hold that truth gently, not in panic but in honesty, something shifts. Failure feels less terrifying because you realize how quickly the moment will pass anyway. Delay feels less attractive because you see how few chances you really have to do what matters. On your last day, you won't care how "impressive" you looked. You'll care whether you loved people well, used your gifts, and told your truth with your life.

Time is the one currency you never get back, and health is the engine that lets you spend it on what you love. When you live as if your days are endless, you postpone the things that actually matter: the walk, the call, the apology, the learning, the sleep that would let you show up fully tomorrow. When you remember that your days are limited, those same acts become non-negotiable. They move from "someday" to "today."

This is not about living in fear of death. It's about letting the reality of death bring your life into focus. Imagine a large hourglass that was flipped the day you were born. The sand runs day and night whether you watch it or not. Once a day, picture that hourglass and quietly remind yourself, "My days are numbered." Let that simple sentence rearrange your priorities. Let it help you choose one thing that truly matters over ten things that only look urgent.

Real-life snapshot

Daniel kept delaying what mattered — time with his kids, his health, his writing. Then a close friend was told he had six months to live. Daniel watched him clear his calendar, write letters to his children, take slow walks with his wife, and live as if every day truly was his last.

Months passed. The scans slowly improved. His friend was given more time — but he never went back to living like his days were endless.

That shook Daniel more than the diagnosis. He began starting each morning with one line: "My days are numbered." He scheduled a weekly family dinner, resumed daily walks, and wrote one paragraph a night, no matter how tired he felt.

Quick science

- Gentle awareness of mortality (processed in a healthy way) can nudge people toward more value-driven, prosocial choices in some studies.
- Aligning daily behavior with core values is associated with better mental health and fewer long-term regrets.
- Reflecting on the finite nature of time can support clearer boundaries and follow-through on health behaviors, especially around work, relationships, and self-care.[92]

Inspiration note

Remembering that life ends can make the part you have more alive.

Today's Invitation

One thing I will do for myself today:

- ☐ Don't postpone it: Do one small thing today that I've been putting off (send the text or make the 2-minute call).
- ☐ Choose one yes + one no: Yes to something that matters (sleep/movement/real food); no to one thing that only feels urgent.
- ☐ Make it real: Take a 10-minute walk and ask one gentle question — what would matter most if this were one of my last ordinary weeks?

Action Step:
Choose the easiest one today. Do it now or set one reminder and do it when it best fits your schedule.

Reflection:
After I took the step today, I felt: ☐ calmer ☐ clearer ☐ steadier ☐ proud ☐ no change yet (effort still counts)

Bottom line

Numbering your days teaches you to live them on purpose.

Your lines

(write one thought, one insight, or rewrite one sentence that rang true)

☐ Done for today

Why this matters
Writing just a few lines by hand locks the concept into memory and gently primes your subconscious mind to adopt and act on it, leading to better recall and follow-through.

DAY 93

"Lost time is never found again."
— Benjamin Franklin

Time is the only resource you can't refill.
Every hour you protect shapes the health you'll live with later.
Boundaries turn "lost time" into "chosen time."

Reflection

If you're trying to restore health — clear brain fog, steady sleep, rebuild stamina — time is your hidden medicine. Without protected time, even the best plan dies on the vine. You know this: you "mean" to walk, cook, stretch, or go to bed earlier, but the day dissolves into email, pings, and "just one more episode." Health isn't just about what you know; it's about what you give time to.

Most modern time loss isn't dramatic. It's micro-fragmentation — tiny slices shaved off your day by distractions. You open your phone "for a second" and, 20 minutes later, you're still scrolling. You respond to every buzz as if it were urgent. You half-work and half-check messages, so both take twice as long. TV was once one show; now it's endless autoplay. The result is a life that feels rushed but strangely unproductive — and no time or energy left for the habits that would change everything.

The fix is not to squeeze more tasks into the day. It's to spend time on purpose. Three small time fences change everything:

- One focus block: Choose one task. Set a timer for 25–45 minutes. Phone out of reach. Then take a real 5–10 minute break.
- Two check-in windows: Pick two times you'll check messages/news. Outside those windows, notifications stay quiet.
- One evening cap: Decide when screens end — or what you'll watch — before you're tired. Then use the reclaimed minutes for sleep, a short walk, or prepping one real meal.

You don't need a new personality to "have more time." You need a few simple structures that stop leaks. When you focus on one thing at a time, name your priorities, fence your phone, and cap TV, hours quietly reappear. Many of them will be exactly what your health has been waiting for.

Real-life snapshot

Leah and Aaron worked at the same company, same role, same workload. By 6 p.m., their days looked completely different.

Leah wasn't lazy — she was responsive. Email, chat, and texts stayed open all day because she didn't want to drop a ball. She'd scroll "for a second" between tasks, then lose her place. Nights ended with TV auto-playing until she was too tired to move. She went to bed feeling behind and told herself, "Tomorrow I'll do better."

Aaron wasn't perfect either — he loved his phone and he could binge a show like anyone. But after a checkup showed his blood pressure was creeping up, he tried one simple experiment: fewer switches, fewer screens, earlier stop times. He worked in focus blocks, checked messages at set windows, and kept his phone out of the bedroom. He still slipped sometimes — but he returned at the next cue instead of writing off the whole day.

Nothing about their job descriptions changed. But six months later, Aaron was leaving work on time most days, walking in the evenings, and winding down earlier. Leah was still "catching up" at 10 p.m., wondering where the day had gone.

Quick science

- Constant multitasking and task-switching increase mental fatigue and reduce efficiency; you lose time and quality every time you jump between tasks instead of focusing on one.
- Protected morning and evening routines (phone-free, calmer activities) help stabilize cortisol rhythm, which supports better sleep, mood, and energy.
- Excess screen time — especially in the evening — is linked with poorer sleep, more perceived time pressure, and lower well-being; setting limits and time blocks reduces stress and improves follow-through on health habits.[8]

Inspiration note

When you don't name your hours, someone else will do it for you.

Today's Invitation

One thing I will do for myself today:

☐ Focus block: Do one 25-minute focus block (one task, no multitasking).

- ☐ Phone windows: Choose two set phone-check windows today.
- ☐ Spend the found time: Use the saved time for one health action (walk, real meal, wind-down).

Action Step:
Choose the easiest one today. Do it now or set one reminder and do it when it best fits your schedule.

Reflection:
After I took the step today, I felt: ☐ calmer ☐ clearer ☐ steadier ☐ proud ☐ no change yet (effort still counts)

Bottom line

Lost time cannot be recovered — but protected time can transform your days.

Your lines

(write one thought, one insight, or rewrite one sentence that rang true)

_____

_____

_____

☐ Done for today

Why this matters
Writing just a few lines by hand locks the concept into memory and gently primes your subconscious mind to adopt and act on it, leading to better recall and follow-through.

DAY 94

"Beware the barrenness of a busy life."
— attributed to Socrates

Busy does not mean full.
A life jammed with activity can still be empty.
Space is where meaning, health, and presence grow.

Reflection

We've been quietly taught that a packed schedule equals importance. Full calendar, full inbox, every slot booked — therefore, you must matter. So we add and add, and almost never remove. We say yes to one more project, one more event, one more late-night message. Notifications pour in without pause. Yet the soul stays strangely empty. Busyness wears the mask of meaning while quietly draining our vitality.

A crowded life leaves no room for depth. You can be in motion from dawn to midnight and still feel like nothing real is happening. Better to do fewer things with full presence than many things with no joy. The nervous system knows the difference. A single unhurried dinner with your family nourishes more than a dozen rushed check-ins. A 20-minute walk without your phone calms more than an hour of distracted "relaxing" in front of a screen.

The shift begins when you start filtering every request through what actually matters to you: your health, your family, your real work, your conscience, your sense of calling. If it doesn't serve those, it becomes a candidate for "no." Not a harsh, defensive no — a clean, kind, unapologetic one. This is a skill, not a personality trait. You can practice it the way you practice anything else. Stand in front of the mirror, meet your own eyes, and say out loud: "Thank you for thinking of me, but I won't be able to do that." Notice that the world doesn't end.

Busyness isn't just a calendar problem; it's a health problem. Chronic overload keeps your stress system switched on, sleep shallow, cravings high, and relationships thin. Empty space is not wasted time; it is where your real life has room to unfold. When you begin to protect pockets of quiet, you don't become less productive; you become more human — and from that place, your yes carries more weight.

Real-life snapshot

Two brothers, Jared and Mark, started adulthood in similar places — same town, similar jobs, same ambition to "make a good life." Over time, their calendars began to look very different.

Jared said yes to almost everything. Extra projects? Yes. Weekend obligations? Yes. Late-night calls from clients? Yes. His calendar looked impressive: back-to-back meetings, volunteer roles, social events, endless "catch-ups." On the outside, he looked successful. On the inside, he felt hollow and exhausted. Meals were rushed, sleep was short, and there was never a moment that wasn't spoken for.

Mark made a quieter choice. Early on, after watching an older colleague burn out, he decided on a few simple guardrails: roughly eight hours of work, eight hours of sleep, and the rest reserved for family, health, and a little time alone. When extra requests came in, he weighed them against those anchors. If something truly mattered or aligned with his values, he said yes. Everything else got a kind, firm no. His life looked less impressive on paper, but he moved through his days with more ease.

At a Thanksgiving dinner years later, their contrast came into focus. When it was time to share what they were grateful for, Mark spoke about his wife, his kids, his health, and the simple joy of having time to be with them. He named long walks, weekend breakfasts, and being present for school events. His voice was steady; his face looked rested.

When it was Jared's turn, he opened his mouth and nothing came out at first. His chest tightened. He realized most of his time had been spent in transit: rushing to the next thing, constantly "on," rarely in his own life. He teared up. "I'm grateful for my family too," he finally said, "but I've been too busy to really be with them. I don't want to keep living like this."

That night, after everyone left, he asked Mark how he had drawn his lines. They sat at the kitchen table and sketched out a different week — one protected evening, one blocked-off weekend morning, one regular walk, one standing "no" to low-value commitments. It wasn't dramatic, but it was a start.

Months later, Jared's calendar still had meetings and obligations, but there were gaps now — white space that didn't used to exist. His blood pressure readings were trending better. His sleep had improved. More importantly, he'd stopped feeling like a guest in his own life. "The first time I said no, I felt guilty," he told Mark. "The fifth time, I felt free."

Quick science

- Chronic overload keeps the stress response activated, raising stress signaling (including cortisol and adrenaline), which over time can impair memory and increase cardiometabolic strain.
- Unstructured, quiet time can give the brain's "default mode network" room to process emotions, consolidate experiences, and support creativity — a kind of mental housecleaning that busyness blocks.
- Carrying too many "open loops" (unfinished tasks, unmade decisions) increases anxiety and is linked with difficulty falling asleep and staying asleep; reducing commitments and closing loops reduces that mental load.[94]

Inspiration note

Your life can't breathe if every minute is spoken for.

Today's Invitation

One thing I will do for myself today:

- ☐ I step out of busy and into living by choosing One Big Thing and letting the rest be secondary.
- ☐ I reclaim my attention by doing one 25-minute monotask block (no tabs, no phone).
- ☐ I give my day room to breathe by creating one buffer (5–10 minutes between tasks, or a real lunch break).

Action Step:
Choose the easiest one today. Do it now or set one reminder and do it when it best fits your schedule.

Reflection:
After I took the step today, I felt: ☐ calmer ☐ clearer ☐ steadier ☐ proud ☐ no change yet (effort still counts)

Bottom line

Empty space is not wasted time — it is where your real life has room to unfold.

Your lines

(write one thought, one insight, or rewrite one sentence that rang true)

_____
_____
_____

☐ Done for today

Why this matters
Writing just a few lines by hand locks the concept into memory and gently primes your subconscious mind to adopt and act on it, leading to better recall and follow-through.

DAY 95

> **"Better is a little with righteousness than great revenues with injustice."**
> — Proverbs

Let money serve your values, not replace them.
Trade meaning for money, and you may quietly trade away health.
Wealth is hard to enjoy without health — and health is harder to sustain without meaning.

Reflection

When money sits above everything else, the body eventually pays the bill.

In a culture that worships hustle, it's easy to treat sleep, relationships, and inner peace as "optional" — something you'll buy back later. Extra shifts, side gigs, endless emails, late calls. The paycheck rises. Meanwhile, sleep shortens, stress climbs, food quality slides, and relationships thin. You look successful on paper and feel hollow in your own skin.

Meaning is like roots. The taller the tree, the deeper the roots must go. Meaning grows out of alignment: your values, your actions, your relationships, and your work all pointing roughly in the same direction.

- Purpose feeds patience.
- Service steadies your hands.
- When choices line up with what you believe, your nervous system relaxes.

Energy that once leaked out as regret or resentment starts flowing into real life. Health isn't just chemistry. It's coherence.

When you live against your own values, your physiology often knows before you do. Heart rate stays higher. Sleep runs lighter. Stress rhythms can flatten. You reach for comfort food, more caffeine, or late-night scrolling to blunt a discomfort you can't quite name.

When you live toward your values — even imperfectly — something deeper softens. It feels like coming home.

Choosing meaning does not mean rejecting money. It means refusing to earn it in ways that bankrupt your body and soul.

Real-life snapshot

Maya worked long shifts and said yes to every extra one. Her bank account grew; her health and mood shrank. She was drained, irritable, and never truly rested.

One day, after snapping at a patient and then at her partner, she wrote down a different question: "What is this money for if I'm too exhausted to live my own life?"

She made three changes: she started protecting family dinners, leaving work on time at least once a week; she visited her mother once a week to ease her loneliness after her father passed; she stopped taking extra shifts and went back to one class at the local dance studio she used to love.

Within weeks, her steps rose without "trying," late snacking dropped, sleep deepened, and her mood lifted. Nothing medically fancy changed. Her meaning did.

A project manager made a similar shift. She swapped ten hours of overtime for coaching youth soccer and Saturday mornings at an animal shelter. Within one season, she fell asleep faster, woke without an alarm, and felt joy return to ordinary days.

Neither woman became poorer in what mattered. They became richer in health.

Quick science

- Chasing only external rewards (money, status) is associated with higher stress and lower wellbeing than pursuing values-aligned goals.
- Living in line with your values supports better nervous-system balance, healthier heart-rate variability, and more sustainable health behaviors.
- Chronic overwork and misaligned goals disturb sleep and stress hormone patterns; setting boundaries and adding meaning-aligned activities help restore recovery.[95]

Inspiration note

Do what you truly love and let money be a close second. Your biology can tell the difference.

Today's Invitation

One thing I will do for myself today:

- ☐ I choose meaning over money by doing one value-aligned act today (something I would still do if no one paid me).
- ☐ I protect what matters by keeping one boundary that helps me stay whole (sleep, family time, or a real meal).
- ☐ I invest in meaning by giving 10 minutes of presence to a relationship that matters (call, text, or time together).

Action Step:
Choose the easiest one today. Do it now or set one reminder and do it when it best fits your schedule.

Reflection:
After I took the step today, I felt: ☐ calmer ☐ clearer ☐ steadier ☐ proud ☐ no change yet (effort still counts)

Bottom line

Choose meaning; protect health. Let money take its proper place — as a tool, not a master.

Your lines

(write one thought, one insight, or rewrite one sentence that rang true)

_____

_____

_____

☐ Done for today

Why this matters
Writing just a few lines by hand locks the concept into memory and gently primes your subconscious mind to adopt and act on it, leading to better recall and follow-through.

DAY 96

> "Don't retire from life — retire into a new pattern of tending."
> — A. Smyrlis, MD

Retirement isn't a finish line; it's a redesign.
When roles vanish, rhythm and health often drift with them.
You still need purpose, challenge, and structure — just in new clothes.

Reflection

Many people dream of retirement as the finish line: no alarm clock, no commute, no meetings. But when work stops, something unexpected often happens. Days blur. There is less reason to get up at a certain time, less built-in movement, fewer people to see.

Without meaning to, you lose three anchors at once: purpose, challenge, and structure.

When those anchors disappear, health often drifts. Sleep slides later. Meals become less regular. Movement shrinks to a few steps between the couch and the fridge. Mood and memory soften. It is easy to blame "age," but sometimes what we label as aging is partly the loss of rhythm and roles.

Designing a healthy later chapter starts with a simple pivot:
Instead of asking, "What am I retiring from?" ask,
"What am I moving toward?"

Your body still wants to be needed. Your mind still wants to learn. Your heart still wants to contribute. Give yourself clear roles that matter: mentor someone younger in your field or community; volunteer once or twice a week in ways that feel meaningful, not draining; become a learner again — a language, an instrument, a craft, a book group. These are not hobbies in the shallow sense; they are new forms of useful identity.

Then, rebuild gentle structure. Treat your days like a well-designed program instead of an endless weekend: a fairly steady wake time, morning light, planned movement (walk/class/simple strength), and scheduled social time — especially if you live alone.

Retirement does not have to be an empty space you fall into. It can be a chapter you author on purpose: roles that matter, rhythms that support your biology, and proof that growth does not end just because one career does.

Real-life snapshot

George worked as an accountant for 40 years. The first month after retirement felt like vacation. By month three, he felt lost. He slept in, grazed on snacks, moved less, and saw his friends mostly through a screen. He was more tired and foggy than when he was working full-time.

His cardiologist gently asked, "What are you moving toward now?"

George decided on three moves: tutor high school students in math twice a week; join a local walking group that met three mornings a week; set a "morning start" at 7:30 a.m. with coffee, light, and a short reading.

Within a few months, his steps climbed, his sleep became deeper, and his mood lifted.

"I thought I needed less responsibility," he said. "What I needed was different responsibility — and a reason to get up."

Quick science

- Loss of structure and roles in retirement is associated with worsening sleep, lower activity, and higher risk of low mood and cognitive decline in some studies.
- Purposeful activity and regular social engagement in later life are linked with better longevity, mood, and brain health.
- Stable rhythms (wake time, light exposure, movement) help preserve metabolic and cardiovascular health at any age.[96]

Inspiration note

Retirement isn't the end of your usefulness; it's the chance to offer your wisdom in new ways.

Today's Invitation

One thing I will do for myself today:

- ☐ Move toward: Take one small step toward a purpose block this week (learn, volunteer, create, or connect).
- ☐ Keep the anchors: Hold gentle structure today (steady wake time, morning light, planned movement).
- ☐ Schedule people: Put one social touchpoint on the calendar, especially if I'm alone.

Action Step:
Choose the easiest one today. Do it now or set one reminder and do it when it best fits your schedule.

Reflection:
After I took the step today, I felt: ☐ calmer ☐ clearer ☐ steadier ☐ proud ☐ no change yet (effort still counts)

Bottom line

Don't retire from life. Retire into a new pattern of tending — your body, your relationships, and the roles that still need you.

Your lines

(write one thought, one insight, or rewrite one sentence that rang true)

_____

_____

_____

☐ Done for today

Why this matters
Writing just a few lines by hand locks the concept into memory and gently primes your subconscious mind to adopt and act on it, leading to better recall and follow-through.

DAY 97

"Health cannot be outsourced."
— A. Smyrlis, MD

Doctors and medicines can help, but they can't live your life for you.
No one else can ride your bike or walk your path.
Only you can keep choosing balance, one wobbly day at a time.

Reflection

We live in a world that quietly whispers: "There will be a pill for that." "The doctor will fix it." "If something breaks, the system will patch it." So we push. We sleep less, move less, stress more, and eat whatever is easiest — and somewhere in the back of our mind we hope that if it goes wrong, medicine will catch us.

Doctors and medications are gifts. They save lives every day. Stents open blocked arteries. Insulin keeps people alive. Antibiotics turn deadly infections into brief chapters. I'm a cardiologist; I've seen miracles in cath labs and ICUs.

But here's the truth: medicine can save you, yet it can't live your day for you. If your daily life keeps pushing against your biology, full health stays out of reach. Health isn't something done to you. It's a balance built with you.

We can diagnose disease, offer tools, and warn you about the cliff. But we can't sleep for you, walk for you, or set your boundaries. We also can't stop you from feeding the same fire we're trying to put out.

We see it all the time: a bypass and "I'm fixed," then the same habits return. A blood-pressure pill becomes permission to live at redline. Reflux meds become a license to eat late and heavy.

It's like asking someone to balance a bicycle for you while you let go of the handlebars. They might hold you for a moment. But when they step away, you fall.

Health is riding the bike yourself. You will wobble. You will drift. You will fall. Everyone does. That's not failure — it's how balance is learned. The skill is returning and adjusting.

Here is the good news: you don't have to be flawless. Your body is remarkably forgiving. It's not your enemy. It's a self-correcting system trying to bring you back to center — if you stop ignoring its signals.

Pain is your body saying, "Something is hurting."
Exhaustion is your body saying, "I'm out of fuel and repair."
Fog is your body saying, "I'm overloaded and under-rested."

You can drown those messages in noise, pills, caffeine, and distraction — or you can listen and adjust. Doctors can help. Medications can buy time. But they can't live your day for you.

Health is built in the small moments: what you reach for under stress, when you turn the lights down, whether you walk or scroll, whether you say yes or protect space. That's a sobering fact — and the doorway to real power.

Real-life snapshot

After his heart attack, Marco lay in the hospital bed and thought, "I hope this fixes me." The procedure went well. His numbers improved. The team did everything right. But at his follow-up visit, his cardiologist looked him in the eye and said: "This opened the pipe. It did not fix your life."

Instead of handing him just a list of medications, they drew a simple picture: a bike. On one wheel: medical care — pills, procedures, follow-ups. On the other wheel: daily life — sleep, food, movement, stress, tobacco/alcohol, relationships.

"If either wheel stops turning," the doctor said, "the bike falls over. I can help with this wheel. Only you can turn the other one."

Marco started small: protecting a real sleep window; walking 10–15 minutes a day; quitting smoking with support; asking his wife to help him keep sweets out of the house.

A year later, his follow-up looked more stable. But more importantly, he felt like he was riding again instead of being pushed in a wheelchair.

Quick science

- Many chronic diseases (like heart disease and type 2 diabetes) are influenced by lifestyle factors such as smoking, inactivity, diet quality, sleep, and chronic stress.
- Medications can reduce risk and manage damage, and daily habits can add meaningful support for energy, symptoms, and long-term health.
- Change doesn't have to be perfect to help; even moderate improvements in movement, sleep, and diet can improve how people feel and can improve some markers over time.[97]

Inspiration note

Your doctor can offer you a map, a lifeline, and a hand up — but only you can walk the path. The miracle is that your body wants to walk it with you.

Today's Invitation

One thing I will do for myself today:

- ☐ Sleep: Protect a real sleep window tonight.
- ☐ Fuel: Eat one real-food meal (protein + plants + healthy fat).
- ☐ Move: Move for 10 minutes today (walk, stairs, or strength).

Action Step:
Choose the easiest one today. Do it now or set one reminder and do it when it best fits your schedule.

Reflection:
After I took the step today, I felt: ☐ calmer ☐ clearer ☐ steadier ☐ proud ☐ no change yet (effort still counts)

Bottom line

You won't build durable health by leaning only on a doctor or a pill. Health is a living balance that no one else can hold for you.

Your lines

(write one thought, one insight, or rewrite one sentence that rang true)

_____

_____

_____

☐ Done for today

Why this matters
Writing just a few lines by hand locks the concept into memory and gently primes your subconscious mind to adopt and act on it, leading to better recall and follow-through.

DAY 98

"Be transformed by the renewal of your mind."
— Romans 12:2

Your mind isn't fixed — it constantly rewires based on what you feed it.
Renewal isn't a mystery; it often comes from repeated better inputs.
When you train your attention, your life quietly changes course.

Reflection

Imagine two versions of the same morning. In the first, the alarm goes off and your hand goes straight to your phone. Headlines, notifications, the market, messages. Your heart rate climbs before you've even stood up. By the time you reach the kitchen, your mind is already buzzing with other people's worries and wins. The rest of the day feels like you're chasing a train that left without you.

In the second, the alarm goes off and you give yourself a different first taste. You drink a glass of water and feel it wake your system. You step toward the window or outside for a few minutes and let real light hit your eyes. You sit down with a short passage that steadies you — a page of something uplifting, a few lines in a journal, a moment of prayer or quiet planning. Only then do you invite the outside world in. The to-do list is the same, but your nervous system is starting from a calmer place.

This is what "renewing the mind" looks like in real life. Not a single grand insight, but small, repeated choices about what you let in first and what you dwell on most. Your brain is always wiring and rewiring. Every morning you're carving a path: toward panic and distraction, or toward steadiness and purpose.

You don't have to build a perfect ritual. You just need a simple one that tells your body and mind, "We start the day on our terms." Over time, those early minutes become a quiet training ground. Worry stops being your default. Focus gets easier. The rest of your health habits finally have a place to land.

Real-life snapshot

Jon used to start every morning the same way: phone in hand, scrolling stock market headlines and social media before he even sat up. By breakfast, his mind was already buzzing with fear, comparison, and urgency. He described his days as "wired and scattered." By evening, he was exhausted but couldn't switch off.

After hearing about the power of a simple morning ritual, he decided to run a 14-day experiment. He set his phone to charge outside the bedroom and made a three-step plan:

1. Water: drink one full glass as soon as he woke.
2. Light + movement: walk outside for 10 minutes in morning light, no phone.
3. Words: sit down with a short, uplifting book and read one page, then jot one line about what mattered that day. Only after that could he touch his phone.

The first few days felt strange and "too quiet." By the end of two weeks, something had shifted. His mornings felt less frantic. His mood steadied. He found it easier to focus on deep work blocks during the day, and his evenings felt less like an adrenaline crash.

Quick science

- Repeated thought patterns strengthen related neural circuits ("neurons that fire together, wire together"), making those patterns easier to return to over time.
- Reducing negative media and social comparison, especially in the morning, can reduce perceived stress and anxiety and support steadier mood.
- Focused work blocks (instead of constant multitasking) can improve cognitive performance, reduce decision fatigue, and increase satisfaction with your day.[98]

Inspiration note

Attention is the steering wheel of your life — wherever you turn it most, you will eventually go.

Today's Invitation

One thing I will do for myself today:

- ☐ Phone later: Keep my phone off for the first 10 minutes after waking.
- ☐ Light + water first: Step toward daylight, then drink a glass of water.
- ☐ Direction first: Write 1–3 priorities so I begin with intention, not reaction.

Action Step:
Choose the easiest one today. Do it now or set one reminder and do it when it best fits your schedule.

Reflection:
After I took the step today, I felt: ☐ calmer ☐ clearer ☐ steadier ☐ proud ☐ no change yet (effort still counts)

Bottom line

Renewal doesn't happen by accident — it happens when you repeatedly aim your attention where you want your life to go.

Your lines

(write one thought, one insight, or rewrite one sentence that rang true)

_____
_____
_____

☐ Done for today

Why this matters
Writing just a few lines by hand locks the concept into memory and gently primes your subconscious mind to adopt and act on it, leading to better recall and follow-through.

DAY 99

> "A meaningful life can only be built from the inside out, never the other way around."
> — A. Smyrlis, MD

First you steady your core self.
Then you tend your immediate environment.
Only then can you shape the world around you in a way that lasts.

Reflection

Most of us are taught to build life outside in. We try to fix work, control outcomes, or rescue the world while running on fumes ourselves. We chase productivity hacks, say yes everywhere, serve everyone, and wonder why our health, patience, and joy keep slipping away.

A meaningful life doesn't work that way. It's built in three circles: Heart, Hearth, and Horizon. Heart is your inner life (sleep, nervous system, habits, self-talk). Hearth is your home climate (the people you live with, the tone, the small rituals that make home feel safe or sharp). Horizon is your outer world (work, service, community — where your gifts meet real needs).

When Heart is neglected, everything feels harder. When Hearth is tense or cold, your whole physiology stays braced. You can still function in the Horizon for a while — but it costs more than it should. It's hard to be kind at work when your sleep is frayed and your home feels like a battlefield.

Inside-out doesn't mean waiting until you are "perfect" before you make a difference. It means you start where your feet are: caring for the body and mind you live in (Heart); calming and nurturing the climate of your home (Hearth); then letting that steadiness flow into your work and service (Horizon).

Service lives in all three circles. You can serve in how you treat yourself, how you show up at home, and how you work. But your job mainly lives in the Horizon. If you build only there and ignore Heart and Hearth, the structure can't hold for long.

As your Heart steadies and your Hearth feels safer, your presence in the Horizon naturally changes. You bring less reactivity, more clarity. You're less desperate for the world to validate you, so you can serve it more cleanly. Your health supports your mission instead of collapsing under it.

Real-life snapshot

Maya and Leo were both busy professionals with two young kids. From the outside, they looked like they were doing everything "right": stable jobs, involved parents, active in their community.

Inside their home, things were frayed. Snapping over small things. Walking on eggshells. Silent evenings. Sleep was restless. They carried that tension into work and came home even more drained.

Maya kept saying, "If work would calm down, we'd be fine." Leo thought, "If the kids were older, this would be easier." Everything felt like a Horizon problem.

One evening, after a pointless argument about dishes, they decided to stop trying to fix everything "out there" and start with Heart and Hearth. They tried a simple 10-minute nightly ritual: lights down and phones away, two minutes each to answer "How are we?", one small fix for tomorrow, one genuine appreciation, and a real hug before bed.

They didn't change jobs. They didn't move. But over weeks, the climate inside their home changed. The air felt less sharp. Mornings were less rushed. Workdays felt lighter because home was no longer a silent battlefield.

"We were so busy trying to manage everything outside," Maya said, "that we forgot to build from the inside. Once we tuned our Heart and Hearth, the Horizon felt different too."

Quick science

- Chronic conflict or coldness at home can raise stress signaling, disrupt sleep, and worsen physical symptoms, even if work stress stays the same.
- Safe, supportive relationships buffer the impact of outside stress and help the nervous system recover faster after hard days.
- Emotional states spill over: improving Heart and Hearth (your inner state and home climate) often improves patience, performance, and decision-making in the Horizon (work and world).[99]

Inspiration note

A symphony tunes to one note before the concert. Tune your Heart and Hearth — then your Horizon can play in harmony.

Today's Invitation

One thing I will do for myself today:

- ☐ Heart: Take 2 minutes to breathe and return to calm.
- ☐ Hearth: Do one small act that makes home feel safer (kind words, a hug, or a tidy corner).
- ☐ Horizon: Do one values-aligned task with full presence (quality over speed).

Action Step:
Choose the easiest one today. Do it now or set one reminder and do it when it best fits your schedule.

Reflection:
After I took the step today, I felt: ☐ calmer ☐ clearer ☐ steadier ☐ proud ☐ no change yet (effort still counts)

Bottom line

A meaningful life is built most reliably from the inside out. Steady your Heart, tend your Hearth, and your work and service at the Horizon will be stronger, clearer, and far more sustainable.

Your lines

(write one thought, one insight, or rewrite one sentence that rang true)

☐ Done for today

Why this matters
Writing just a few lines by hand locks the concept into memory and gently primes your subconscious mind to adopt and act on it, leading to better recall and follow-through.

DAY 100

"Aim for love, and health will often follow."
— A. Smyrlis, MD

The deepest health decisions aren't about numbers.
They're about who you're becoming and who you're loving.
When love leads, your choices often start to change.

Reflection

At the deepest level, health is not about chasing numbers. Blood pressure, weight, labs, steps — they matter. But they are not the whole story. You can "hit your numbers" and still feel empty, frantic, or cruel to yourself.

Real health is learning to live in love's balance — giving and receiving, effort and rest, honesty and compassion, boundaries and mercy.

When you act from love — love for God, for your family, for the life you've been given — your choices shift naturally.

You stop starving or punishing your body to impress someone else. You start feeding it because you want to show up for the people you love. You stop driving yourself into the ground to look "disciplined." You start resting because your work and your relationships deserve a clear mind and a steady heart.

Your body stops being an object to force and becomes a partner in service.
That is where courage comes from.
That is where consistency lives.
That is where peace begins.
A simple way to live this out is to ask, in small moments:
"What would love choose here?"
Not fear. Not ego. Not convenience. Love.
Over time, that question will quietly reshape:

- what you eat and why
- how you move and rest
- how you talk to yourself
- how you respond to others

Not perfectly. Not all at once. But consistently enough that your life starts to feel more like it's coming from you instead of happening to you.

Real-life snapshot

Anthony spent years trying to "get in shape" from a place of self-disgust. Every diet, every workout was fueled by hatred for his body and comparison to others. He lost weight quickly, then gained it back. His labs swung. His mood did too.

One day, in a moment of honest prayer, he wrote:

"Lord, help me treat this body like a gift, not an enemy."

He started asking one question at key moments — at meals, at night, and at work: "What would love choose here so I can show up well?"

He still had days of stress and imperfection. But over months, something shifted:

- He ate fewer extremes and more real meals.
- He slept earlier more often.
- He walked to clear his head instead of scrolling.

Quick science

- Health behaviors driven by intrinsic motives (love, values, purpose) are more likely to stick than those driven only by fear or shame.
- Compassion — toward self and others — is linked with lower stress and better emotional regulation.
- Feeling connected to something larger than yourself supports resilience and makes long-term changes more sustainable.[100]

Inspiration note

Fear can scare you into a few changes. Love can walk with you for a lifetime.

Today's Invitation

One thing I will do for myself today:

- ☐ Ask the question once: What would love choose here?
- ☐ Do one gentle act: Sleep, a real meal, or movement.
- ☐ Use a kinder voice: Speak to myself with compassion while I change.

Action Step:
Choose the easiest one today. Do it now or set one reminder and do it when it best fits your schedule.

Reflection:
After I took the step today, I felt: ☐ calmer ☐ clearer ☐ steadier ☐ proud ☐ no change yet (effort still counts)

Bottom line

The push of fear is loud and short-lived; it pales in comparison to the pull of love.

Your lines

(write one thought, one insight, or rewrite one sentence that rang true)

_____
_____
_____

☐ Done for today

Why this matters
Writing just a few lines by hand locks the concept into memory and gently primes your subconscious mind to adopt and act on it, leading to better recall and follow-through.

DAY 101

"Ask and you will receive; seek and you will find."
— Jesus (Matthew 7:7)

Health is not perfection — it's returning to the basics again and again.
If you seek what heals, you can find your way back.
One small, faithful step at a time.

Reflection

You've spent this book thinking about sleep, food, light, movement, stress, boundaries, and habits. All of that matters. But underneath it all is a deeper question: what is my life for — and how do I stay steady when it's hard?

That's where prayer lives.

Prayer is not a performance. It's a turning. It's the moment you admit, I can't hold all of this alone. Help me. Guide me. Use me. When you pray, you step out of the swirl and back into the center. Your breath slows. Your shoulders drop. Your attention returns to what actually matters.

Prayer also names what's real — fear, gratitude, confusion, hope — without pretending. And it reorients you toward love: toward the people you're responsible for, the work you're called to, and the kind of person you want to be. It reminds you that you are more than your lab results and your to-do list.

From a health perspective, prayer (and related practices like quiet reflection, meditation, worship, or honest journaling) can help the nervous system settle and can make it easier to choose wisely when you're tired or stressed. It doesn't erase suffering. It gives you a place to stand inside it.

You don't have to pray perfectly, or long, or with fancy words. A few honest lines can realign a whole day:

Thank you for _____.
Help me with _____.
Show me how to love well today.

This book was never about chasing perfection. It was about remembering you are not broken, that change is possible, and that you can walk the path one day at a time — with help. Prayer is one of the simplest ways to keep that hope alive.

Real-life snapshot

Alex was in their mid-40s, working a demanding job and raising two kids. On paper, life looked good. Inside, it felt like everything was fraying.

Mornings started with heavy fog and two strong coffees. Evenings ended with scrolling, late-night email, and "just one more" episode. Sleep was broken. Energy crashed mid-afternoon. Little things set off a sharp temper — snapping at the kids, feeling irrationally angry in traffic, resenting coworkers over small requests.

Lab work was "borderline" in too many places: edging toward high blood pressure, creeping blood sugar, rising weight. Alex felt like a stranger in their own body: "I'm too young to feel this old."

A friend shared two things at once: a simple health book and an invitation to pray together once a week. Nothing dramatic. Just: "Let's try some small changes — and talk to God about it."

Alex started with tiny bricks: protecting a basic sleep window and charging the phone outside the bedroom; a 10-minute walk after dinner instead of collapsing onto the couch; one home-prepped lunch instead of relying on cafeteria food; and a three-line prayer before bed: thank you, help me, show me how to love well tomorrow.

They didn't "fix" everything. Some weeks were messy. But over a few months, the fog began to lift. Sleep deepened. The edge came off the temper. The numbers on the lab sheet nudged in a better direction.

Eventually, Alex noticed something else: coworkers and friends were describing the same exhaustion and the same 3 a.m. wake-ups. Instead of preaching, Alex quietly shared what had helped: a little structure, a little kindness to the body, and simple, honest prayer. They started a once-a-week "walk and pray" lunch with a colleague who was struggling.

"I still have hard days," Alex said. "But now, when I fall, I know how to get up. I know Who to ask, and I know a few steps to take. And I can help other people find their footing too."

Quick science

- Regular spiritual practices (prayer, meditation, reflective worship) are associated with better coping, lower perceived stress, and greater resilience in many studies, especially during illness or loss.
- Quiet, reflective practices can lower heart rate and blood pressure in the moment and may support better sleep over time.

- Feeling connected to something larger than yourself (God, meaning, purpose) is linked with better mental health and can support sustained healthy behavior change.[101]

Inspiration note

You don't have to fix everything. You have to show up, ask for help, and take the next loving step.

Today's Invitation

One thing I will do for myself today:

- ☐ Gratitude: Write one honest thank-you line before bed.
- ☐ Ask for help: Name one burden I'm carrying and ask for help with it.
- ☐ Take the next step: Choose one small faithful action for tomorrow and set a reminder now.

Action Step:
Choose the easiest one today. Do it now or set one reminder and do it when it best fits your schedule.

Reflection:
After I took the step today, I felt: ☐ calmer ☐ clearer ☐ steadier ☐ proud ☐ no change yet (effort still counts)

Bottom line

Health is the foundation that lets you live, love, and serve. Hope says it's not too late. Love says it's worth the work. Direction says the compass is inside you now. Small faithfulness says one day at a time is enough. Prayer is one of the simplest ways to keep all of that alive in your heart.

Your lines

(write one thought, one insight, or rewrite one sentence that rang true)

_____
_____
_____

☐ Done for today

Why this matters
Writing just a few lines by hand locks the concept into memory and gently primes your subconscious mind to adopt and act on it, leading to better recall and follow-through.

PART III
THE COMPASS EXPLAINED

CHAPTER 12
Your Energy Grid

How Your Body Makes Power (and How Life Quietly Steals It)

There is a moment in almost every person's journey when they say some version of, "It feels like my battery just doesn't hold a charge anymore." They try to sleep more, eat better, drink more water, take supplements, push through workouts, or rest for entire weekends — and still their energy feels thin. Not gone, but unreliable. Not broken, but inconsistent. And underneath it all lives the quiet fear that something fundamental inside them has changed.

They start to believe they've **lost their spark**. But that isn't what's happening. Your spark is still there — it's being smothered. And the thing smothering it is not your character, not your age, not a personal weakness; it's the slow, invisible dimming of your internal power grid.

Your body runs on billions of microscopic power plants called mitochondria. They take the food you eat, the oxygen you breathe, and the signals your body gets from light, movement, and timing — and convert all of that into energy your body can actually use. When these power plants hum, you feel it everywhere. Your thoughts are sharper. Your patience is longer. Your sleep is more restorative. Your mood feels sturdier. Your body feels able.

When they struggle, you feel that too.

Fog.

Heaviness.

Irritability.

Low resilience.

Restless sleep.

A sense that you're running below your potential.

The most important truth you need to hear is this: **your power plants didn't slow down because they're old — they slowed down because they're overwhelmed.**

Most people don't realize how much these tiny structures depend on rhythm. They need consistent sleep to repair. They need morning light to time their activity. They need steady meals — not perfect meals — to give them what they need to build energy. They need movement woven throughout the day to circulate nutrients and clear waste. And they need periods of true rest so the "repair crews" inside the body can come out and do their work.

When life becomes chaotic — too many late nights, too much sitting, too much stress, too much processed food, too much pollution — these power plants become confused, dysfunctional, and under-resourced. They're not broken. They're starved for the conditions that keep them strong.

Many people lose power because, as we discussed, the timing of their day has unraveled. Their energy machinery never gets a clear signal for "Go now" or "Rest now," because their sleep schedule is irregular.

Others lose power because of supply issues. They aren't getting enough protein, minerals, healthy fats, or colorful foods to give their power plants the raw parts they require. Low iron, low B vitamins and vitamin D, low magnesium — all common — quietly thin your energy long before labs show anything "abnormal."

Still others lose power because of **quiet inflammation** — the slow, smoldering kind that comes from gut irritation, sinus congestion, gum or joint inflammation. Inflammation doesn't always feel dramatic, but it blankets your power plants like smoke. They can survive in smoke — but they can't thrive.

And then there are the people who lose power because they're doing everything "right," but too much of it. Overexercising. Undereating. Working late. Forcing productivity. Living in a constant "output" state with no room for recovery. They think more effort will fix the fatigue — but their system needs less fire and more air to burn efficiently.

You may recognize yourself in one of these stories.

Or a little in all of them. The point isn't to label yourself — it's to understand your energy with compassion, not criticism.

I often think of what one of my patients, Anthony, said after he realized what caused his low energy problems and addressed it. He had spent years feeling exhausted, dragging himself through work, and propping himself up with caffeine. Nothing he tried worked. Then he made a few simple but consistent changes: morning sunlight and a vitamin D supplement for his low levels, protein with breakfast, a 10-minute walk after lunch, earlier dinners and a calmer evening routine. One day he walked into my office and said, "It feels like the lights turned back on inside me!"

This is what happens when the energy grid wakes up.

It doesn't require dramatic changes.

It doesn't require perfection.

It requires better signals — gentle ones — delivered consistently enough over weeks for your body to trust them again.

It simply needs the conditions that let those power plants turn back on.

One more piece matters here: **your body loves waves, not flat lines**. Nothing in nature runs flat. Light and dark, work and rest, feast and fast — all arrive in cycles. Your biology expects the same. When every day looks identical — same stress, same workload, same food, same intensity — your systems tire out.

Think of it more like gentle tides than a straight line. Some days emphasize effort (a strength day, a focused work block, a longer walk). Other days emphasize recovery (lighter movement, more time outside, earlier bedtime, playful time with people you love). Even supplements and workouts often work best in pulses — periods "on" and "off" — rather than the same strain every day. Waves prevent plateaus and protect you from overusing joints, pathways, and willpower.

In the **101-Day Guided Journey**, you'll learn exactly how to restore these conditions — not in overwhelming ways, but in human ways. Ways that fit around your life, your responsibilities, your limitations, and your needs.

Before we move forward, I need you to hold one simple truth close:

Your low energy is not your identity — it is a signal.

And every signal can be answered.

Your energy grid can wake up again.

Piece by piece.

Cue by cue.

Day by day.

And when it does, the life you've been trying so hard to push through will start to feel liftable again — not because you're forcing it, but because your body is finally working with you instead of against you.

CHAPTER 13
The Domino Game

How to Start Without Overhauling Your Life

By now, I hope you feel something you may not have felt in a long time: **Relief**. Not because your symptoms have vanished, but because, for the first time, they finally make sense. You're not imagining your exhaustion. You're not weak for feeling foggy. You're not lazy for wanting rest. You're simply out of rhythm — and rhythm is one of the most reversible things in human biology.

Before we move forward into the more practical chapters — Sleep, Movement, Food — I want to give you a truth that will shape everything that comes next: **you do not need to fix your entire life**. You need to shift one lever. One tiny domino. One gentle signal that tells your body, "We're coming back into alignment."

Your biology doesn't respond to intensity. It responds to consistency.

The most common mistake people make at this stage is trying to overhaul everything at once — new diet, new sleep schedule, new workout plan, new supplements, new rules. They sprint out of the gate full of hope, then burn out within days because the plan demands more than a tired body can give.

That's not how healing works.

Healing begins with one small change repeated lovingly, not forcefully — the same way you would steady the hand of a child learning to walk.

For many people, that first domino is morning light — stepping outside for ten minutes after waking. For others, it's an earlier dinner so digestion doesn't steal the night. For others, it's a calmer wind-down, softening the evening so the body can land in bed. For others still, it's simply a consistent wake time, the anchor that tethers the whole day.

Whatever your first lever is, choose something small enough that you can keep it even on your hardest day. Healing is not about heroic effort. It's about teaching your nervous system, gently and repeatedly, that it can trust you to take care of it and the world is not a threat.

Once you restore even one rhythm — sleep, light, food timing, or small bits of movement — you begin a quiet chain reaction. At first, it feels like a lot of effort for a small result. That's normal.

Think of a rocket leaving the ground. Almost all of its fuel is burned in the first few minutes, just to break free from gravity. After that, momentum carries it forward with far less energy. The hardest work is at the beginning stages.

Your health changes work the same way. The first new habit — the first steady rhythm — is your "lift-off fuel." It takes more focus at the start. But once that rhythm is in place, the others get easier.

It's also like a big puzzle: at first, every piece feels confusing. After some effort, you cross a tipping point — enough pieces are in place that the rest starts to click faster and easier.

As your first rhythm settles in, sleep steadies. Cravings soften. Mood brightens. Your mind feels less crowded. Decisions feel less impossible. The day becomes more navigable because the "gravity" you were fighting has finally begun to let go.

The hidden delay — why it feels slow (and why that's normal)

Everything in nature follows the same non-negotiable laws.

You can't plant a seed and get a tree the next morning.

Planting a new habit is the same. At first, nothing seems to be happening on the surface. The "roots" are forming underground — wiring in your brain, tiny shifts in hormones, quiet repairs in your cells.

Too many of us get impatient in this phase. We decide nothing is working, so we pull the little shoot up to "check on progress": we stop, restart, change plans, or tear everything up. In doing that, we interrupt the very roots that were just starting to take hold.

It is important to expect this natural delay instead of being surprised by it.

- Expect sleep to begin improving after two to four weeks of a steady wind-down and consistent wake time.
- Expect daytime energy to feel more stable over four to six weeks of morning light, better food timing, and daily movement.
- Expect body composition and deeper stamina to shift over eight to twelve weeks of rhythm.
- Expect a basic gut reset (as we'll see later) to need about six to eight weeks of "remove, repair, reseed, replace."

Think of it like planting a small tree: the first month is roots. The next months are trunk and branches. The fruit comes later.

Mark a 30-day check-in on your calendar now and judge your plan then — not after three "perfect" days.

Consistency beats intensity.

Keep the edges firm — morning light, last bite, lights down — and let the middle be human. You'll get there.

Before you turn the page, I need you to pause and write one soft intention — not a vow, not a rule, not a promise to become a different person, but a quiet orientation toward healing:

"I will change one thing — and trust my body to meet me there."

That's all it takes to begin.

Your body will do the rest.

Let's start with the first domino.

CHAPTER 14
Sleep

The First Domino

Most people think sleep is what happens when the day is over and "nothing important" is going on.

The science says the opposite.

When you sleep, your body runs the most powerful health program you own. Every night, if you let it, sleep quietly resets how you handle sugar and food, repairs your heart and blood vessels, trims and balances stress hormones, reloads your immune system, and gently works on the emotional weight of what you've lived through.

If sleep were packaged as a pill, it would be the most prescribed, most expensive drug in history. Instead, it's already in your hands — and even if it's been a mess for years, it can be repaired.

There is a famous natural "experiment" that happens once a year in many countries: the clock change for Daylight Saving Time.

In the spring, most people lose just one hour of sleep opportunity. Researchers looking at millions of hospital records have found that, on the very next day, heart attacks jump by around twenty percent. In the fall, when people gain an hour, heart attacks drop by a similar amount. Strokes and car crashes follow the same pattern.

One hour. One night. Enough to move heart attacks and accidents across a whole population.

I'm not telling you this to scare you. I'm telling you this to show how powerful sleep is. If losing a single hour on a single night can tip things in the wrong direction, imagine what better sleep — protected night after night — can do for you over a year or a decade.

You can't go back and erase every bad night. But from tonight forward, you can start tipping the scale in your favor.

Sleep and sugar are tied together much more closely than most people realize.

In lab studies, even one week of short sleep makes healthy young people's bodies act "prediabetic." Their cells become more resistant to insulin, the hormone that moves sugar out of the blood and into cells. The same meal suddenly produces a higher sugar spike.

At the same time, two hunger hormones drift in the wrong direction: ghrelin, the "I'm hungry" signal, goes up; leptin, the "I'm satisfied" signal, goes down.

The tired brain starts calling for quick carbohydrates and sweets — not because you are weak, but because your chemistry is shouting for fast fuel.

When sleep is steady instead of shredded, these signals are calmer and clearer. Your body uses insulin more efficiently. You feel more satisfied by real meals. It becomes easier to say no to junk food without a wrestling match in your head.

This is why, in this book, we put sleep before the "perfect diet" or the "ideal workout." If you try to fix food and exercise on a sleep-starved brain, you're rowing upstream all day.

Your immune system has night shifts and day shifts too.

At night, especially during deeper phases of sleep, your immune cells patrol more effectively. Natural killer cells and T cells — the ones that find virus-infected cells and early cancer cells — become more active and accurate.

After just one night of drastically shortened sleep, some studies have shown that natural killer cell activity can drop by more than half the next day. Over the long term, large population studies have linked chronic short sleep with higher rates of several cancers. The World Health Organization has gone so far as to classify long-term night-shift work as a "probable carcinogen," in part because of what it does to sleep and circadian rhythm.

This does not mean one bad night will cause disease. It means that, over time, steady sleep gives your immune system more full nights to repair and patrol. Your cancer-fighting cells are not gone. Many of them are simply over-tired. Sleep is how you hand them their weapons back.

You can't rewrite your years of residency, call shifts, or newborn nights. But you can absolutely stop adding extra strain now and begin handing your immune system better nights going forward.

Your brain loves sleep more than any other organ.

During deep non-REM sleep, short-term memories from the day are sorted and filed. Some are stored. Many are gently deleted. Your brain also runs something like a rinse cycle: fluid washes through and helps clear away metabolic waste, including some of the amyloid proteins linked with long-term cognitive decline and Alzheimer's.

Then comes REM sleep, the dream-rich stage, and something very special happens there.

In REM sleep, your brain replays emotional experiences with the stress chemistry turned down. You keep the story of what happened, but the sharp edge of the feeling can soften. It is like overnight emotional therapy:

- the memory is kept,
- the raw charge is slowly reduced.

When REM sleep is repeatedly disrupted — especially after traumatic experiences — those memories can stay "hot." They don't get processed and filed away as effectively. That is part of why poor sleep and nightmares are so tightly tied to persistent post-traumatic stress.

Sleep does not magically erase trauma. But without enough REM, the emotional knot is much harder to loosen. With better sleep, your brain finally gets more chances to work on those memories in the background, while you rest.

Even on ordinary days, you feel the difference. With good sleep, you wake clearer. Your patience is longer. Small hassles feel small again. With bad sleep, you forget simple things; minor problems feel enormous; noise and conflict feel unbearable. Over years, this raises the risk of anxiety, depression, and cognitive decline — not because you're weak, but because your brain is missing its nightly maintenance window.

You are not "losing your mind." Your brain simply needs more of the kind of sleep it can actually work in.

Your heart and blood vessels also depend on your nights.

During healthy sleep, your blood pressure naturally dips. This "nighttime dip" is one of the most protective things your cardiovascular system does. Your blood vessels relax and repair tiny areas of wear and tear. Your heart rate slows and deepens, giving the muscle more time to rest between beats.

When sleep is short or broken, night after night, that dip flattens. Blood pressure tends to stay higher. The lining of your blood vessels sees more inflammation and stress. Over years, the risk of hypertension, rhythm problems, and heart events climbs.

No one bad week "ruins" your heart. But every stretch of better sleep is a quiet investment in your future heart health, just as real as a medication—and often more powerful.

Many people try to get healthy by focusing on food and exercise alone. Those matter deeply. But many of your repair and growth hormones only come out fully when you sleep.

In the deeper parts of the night, growth hormone pulses — not to make you taller, but to help repair tissues, maintain muscle, support cartilage and bone. Testosterone and other sex hormones recalibrate, supporting strength, libido, and stable mood. Tiny muscle tears from daily use and exercise are patched. Connective tissues receive the signal: "Keep this, we still need it."

Without robust sleep, it becomes harder to build or maintain muscle, even if you exercise. Injuries linger. Body composition drifts toward more fat and less lean tissue, even when you haven't changed your diet much. For many people, the first "fitness change" their body truly needs is not a harder workout, but deeper, more regular sleep.

At this point, you might feel a mix of awe and worry.

Awe at what sleep does. Worry about what your past nights might mean.

This is where I want to take your shoulders down a notch.

First, the risks we've been talking about are about patterns over many years, not isolated nights. Your body is not keeping a scorecard on a single call, a few years of training, or a rough patch with your children. It responds to trends, and trends can change.

Second, the body is remarkably forgiving. Blood pressure can come down. Insulin sensitivity can improve. Natural killer cells can rebound. Nightmares can soften. You are not stuck with the fallout of your worst seasons forever.

You cannot rewrite the years behind you. You can radically improve the nights ahead of you.

When people are desperate, they quite understandably look for quick fixes. Sleeping pills are often sold as that fix.

It's important to know what they are and what they are not.

Many common prescription sleep medications are sedative-hypnotics. They are very good at one thing: sedation. They can knock you out. But sedation is not the same as natural sleep.

Under many of these medications, the brain does not reliably generate the same deep, slow brain waves of healthy non-REM sleep or the normal pattern of REM sleep. On a sleep study, it can look like a lighter, more fragmented version of sleep. Many people also feel groggy, foggy, or "off" the next day.

If we go back to our "night-shift crew" image, you can think of it this way: natural sleep is like opening the doors and letting the full crew in with the right tools, in the right order, for as long as they need. Drug-induced sedation is more like turning the lights off, shoving everyone into the building at once, and asking them to work without the right tools or sequence. The lights may be out, but the real job can't be done properly that way.

There are times when short-term medication is very appropriate — severe acute insomnia, intense situations where nothing else is available, or moments when it genuinely helps reset your sleep rhythm. That is a decision to make with your prescriber. If you're already taking one of these medicines, it's important not to stop suddenly or on your own; always talk with your prescribing doctor before making any change.

But the goal of this book is to help you rebuild the architecture of real sleep so your brain and body can work the way nature intended. The crew doesn't just need eight hours in the building. They need the right sequence and depth to actually repair you.

Let's pull all of this together.

In one ordinary night of good sleep, your body resets your blood sugar, appetite, and weight signals; lowers your blood pressure and repairs your blood vessels; re-arms your immune system to better fight infections and survey for cancer; rinses and organizes your brain; files memories and turns down the volume on painful feelings; and restores the hormones that protect muscle, bone, mood, and drive.

All while you are lying there, doing "nothing."

Sleep is not a luxury.

Sleep is not laziness.

Sleep is how your body keeps you alive and whole.

And — this is the part I most want you to carry — sleep is trainable.

You can learn, step by step, to:

- send your brain clearer day-and-night signals,
- design evenings your nervous system actually trusts,
- protect the hours when your best repair work happens,
- and give your body a chance to remember what it already knows: how to sleep.

If your nights have been restless, broken, unpredictable, or lonely, you have every reason to feel discouraged. But your story is not over.

Your nights still want to repair you.

Your body still wants to exhale.

Your deeper self still wants to sleep.

In the pages ahead — and especially in the journey section — we'll turn sleep from a source of frustration into your first domino, the one that makes every other change easier.

One cue at a time.

One night at a time.

One nervous system learning, again, how to rest.

CHAPTER 15
Movement

Your Daily Dose

Most people think exercise is something you "add on" if you have time — a gym plan, a class, a program to burn calories or earn dessert.

The science says something very different.

Movement — especially simple walking and gentle jogging — is one of the most powerful brain and mood medicines we have. Regular movement rewires how your brain handles stress and anxiety, grows and protects memory centers, can meaningfully reduce symptoms of mild to moderate depression in many people — sometimes comparable to medication in studies — and helps steady attention, impulse control, and mood across the neuropsychiatric spectrum.

If this same effect came in a pill, it would be on every billboard in the country. Instead, it's sitting there in your shoes.

And like sleep, even if your relationship with movement has been painful or complicated for years, it can be rebuilt.

Jennifer's story: from punishment to medicine

Jennifer is forty-four. She works at a desk and has spent half a decade trying to "get in shape" the way modern life teaches us.

Every January looked the same.

She'd join a gym with good intentions.

She'd go to intense classes three or four times a week.

She'd feel wrecked, sore, and exhausted.

She'd miss a week because of pain or a deadline.

Then she'd stop going and feel guilty every time she drove past the building.

Three years, three memberships, same story.

Her baseline wasn't unusual: around 2,500 steps a day, a heavy slump around three in the afternoon, rising blood pressure, and a feeling that even one flight of stairs asked more of her than it should. She didn't hate exercise; she hated what those versions of exercise did to her.

"My body just doesn't like it," she told me, half joking, half ashamed. "Maybe I'm just not an exercise person."

"Or," I said gently, "maybe your body doesn't like being attacked."

We backed up and asked a different question:

"What if movement wasn't punishment?

What if it felt like something your body could trust?"

So Jennifer did something almost embarrassingly simple. She bought a cheap step counter and spent a week just watching it. No judgment. No goals. Just data. Her average was 2,500 steps.

"That's your weather report," I told her. "Now we'll change the season."

We started by adding roughly 1,000 steps a day — ten to fifteen minutes of extra walking, broken into small pieces: a five-minute loop after lunch, a walk while making a phone call, a lazy lap around the block after dinner. As it got easier, we added more in small, realistic increments. Nothing fancy. Nothing heroic. Rule number one: you're not allowed to hurt yourself.

Three weeks later, Jennifer was averaging around 8,000 steps. She felt less foggy in the afternoons. Her mood was lighter. She still hadn't set foot in a gym.

"Twelve weeks," I told her. "Let's see where you land."

By then she hovered near 10,000 steps on most days — not as a project, but as her new normal. Her evenings no longer felt like collapse; they felt like landing. Her blood pressure started to drift down. Her sleep deepened. What surprised her most wasn't the numbers; it was how different her brain felt.

"The craziest part," she said, "is how calm I feel after walking. My head used to spin by mid-day. Now, ten minutes outside and it's like someone opened a window in my mind."

Movement didn't turn her into a fitness influencer.

It turned her into someone who could think, feel, and cope again.

What walking and jogging do to your brain

When you move your body, your brain gets a chemical and structural upgrade.

Aerobic movement — walking with some purpose, easy jogging, light running — increases a protein called BDNF: brain-derived neurotrophic factor. One psychiatrist who's written about this calls it "Miracle-Gro for the brain," and I couldn't agree more.

BDNF helps brain cells:

- grow new branches,
- strengthen existing connections,
- and even support the birth of new neurons in key areas like the hippocampus — a region crucial for memory and mood.

In older adults, regular aerobic exercise has been shown to increase hippocampal volume and improve memory, effectively reversing some of the shrinkage that comes with age.

At the same time, movement lights up and tunes the prefrontal cortex (focus, planning, impulse control), the hippocampus (learning, memory), and circuits that regulate fear and threat signals.

In plain language: walking, jogging, and running literally reshape and refuel the parts of your brain that help you think clearly and stay emotionally steady.

Creativity and problem-solving: why ideas show up on walks

This book was, in many ways, written in my walking shoes. There's another gift movement gives your brain that most people don't know about: creativity.

In simple experiments, people asked to come up with new ideas did far better when they were walking than when they were sitting. Their creative output jumped dramatically — not because they were trying harder, but because the act of walking seemed to unlock more flexible, divergent thinking.

You've probably felt this yourself: the solution that appears on a walk, the fresh angle that shows up while you're pacing on the phone, the knotty problem that suddenly loosens halfway around the block.

Walking doesn't just clear your head. It helps your brain make connections it couldn't see when you were glued to a chair.

Mood, anxiety, and trauma: why movement works where pills can't reach alone

Antidepressant medications mostly lean on a few specific neurotransmitters — for example, serotonin or norepinephrine. They can be life-saving and absolutely have their place, especially in moderate to severe depression.

Exercise, by contrast, tunes the whole orchestra.

Regular movement increases or balances:

- serotonin (mood, calm, sleep),
- dopamine (motivation, attention, pleasure),
- norepinephrine (focus, energy),
- endorphins and endocannabinoids (natural pain relief and "inner quiet"),
- and BDNF, which supports long-term brain health and plasticity.

Clinical trials and meta-analyses show that regular aerobic exercise can significantly reduce symptoms of depression and anxiety — in many cases performing about as well as antidepressant medication for mild to moderate depression, and enhancing the effect when the two are combined. For some people, exercise is enough on its own; for others, it makes medication work better.

For trauma and PTSD, movement matters too. Exercise doesn't erase painful memories, but it:

- lowers baseline stress hormones,
- improves sleep (which, as you saw in Chapter 14, is critical for emotional processing),
- and builds a stronger, more resilient brain network to handle triggers.

That's something no pill can fully replicate, because exercise isn't inserting one chemical; it's rebalancing the entire system from the ground up.

A very important note: if you are on antidepressants, mood stabilizers, or other psychiatric medications, do not change or stop them on your own. Movement is not an either/or. It is a powerful addition. Any medication decisions should be made slowly and safely with your prescriber.

Movement and the rest of your body (the short version)

You've already seen how sleep touches everything. Movement is the same.

Even simple walking:

- lowers blood pressure and improves artery flexibility,
- helps muscles soak up blood sugar so your pancreas doesn't have to shout with insulin,
- reduces inflammatory markers over time (less nasal congestion, fewer joint and back flares),
- improves balance, joint lubrication, and bone strength,
- and deepens sleep — which then amplifies all the benefits again, pushing your body into a virtuous cycle.

You don't need to memorize the mechanisms. The point is this:

Every time you move, you're not just "burning calories." You're sending a whole-body message:

"I am alive. I am using my body. Let's keep it strong and responsive. I want this body to carry me through my demanding days and well into my later years."

Your body hears that message more clearly than any speech you could give it.

"But I'm not a runner" — how to build this without breaking yourself

A lot of people read about the benefits of exercise and do what Jennifer did the first three times: launch into a plan that is way too hard for their current body, drown in soreness and shame, and then stop.

We are not doing that.

Think of movement in three gentle gears.

Baseline walking – your daily floor.
First goal: notice your current average (step-counter wristband or phone). Next: add 500–1,000 steps most days — about 5–10 minutes of extra walking. Spread it out after meals, between tasks, or while on calls. This is about being less still, not about "training."

Purposeful walking / easy aerobic – your brain tonic.
Aim for most days to include at least one 10–20 minute walk where you feel "a bit warm, breathing a little faster, but can still talk." This is the zone where BDNF and mood benefits really begin to show up over time.

Jogging and running (optional, slow transition) – your extra.
If walking feels natural and your joints are happy, you can experiment with tiny jog intervals: 30–60 seconds of very gentle jog, followed by a few minutes of walking, repeated a few times. Build slowly over weeks, not days. Your joints, tendons, and heart all need time to adapt. If pain shows up (sharp, in a joint, or lasting more than a day), back off. Pain is feedback, not a test of character.

Healthy movement doesn't mean marathons. It means stairs don't intimidate you. It means you can carry groceries or a sleepy child without feeling wrecked. It means you can get off the floor without planning your strategy. It means your legs feel warm and alive during the day, not stiff and heavy. It means that when you stop moving, you feel better, not broken.

The quiet superpower of walking after meals

There is one habit so simple and powerful that I want to name it clearly:

Walking after meals is one of the quiet superpowers of movement.

A 5–15 minute walk after eating:

- flattens sugar spikes,
- smooths afternoon crashes,

- helps digestion move along,
- steadies your mood,
- and sends your brain a signal of "we are not stuck; we are moving through life."

For people with prediabetes or type 2 diabetes, studies show that these short post-meal walks can significantly reduce post-meal glucose spikes and, over time, help improve long-term markers like HbA1c when combined with other lifestyle changes. For some, this is a key part of moving blood sugars back out of the "danger zones" toward safer ranges.

If you are on insulin or other blood-sugar-lowering medications, talk to your clinician as you add more walking — your doses may eventually need to be adjusted to avoid lows. That is a good problem to have, but it needs to be handled safely.

For many of my patients, three small walks a day have done more for their blood sugar, energy, and mood than any single intense workout ever did.

Awe, not guilt

By now, I hope you're starting to feel about movement the way you began to feel about sleep:

A little awed.

Maybe a little frustrated at how long no one told you this.

If someone could patent your daily walks, you would see commercials for them every night. Modern medicine often bends toward easier, "effort-free" solutions because that's what the system knows how to sell and bill for. A pair of shoes and a sidewalk don't make anyone rich.

That is a systems problem. It is not your failure.

Guilt has no place here. Awe and hope are appropriate. You have just learned that something very simple — walking, moving, using your body as it was designed to be used — can change your brain, your mood, your blood sugar, your sleep, and your future in ways no pill can fully match.

You don't need a perfect training plan.

You don't need to become "a runner."

You don't need to punish yourself for all the years you sat.

You need small, steady steps — steps that feel like kindness, not punishment.

Your brain is built to respond.

Your mood is built to brighten.

Your body is built to move.

And movement — simple, ordinary, human movement — is how you open that door and walk back into your own life.

CHAPTER 16
Food

Instructions for Your Brain, Energy, and Sleep

Food is not just fuel and building blocks; it is instruction.

Every bite you take tells your body what to do next: wake up or wind down, store or burn, calm or inflame. Over time, the pattern of those instructions becomes your everyday reality — your mental clarity, your cravings, your sleep, your mood, your weight, and even your sense of self.

Leah's story

Leah's days were proof of this. At thirty-nine, she led a busy team at work and carried a mental to-do list that never seemed to end. She prided herself on her resilience. But most weekdays followed the same exhausting pattern.

She would start the morning with cereal or a bagel and a large latte swirling with flavored creamer. By mid-morning she reached for a granola bar, because her energy was dipping and "there wasn't time" for anything else. Lunch was a sandwich and chips eaten in front of her laptop. In the afternoon, she reached for cookies "for focus." Dinner arrived late — usually pasta, bread, and wine, her way of unwinding and rewarding herself for getting through the day.

By 2 a.m., she was awake. Again.

Brain buzzing.

Heart not exactly racing, but not quiet either.

She would lie there, staring into the dark, thinking, Why can't I just sleep?

Morning felt heavy and thick. She woke as if someone had stolen the recharge she was promised. Coffee became less of a choice and more of a survival strategy.

"I don't understand," she said. "Why do I feel lightheaded and drained two hours after I eat… and then need to eat again just to function?"

The answer wasn't that she was weak.

The answer was that her food was issuing confused instructions.

She wasn't eating "junk" in the way most people use the word. She was eating confusing food — meals and snacks that spiked her blood sugar too high, followed by a crash that forced her brain to ride wave after wave of instability all day long. Her body never had the chance to settle into a steady rhythm, because it was constantly reacting to peaks and dips.

Fast carbs — cereal, bread, pastries, crackers, juice, sweet coffee drinks — throw sugar into the bloodstream quickly. Insulin surges to push that sugar into cells. Sugar then falls just as fast. On paper, this looks like a spike and dip. In a human life, the dip feels like shakiness, irritability, fog, and that vague, gnawing sense of "needing something" without knowing what.

When this pattern repeats all day, you live on a spike-and-crash loop. Your brain never finds steady footing.

The opposite of this is not suffering, restriction, or perfection. The opposite is steadier instruction: protein, fiber, healthy fats, and smarter timing. These give smaller rises, slower falls, and longer, smoother stretches of energy. They say to your body:

"It's okay. You're safe. You have what you need.

You don't need to ring the alarm bell every two hours."

When we talked with Leah, we didn't introduce a "diet." We introduced a different kind of day.

Instead of starting with sugar and caffeine alone, we anchored her first meal with protein — eggs and vegetables, or Greek yogurt with nuts or seeds and berries, or leftovers from last night's dinner on a bed of greens. Lunch shifted from chips and a sandwich to something her body recognized as substantial: protein, plants, healthy fat. The afternoon cookie became optional rather than automatic. If she was truly hungry, we replaced it with something that actually carried her forward — yogurt and seeds, an apple and a handful of nuts or seeds, carrots and hummus.

Most importantly, we moved most of her starch — pasta, potatoes, rice, bread — toward dinner, where it could act like a gentle brake on her nervous system instead of a roller coaster in the middle of the workday. We didn't "ban" anything. We simply reassigned it.

Six weeks later, she said, "My 10 a.m. crash is gone. I don't need emergency sugar. I'm sleeping through the night. I had no idea food timing mattered this much."

Food is language. For years, Leah's body had been listening to a frantic, choppy dialect of spikes and crashes. Once the messages softened and slowed, her system listened differently.

Food and sleep: why timing matters

This isn't only about daytime energy. It's about sleep.

Big sugar swings late in the evening can fragment sleep, trigger night sweats, and cause the 2 a.m. wake-ups that so many people blame on "stress alone." A large, rich, late dinner tells your body, "We're still in the middle of the day," while your brain is trying to say, "We're done."

A steady food rhythm — a first meal that partners with your natural morning wake signal, daytime meals spaced far enough apart to let insulin rest, and an evening meal that satisfies but doesn't overwhelm — sends a different message:

"You're allowed to rest now. The work is done."

Your body doesn't need perfection. It needs:

- a steady, balanced first meal that tells your system, "We're safe. We can start the day without panic,"
- gaps between meals so insulin and the gut can recover, instead of living under a constant drip of "just one more bite,"
- caffeine kept earlier in the day (generally avoiding it 8–10 hours before bed), so your sleep chemistry isn't fighting a stimulant all night, and
- water layered in between meals, so you're not chasing thirst with food.

Layer in water between meals — our brains often confuse thirst, tiredness, and hunger. Often, a glass of water and a short pause will make your next food choice clearer.

Your food rhythm in one glance

Here is the basic map you can hold in your head:

- Morning: more protein, fiber, and healthy fats; less sugar. Think: "steady, not spiky."
- Daytime: clear meals every 3–4 hours; minimal grazing.
- Evening: satisfying but not huge, earlier rather than right before bed; starch moved more toward dinner than breakfast.
- Always: mostly real food that once grew, swam, or walked; ultra-processed foods as the exception, not the backbone.

If you do nothing else but move gently toward this rhythm, your brain, energy, and sleep will feel it.

Ultra-processed foods: when convenience becomes a risk signal

Before we go further, it's worth giving one group of foods its own spotlight: ultra-processed foods, often shortened to UPFs.

UPFs are not just "processed" in the everyday sense (like frozen vegetables or canned beans). They are industrial formulations built from refined ingredients, additives, and flavorings, often with little resemblance to whole food. A simple rule of thumb:

If it has a long ingredient list full of things you don't keep in your kitchen — emulsifiers, colorings, "natural flavors," stabilizers, gums — it's probably a UPF.

Common everyday examples in the U.S. include:

- sweetened breakfast cereals and cereal bars
- soda, energy drinks, bottled "teas" and flavored coffee drinks
- packaged cookies, cakes, pastries, donuts
- chips, cheese puffs, flavored crackers
- fast-food burgers, chicken nuggets, and many drive-thru sandwiches
- frozen pizzas, instant noodles, boxed "helper" meals, microwave dinners
- highly sweetened or dessert-style yogurts and puddings
- many protein bars and "meal replacement" shakes that are more candy than food

These are simply what many people eat most days. The problem is not one snack or one takeout meal. The problem is when these foods quietly become most of the diet.

Beyond blood sugar spikes, UPFs may irritate and weaken the gut lining over time, like tiny fingers picking at the stitching of your intestinal wall. That irritation can keep your immune system on high alert and your brain in a low-grade fog.

Large cohort studies and meta-analyses have added another layer: **the more of your daily calories that come from UPFs, the higher the long-term risk of several major diseases.**

Across multiple European and international cohorts, researchers keep seeing a similar pattern:

- For roughly every 10% increase in the share of daily calories from ultra-processed foods, the risk of outcomes like overall cancer and early death rises by about 10–15%, even after adjusting for weight and other factors.

- Higher UPF intake has also been linked with faster cognitive decline and higher dementia risk in several large cohorts.

These are associations, not courtroom proof of direct causation. But when many different studies, in many different populations, keep showing the same dose–response pattern — "more UPF, more trouble" — it's wise to pay attention.

A simple way to frame it:

For every step your diet takes toward more ultra-processed food, the long-term risk curves bend a little further in the wrong direction.

For every step you take back toward real food, those curves can begin to bend back.

The goal is not to never touch another packaged product, or to panic over an occasional frozen pizza. The goal is to change the base of your diet.

Let foods that once grew, swam, or walked be the main characters of your day. Let ultra-processed foods be occasional side characters, not the core of every breakfast, snack, and dinner.

Food is also connection — culture, comfort, celebration. The point is not to turn every meal into a lab experiment. It's to build an everyday pattern that keeps you clear and steady, so you can actually enjoy the treats and celebrations when they come.

Eat the rainbow (color means something)

Food colors are not accidental and not decoration; nothing in nature is. They are clear signals from plants that nourish, train, and protect your cells.

- Red foods often bring compounds like lycopene.
- Orange and yellow foods carry carotenoids and other calming, antioxidant helpers.
- Greens bring sulforaphane and other detox allies.
- Blues and purples carry anthocyanins and resveratrol.
- Whites and deep reds carry ellagic acid and related defenders.

You don't need to memorize the chemistry. Your job is to invite variety.

Aim for at least five colors across most days of the week. Think: tomato or watermelon, onions or apples, a heap of dark greens or broccoli sprouts, a bowl of berries or grapes, and a handful of pomegranate seeds.

As color stacks up, cravings often quiet, and your internal defenses get daily practice instead of once-in-a-while drills.

The idea of "metabolic winter": giving healthy cells the edge

Cells that drive trouble — many pre-cancerous and cancerous cells, and certain inflammatory cells that fuel autoimmune disease and arthritis — tend to rely heavily on easy sugar. These cells seem less resilient during "leaner" times.

A life of constant snacking and sweet drinks keeps insulin high and keeps that easy fuel coming. That pattern tilts the terrain in the wrong direction. I am not implying that sugar alone causes cancer, but large cohort studies have shown that diets higher in ultra-processed, sugar-rich foods are associated with higher rates of cancer, cardiovascular disease, and dementia. The link is strong; the exact cause-and-effect is still being worked out.

Short, regular seasons of lower insulin — what we might gently call **"metabolic winter"** — tend to favor healthy cells and strain the more vulnerable ones. You don't need extreme fasting or heroic cleanses to help your terrain.

For many people, simply:

- eating in an 8–10 hour daytime window most days, and
- closing the kitchen about three hours before bed

creates 14–16 hours where sugar and insulin can drift lower and your body can enter repair mode.

Build meals around protein and plants first, then add a moderate amount of starch if you still truly want it. That alone moves you toward a quieter metabolic landscape.

If you have a cancer history, are in active treatment, are very underweight, pregnant, on insulin or certain diabetes medications, or live with a complex medical condition, talk to your care team before making major changes. The point is not punishment or deprivation. It is giving healthy cells the edge, week after week, by not bathing every waking hour in sugar.

How you cook your food is as important as what you eat: low-toxin cooking

High, dry heat makes tasty brown crusts — but it also makes by-products your body has to mop up, including compounds that can damage DNA and quietly add to your disease and inflammation load.

Common examples include:

- grilling fatty meats over open flame, where dripping fat hits hot coals or burners, creating smoke rich in PAHs (polycyclic aromatic hydrocarbons) that then stick to the surface of the meat
- pan-frying or deep-frying at very high temperatures, which can form HCAs (heterocyclic amines) and AGEs (advanced glycation end products)

Moist and lower heat keep dinner closer to "therapeutic" instead of something your system has to defend against.

Let steaming, poaching, boiling, and braising be your defaults. If you love a sear, do it quickly in a hot pan, then finish the food low and slow in the oven or in a covered pan.

A simple 30-minute marinade with citrus, herbs, garlic, or turmeric before cooking has been shown to dramatically cut the harmful compounds that form on the surface of meat or fish.

Keep oils below their smoke point; when oil smokes, you are making compounds you don't want to breathe or eat. On the grill, use indirect heat when you can, keep flame off fat drips, and cut away blackened char instead of eating it. You still get flavor and tenderness — just with less "smoke for your cells" and more room for repair in every bite.

Supplements: to take or not to take?

In an ideal world, we would not need supplements at all.

If you ate a varied diet built from animals raised on real pasture in real sunlight, eating what they were designed to eat; if your fruits and vegetables were grown in mineral-rich soil without chemicals; if you spent generous time outdoors, slept deeply, and moved your body every day — your food and your environment would likely cover everything your cells need.

That world is not the one most of us live in.

Modern life has bent the terrain. Agricultural soil, after decades of intense cultivation and chemical use, is often less mineral-rich than it once was. Many crops are bred for yield, storage, and appearance more than micronutrient density. Animals are frequently fed grains and soy instead of grass, and many see far less sun than their wild counterparts. We spend much of our time indoors, under artificial light, moving less than our grandparents did.

In short: the average plate tends to deliver fewer nutrients at the very same time that our stressed, sleep-deprived, overextended lives demand more.

In that context, the question is no longer, "Should a human ever need supplements?" but rather:

"Given the world I actually live in, can some carefully chosen supplements help close the gap?"

For many people eating a standard modern diet, my personal opinion is yes.

A high-quality multivitamin can be a simple safety net — not a license to eat poorly, but a way to help cover common gaps in everyday intake. Beyond that, a small set of targeted supplements may be reasonable for some people, especially when food quality, gut health, stress, or sleep are not where they need to be. The key is fit: choose what's appropriate for you, and confirm doses and interactions with your clinician.

- **Magnesium glycinate** can support muscle relaxation and nervous-system calm in the evening, and for many patients it becomes a gentle ally for sleep.
- **Apigenin** (often from chamomile) can also be a gentle sleep support for some people, especially when the mind feels "tired-but-wired." It's best used as a bridge while you build better light, wind-down, and timing cues. Start low, and pay attention to next-day grogginess.
- **CoQ10** helps with cellular energy production and can be particularly relevant for people on certain medications or under high metabolic demand.
- **Omega-3s** (fish oil) help counterbalance the heavy dose of omega-6 fats in the standard American diet and support brain, heart, and anti-inflammatory pathways.
- **Probiotics** can help restore some of the microbial diversity our grandparents got for free from soil, unprocessed foods, and less-sanitized environments.

None of these are magic pills. They are more like extra tools, helping a body that is doing its best in a demanding environment.

Timing matters as much as dosing. Your body is not a bucket you simply pour nutrients into; it runs on rhythms. Taking supplements in harmony with those rhythms makes them more effective and usually easier to tolerate.

- Alerting or energizing tools — like vitamin D, CoQ10, and many B vitamins — belong with daylight and food, usually in the earlier part of the day, so they support natural wakefulness instead of interfering with sleep.
- Calming tools, like magnesium glycinate and apigenin, fit better in the evening, roughly an hour before bed, as part of a wind-down routine.
- Omega-3s are often best taken with a meal that contains some fat, which can help absorption and reduce any aftertaste.

- Probiotics can be taken either in the morning or evening depending on the product and the individual, but they tend to work best when taken consistently, not sporadically.

Quality matters too. Many supplements on the shelf are more candy than care: loaded with sugar, artificial sweeteners, dyes, and unnecessary fillers. Some use the cheapest synthetic forms of vitamins, which your body may not handle as gracefully.

I generally recommend avoiding products that:

- look or taste like dessert,
- have long lists of additives, or
- rely heavily on "proprietary blends" without clear amounts.

Whenever possible, choose products that use forms of nutrients closer to those found in food and that are manufactured by companies that test for purity and potency.

Even good supplements are not neutral. They are active tools. They can interact with medications, medical conditions, and each other. Apigenin can be calming, so use extra caution if you are already taking sedating medications, and avoid stacking multiple sleep aids unless your clinician advises it. If you are pregnant, breastfeeding, on blood thinners, on diabetes or blood pressure medications, living with kidney or liver disease, dealing with heart rhythm issues, or under treatment for cancer or autoimmune disease, you should not build a supplement plan alone. This is where a thoughtful conversation with a clinician who understands both your medications and your goals is essential.

If you have to choose, spend more on real food and sleep first, supplements second. No capsule can replace a colorful plate and a decent night of rest to restore energy.

The goal is not to live "on supplements." The goal is to use them, when needed, as bridges — tools that support you while you improve food quality, mend your gut, restore your sleep, and reshape your daily rhythm. Over time, as your plate becomes more colorful, your cooking gentler, your sleep deeper, and your stress better managed, your need for certain supplements may decrease. That is success.

In a perfect ecosystem, food would be enough. In our current ecosystem, a small, carefully chosen set of supplements — used with respect for circadian timing, in clean forms, and in partnership with real food — can help close the gap between the world we live in and the level of health your body is capable of.

Rule of thumb: change one thing at a time — add only one new supplement for 7–10 days before adding another, so you can tell what's helping (or hurting).

CHAPTER 17
Gut Health

Soil Before Seeds

By now you've seen how powerfully food can shape your day — how timing and composition can steady your energy, calm your cravings, and soften those 2 a.m. wake-ups.

But there's a truth I can't leave out, because I see it almost every week in clinic: Sometimes, even when you're eating "better," you still don't feel right.

The bloat doesn't fully go away.

The fog doesn't fully lift.

Your sleep improves, but not as much as you hoped.

Your skin is still angry.

Your afternoons still swell with discomfort.

When I see that pattern, I stop and take one more step back.

Because when the soil is irritated and unbalanced, even good seeds struggle.

Maya's story

Maya is one of those people. At forty-one, she decided to restore her health and had already made serious changes. She cut back on sugar. She cooked more at home. She swapped soda for sparkling water. On paper, she was "doing the right things."

But every afternoon, like clockwork, her belly would swell. Her waistband felt tighter. A heavy fog rolled into her mind, making it hard to string thoughts together. In the evenings, her skin flared — small red patches across her chest and arms, itchier on stressful days, unpredictable but familiar. Most nights she woke around 2:30 a.m. feeling uncomfortable and oddly alert, heart a little faster than it should be.

"I'm eating healthier," she said, "but I still feel inflamed. Bloated. Foggy. Is this just my body now?"

We didn't start with exotic tests or long supplement lists. We started with a gentler question:

"What kind of soil are we asking your food to land in?"

Filter, garden, phone line

Your gut is not just plumbing. It's a filter, a living garden, and a phone line to your brain — all at once.

The filter is your gut lining.

It is unbelievably thin — just a single layer of cells standing between the outside world and your bloodstream. When that lining is healthy and tight, it lets through what you need (nutrients, water, small molecules) and keeps back what you don't (undigested fragments, microbial debris, irritants).

When it gets worn down, scraped, or loosened, tiny bits slip through that shouldn't. Your immune system sees them and raises its voice.

You feel that raised voice as tiredness, fog, joint aches, skin changes, and a jittery, unsettled feeling you can't quite name.

Researchers sometimes call this "metabolic endotoxemia" — in plain terms, tiny fragments from gut bacteria slipping into the blood and turning on a slow, body-wide alarm. You don't spike a dramatic fever. Instead, you get post-meal fog, cravings, and "I need coffee now" crashes after what looks like an ordinary lunch.

Many people call this "leaky gut." Imagine your gut as security at an airport. When the screening is tight, only the right passengers get through. When the screening gets sloppy, the wrong things slip past and stir up trouble on the other side. Some of those "wrong passengers" are modern food additives, pesticide residues, bits of bacterial debris, and other environmental toxins. Once they're past security, they can quietly hijack the flight plan of your day — inflaming your system and holding your energy, mood, and sleep hostage.

The garden is your microbiome.

This is the community of trillions of microbes that live along the lining, forming something closer to a living city than a simple patch of soil. When you feed them well, the "city" runs smoothly. The right microbes act like skilled workers and calm security guards: they help digest your food, make healing compounds that cool inflammation, support your immune system, keep the gut lining tight, and send steady messages that calm and regulate your nervous system and brain.

But when the main fuel is ultra-processed food, sugar, alcohol, and constant snacking, that city starts to fall apart. The helpful residents shrink back, and the rowdy ones move in. The garden becomes overrun with weeds — gas-producing, inflammation-stirring species that bang on the walls, irritate the lining, and keep your immune system on edge.

You don't just get bloating; you get a nervous system that feels jumpy, a brain that feels foggy, and a mood that feels hijacked by something you can't quite see — because, in a way, you are living in a body ruled by the wrong microbes.

The phone line is the gut–brain axis.
Your gut and brain are in constant two-way conversation. They speak through nerves (especially the vagus nerve), hormones, immune signals, and small molecules.

When your gut is calm, the messages sent to your brain are steady and clear. You feel more grounded, your mood feels more stable, and sleep comes more naturally. When your gut is irritated, the messages become noisy and jagged. You might feel jumpy or low with no obvious trigger. You might wake at 2 or 3 a.m. with vague unease or an undefined sense of "being off."

This is why nervous-system work — breathing, gentle movement, therapy, feeling safe — is gut work too. You can't fully heal the lining while living in a constant fight-or-flight state.

Maya's afternoons and nights were classic: a gut that was overwhelmed and inflamed, sending distress signals she felt as bloating, fog, skin flares, and broken sleep.

This wasn't "in her head."

It was in her gut.

Once we understood that, our goal was not to punish her with restrictions. It was to soothe, feed, and rebuild.

She didn't have to be perfect. She simply needed fewer irritants and more support.

How we helped Maya's gut

We eased out the loudest offenders in her diet, not forever, but long enough to let her gut take a breath: fewer packaged snacks, sweets, sugary drinks, and flour-heavy foods; gentler meals built around protein, plant fiber, and natural fats.

We shifted away from all-day grazing, because the gut absolutely needs breaks between meals to sweep, repair, and reset. When food drips in from morning to night, the housekeeper never gets a chance to clean.

We also shifted the order of her meals. Whenever she could, she started with vegetables or a small salad — letting fiber "hit first" so sugar and starches arrived more slowly. We added a spoonful of fermented foods she tolerated most days — a bit of yogurt, kefir, or sauerkraut — to gently nudge her microbes in a healthier direction.

After her main meal, she began walking for ten or fifteen minutes. That short, easy walk was not about burning calories; it was about helping blunt the sugar spikes that had been feeding the wrong bacteria and crashing her energy — and, over time, supporting a calmer barrier.

We brought in small, bitter foods — a few leaves of arugula or broccoli rabe, a squeeze of lemon with olive oil before dinner — not as a ritual of suffering, but as a tonic. Bitter flavors wake up digestive juices, signal "we're about to eat," and help move food through in a calmer way.

We paid attention to timing. Her biggest meals moved earlier in the evening. The kitchen closed about three hours before bed. That simple shift — not lying down on a full, acidic stomach — took a surprising amount of pressure off her sleep.

In other words, we began to heal that space by calming, feeding, and re-timing: calming the insults, feeding the right microbes, and re-timing when and how food arrived.

Four to six weeks later, she looked like a different person. The change wasn't cosmetic; it was in her eyes.

"The swelling is gone," she said, resting a hand on her belly. "My skin is calmer. My brain feels like it belongs to me again. And I'm sleeping."

Her afternoons were steadier. Her post-meal crashes softened. The 2:30 a.m. wake-ups became the rare exception instead of the rule. That is what it looks like when the alarm starts to turn down.

Gut healing is rarely dramatic in the moment. It is slow, quiet improvement — a little less bloat here, a little more clarity there, one fewer night-wakening, a softer sense of inflammation in your own skin. But over time, the accumulation of these small changes is enormous.

Most people feel the first shifts within 4–8 weeks. Deeper calm and resilience can take months. That's not failure — that's biology rebuilding at the speed of tissue.

How does the gut get into trouble in the first place?

Again, not usually in dramatic ways. More often, it's the small, repeated insults:

- ultra-processed foods loaded with sugars, emulsifiers, artificial ingredients, and refined flours that spike blood sugar and feed the wrong microbes
- constant snacking that never lets the gut rest between meals
- late, heavy dinners that keep your digestive tract busy long after your brain wants to sleep
- frequent use of NSAIDs (ibuprofen, Motrin, Aleve, etc.), alcohol, or other irritants
- high stress, low sleep, or shift work that keeps the nervous system on edge and the gut lining bathed in stress signals

For some, specific foods like gluten, wheat, casein (milk protein), or certain fermentable carbs (FODMAPs — fibers and sugars that some guts struggle to break down) act as louder triggers. For others, dairy causes congestion, skin changes, or digestive discomfort.

But I want to be very clear: not everyone needs to be gluten-free or dairy-free. What matters most is your pattern. Your signals. Your unique roots.

It is always wise to rule out serious gut conditions with your clinician if you have red-flag symptoms — blood in the stool, black or tarry stools, unexplained weight loss, persistent severe pain, vomiting, or a family history of inflammatory bowel disease or colon cancer. Those need medical attention, not a self-guided reset.

But for many people, especially those whose tests are "normal," the gut trouble lives in this functional space: a barrier that's a little too loose, a garden that's a bit overgrown with weeds, and a phone line to the brain that's too noisy.

Your gut is not your enemy. When it's loud, it's asking for help. When it's inflamed, it's not misbehaving — it's defending itself.

Once you begin to treat it like a living ecosystem — something to protect and nourish rather than fight — everything that sits on top of it works better. Food plans make more sense. Sleep improvements land deeper. Your nervous system feels safer. Your brain feels clearer. Your evenings feel calmer. Your nights feel quieter. Your mornings feel softer.

Food matters, deeply. But food cannot do its full job in a gut that is overwhelmed. That's why we address them together: first by stabilizing your instructions (what and when you eat), and then by tending to the soil (how your gut receives it).

Your gut doesn't need perfection. It needs less chaos and more care. And once it begins to heal, you may finally feel a sensation you've been missing for a long time: a quiet, deep "okay" in your belly — the kind that your mind can finally trust.

How you eat matters too

So far, we've talked about what and when you eat. There is another piece that is often overlooked: how you eat.

Many people eat most of their meals:

- standing up,
- in the car,
- or in front of a screen, half-focused on a spreadsheet, show, or phone.

From your gut's perspective, that looks and feels like stress. Your body reads speed, divided attention, and a flood of information as "we might not be safe." Digestive processes are dialed down; fight-or-flight is dialed up.

Whenever you can, give food its own protected space and time:

- Sit down for meals without your computer in front of you.
- Put your phone away or face-down.
- Take a breath or two before you start.
- Chew more slowly than feels "natural" at first.

This is not about perfection or rituals. It's about sending a clear signal: "We are safe enough right now to digest. We don't have to gallop this down and run."

Even a five- or ten-minute window where you honor a meal as its own activity — not multitasking fuel — can make a quiet difference to how your gut experiences the same food.

A brief note on "gut renovation" protocols

If you've read or heard about functional medicine, you've probably come across gut "reset" or "renovation" plans. Most of them share the same basic idea: give the gut a season of protection and focused support so the lining can tighten, the microbes can rebalance, and the alarm can turn down.

In practice, these plans often last around three months and include three main moves.

1. **Remove common irritants.**
   For a defined period, many protocols ask you to step away from the loudest triggers: gluten-containing grains, most dairy, ultra-processed foods, excess sugar, alcohol, and sometimes coffee for people who are very sensitive or reflux-prone. The goal isn't to label these foods as "evil forever," but to lower the daily hits on an already inflamed lining so it can breathe.

2. **Repair and feed the lining.**
   This is where targeted supplements can sometimes help. L-glutamine is an amino acid your gut cells use as fuel and is often used to support barrier repair. Butyrate, a short-chain fatty acid your own microbes make when they ferment fiber, helps nourish colon cells, cool inflammation, and support a tighter barrier. You can support butyrate naturally by eating more diverse fibers and, for people who tolerate it, by using foods like ghee

(clarified butter), which contains small amounts of butyrate along with healthy fats.

Some people also use zinc carnosine, soothing herbs, or carefully chosen probiotics — but these really need to be matched to the person, not copied from a list on the internet.

3. **Re-time eating to match your biology.**
   Many gut-focused plans use gentle time-restricted eating, such as a 16:8 pattern (eating within an eight-hour daytime window and allowing roughly sixteen hours overnight without calories). When it's a good fit, this gives the gut a longer daily window to sweep, repair, and reset, and can lower the constant insulin and sugar exposure that keep the alarm turned on.

For others, a slightly wider window (12:12 or 14:10) is safer and more sustainable, especially if there are blood sugar issues, pregnancy, a history of disordered eating, or significant underweight.

Done well, these protocols are not about starvation or punishment. They are about giving the gut a season of calm: fewer irritants, more nourishment, and clearer rhythms.

But they are also not one-size-fits-all. Medications, weight, other diagnoses, and your history all matter. If you are considering a more intensive gut renovation — taking supplements like L-glutamine, using concentrated butyrate products, or trying a strict 16:8 pattern — it is wise to do it under the guidance of an experienced health professional who understands both functional medicine principles and your medical story.

The goal is not to live in a permanent elimination diet. The goal is to give your gut enough support that, over time, you can enjoy a wider range of real foods in a body that feels calmer, clearer, and genuinely safe from the inside out.

CHAPTER 18
From Redline to Rhythm

Stress, Screens, and How to Stop Running on Empty

Most people don't need to be told they're stressed. They already know. What's harder to see is how that stress is living inside their body — how it shapes their sleep, cravings, mood, memory, and ability to recover from even small setbacks.

They know they're "always on." They just don't know how to turn "off" without feeling like everything will fall apart if they do.

Robert is fifty and runs construction projects. His days begin before dawn and rarely end before dark. He wakes to emails in bed, checks weather and schedules over coffee, fields texts from subcontractors during his commute, and steps onto the job site with three voicemails already waiting for him. By nine in the morning, his jaw is tight, his shoulders are near his ears, and his mind feels like a dozen browser tabs — all open, none fully loading.

By mid-afternoon, he becomes short and impatient. By evening, he is both wired and exhausted — scrolling, snacking, replaying arguments, mentally revising tomorrow's plan. At night, he falls asleep with his phone inches from his face, only to wake at three a.m. thinking about bills, delays, and people depending on him. He stares at the ceiling, then "just checks email" to feel less helpless.

His labs are starting to whisper. His blood pressure is edging up. His cholesterol is creeping. His fasting sugar isn't quite "bad," but it isn't entirely reassuring either. "I'm always on," he tells me. "If I let up, everything falls apart."

He doesn't need a lecture on deep breathing or a command to "stress less." He needs to understand his engine.

Stress is not the enemy. Mismanaged stress is. A better word for stress is activation.

Your stress response is like an engine with multiple gears. Short bursts of activation are not only normal — they're healthy and vital. They mobilize energy, sharpen focus, and help you perform when a problem needs solving or a challenge needs meeting.

The issue arises when that engine never drops the RPMs, when every email, every notification, every minor inconvenience, every thought of tomorrow keeps your nervous system hovering near redline.

Robert is not broken. He's been living with his foot welded to the gas pedal for so long that he can't remember what "idle" feels like.

Then there's Nadia, forty-six, an architect who built her identity around relentless output. She worked late nights "just to be safe," ate lunches at her desk, and spent Saturdays "catching up." She believed rest was something you earned by finishing everything — and she never finished everything. Her body kept score with migraines, neck and back tension, and crushing exhaustion that refused to translate into deep sleep.

She took a week off once and mostly slept. Two weeks after returning to "normal," all the same symptoms roared back.

"If I stop pushing," she said, "I'll fall behind. Everyone else is going full speed."

Her rhythm had flattened into one long, endless push. No waves. No exhale. No off-switch. Just a straight line.

But biology doesn't run on straight lines.

It runs on waves.

Your heart beats in pulses — squeeze, relax.

Your breath flows in and out — inhale, exhale.

Your brain works in cycles of deep focus and natural dips.

Your gut works after meals and cleans between them.

Your hormones rise and fall by day, month, and season.

When your life honors those waves, your system has a chance to repair. It's the difference between hacking all day with a dull saw and taking time to sharpen it. Abraham Lincoln is often quoted as saying, "Give me four hours to cut down a tree, and I will spend the first three sharpening the saw." Respecting rhythm is how you sharpen your saw in real life.

Stress comes in manageable bursts; recovery follows. You can push hard and then genuinely rest. You fall asleep without feeling like your nervous system is screaming. You wake tired some days, yes, but not endlessly exhausted.

When your life crushes those waves into a flat line of "always on," everything blurs and dulls.

You become half-tired, half-wired.

Small setbacks feel like collapses.

You don't bounce back — you drag back.

Robert and Nadia look different on the outside, but inside they share the same problem: no gears.

In the modern world, stress is no longer a sharp spike followed by recovery like it was for millennia — it's a low-grade hum carried in your posture, your breath, your pulse, your inbox, and your pillow.

Screens don't help. They drip stimulation into your brain from the moment you open your eyes to the moment you close them — news, arguments, to-dos, notifications, tiny hits of dopamine over and over again until you feel tired but not satisfied, busy but not productive, connected but not truly present.

Your brain's reward system — the circuitry that uses dopamine to motivate you — becomes trained on crumbs: likes, pings, scrolls, jumps, sugar, caffeine. None of these are evil. They just become constant. And anything constant loses its impact.

Over time, your internal bar rises. You need more stimulation to feel the same "okay." Coffee doesn't work as well as it used to. Scrolling stretches longer. Real-life pleasures like a quiet walk, a deep conversation, or an hour of true focus feel oddly flat because your brain is used to quick, frequent hits.

On top of this, your focus system — which was built to give you stretches of single-task attention — is constantly being shredded into fragments. Every tab you flip to blindly, every notification you answer immediately, every "just checking" your phone for no reason, costs you. Not because you're morally failing, but because brain chemistry and energy resources are finite.

Switching focus costs energy. Frequent switching costs a lot of energy. By the end of the day, you feel like you've driven in stop-and-go city traffic: always moving a little, never getting far, completely drained.

None of this happened because you lack discipline. It happened because the modern environment is designed to hijack your brain's stress, reward, and attention systems. Your job is not to eliminate stress or screens. Your job is to take back the steering wheel.

Dopamine: earned vs. bought

Dopamine is your brain's "that mattered" signal. You can earn it through effort — or buy a quick hit with sugar, alcohol, or endless scroll. The quick route feels good for a moment, then flattens your ability to feel good without it. The earned route starts rough but restores motivation, pleasure, and pride.

A simple reset: put a small effort before each reward.

- Ten minutes of walking or one focused task before coffee.
- Finish a tough email before a treat.
- Delay a craving by ten minutes and step outside for three slow breaths; most urges fade.
- Keep your biggest treats earlier in the day and after real food, not late at night alone in the dark.

Over days, you'll notice less "itch," more calm, and the return of simple joys — sun on your skin, a clear thought, a good laugh — without needing to push the brain's gas pedal all day.

When I work with people like Robert and Nadia, I don't tell them to quit their jobs or throw their phones away. I help them learn the gears.

They start by discovering what "brake" feels like in their bodies. Not a vacation, not a weekend away — a sixty-second brake they can access anytime. Slow breathing. Shoulders softening. Jaw unclenching. One minute before the first big task of the day, one minute before lunch, one minute before bed. Not a grand ritual. Just a signal to the nervous system: we can afford to shift down for a moment.

Then we help them reclaim their attention. This doesn't require a monastery. It requires boundaries.

Instead of living in a blur of constant checking, they choose a small number of times each day when they will open their inbox, answer texts, or handle messages — and let everything else wait. They protect at least one block of time — forty-five to ninety minutes — where they do one thing only: one task, one screen, one direction.

When distractions arise, they write them down instead of acting on them. They turn notifications off by default and let only true emergencies break through. They treat their attention like a resource, not like an open trash can.

Over time, their days feel less like city traffic and more like highway: fewer starts and stops, more steady progress, less white-knuckle driving.

Finally, we tune their rhythm. Instead of pushing their hardest work into the latest hours of the day — when their biology is trying to wind down — we shift as much as possible to the first half, when cortisol and alertness are naturally higher. We place physically demanding workouts earlier, when the stress they induce will be processed and integrated by a system that's awake. In the evenings, we favor gentler movement, slower conversation, softer light.

None of this erases stress.

It simply gives it shape.

Stress becomes a wave you can ride rather than a tide that drags you under.

Nadia learned to build waves into her life on purpose. She still works hard. She still cares about her craft. But she now structures her weeks with focus blocks and real breaks. She protects one true day off — inbox closed, no "just checking." Once a month, she has a lighter "deload" week where she reduces the intensity of her training and aims to finish projects rather than start new ones. She moved dinner earlier, set a consistent sleep window, and gave herself five minutes most evenings to breathe slowly with the lights dimmed.

Three months later, she didn't tell me she had less stress. She told me something much more important: "I get more done now, but it doesn't feel like drowning. I don't fear a bad week anymore. I know how to recover."

That is resilience.

Resilience is not never falling. It's recovering more gently and more quickly. It's knowing how to come back from stress instead of staying stuck inside it.

You will never have a stress-free life. You don't need one.

What you need is:

A nervous system that knows what "brake" feels like.

Attention that isn't spent on crumbs.

Days that move in waves, not in a continuous line.

Evenings that let you step out of the driver's seat instead of falling asleep in it.

As you move through this book, you'll see how sleep, movement, food, gut health, and stress all interlock. For now, remember this simple truth:

You don't have to earn rest by breaking yourself.

You don't have to justify boundaries with collapse.

You don't have to live with your foot on the gas to be worthy or reliable or successful.

Your brain, your body, your heart — they all need rhythm.

And rhythm is something we can rebuild, together, one small gear shift at a time.

CHAPTER 19
Hidden Saboteurs

The Things You Can't See But Your Body Can

The Backpack You Didn't Know You Were Wearing

Imagine you're wearing a backpack.

Every time you drink water with PFAS or lead, a small stone goes in.

Every time you breathe dust laced with flame retardants or pesticides, another stone.

Every time you microwave in plastic, cook on flaking non-stick, or breathe heavy fragrance, more stones.

One stone? No problem.

Ten stones? Still fine.

Hundreds of stones over ten or twenty years?

Now your shoulders ache, your steps feel heavier, and a walk that used to feel easy suddenly feels like a climb. You didn't become "weak." The load quietly increased.

Some people have sturdier straps and stronger backs; others are more like the canaries miners once used to detect danger early. These "sensitive" people — the ones who get headaches in new buildings, feel sick around strong perfumes, or crash with brain fog after shopping in the cleaning aisle — are not fragile. They are early warning signals for the rest of us.

For an extreme example of what a suddenly overloaded backpack can do, think of the 9/11 responders who worked at Ground Zero. The dust cloud they breathed was not ordinary dust; it was a highly alkaline mix of pulverized concrete, glass fibers, asbestos, heavy metals, and combustion by-products. Many worked for weeks or months in that environment with little or no respiratory protection. In the years that followed, large health registries found high rates of chronic cough, sinus and reflux problems, asthma, sleep apnea, PTSD, and, over time, excess cancers in these workers — especially in those with the heaviest dust exposure. Their backpack wasn't loaded over decades; it was filled almost overnight.

Most of us will never face that kind of single, catastrophic exposure. But their experience reminds us that **what's in the air, water, and dust around us matters** — and that the body can only carry so much before systems start to show strain.

You cannot remove every stone. That's not the goal.

The goal is to lighten the backpack enough that your built-in detox systems can keep up again.

Your liver, kidneys, lungs, gut, skin, lymphatics, mitochondria — these are not fragile organs. They are robust, adaptive, and wired to protect you. But modern life throws more at them than they were designed to handle.

You don't need a "cleanse" as much as you need a quieter environment to live in.

Claire's story

Claire was, on paper, a "success story."

She had cleaned up her sleep, started walking after meals, cooked more at home, and pulled her evenings back from the edge of overload. Her numbers improved. Her weight stabilized. Her sleep was better than it had been in years.

And yet, by lunchtime, it still felt like someone had packed sand around her brain.

Most days, a dull headache slid in around noon. By mid-afternoon, she found herself rereading the same sentence three times. At night she was "tired but wired" — too wound up to fully rest, too drained to feel like the person she used to be.

"I guess I'm just getting older," she said at first.

Then she blamed coffee.

Then she blamed herself.

Her labs were "normal." Her scans were "normal." Her sleep tracker looked "fine."

But her life wasn't.

We had already worked on the obvious roots — sleep, food, movement, stress. So I asked a different question:

"Walk me through your day — not just what you do, but what you live in."

That's when the picture changed.

Her office looked beautiful if you only used your eyes: bright white walls, a stylish plastic fiddle-leaf fig, soft gray carpet that somehow never stained, and a plug-in that promised "ocean breeze" but smelled like a department-store perfume aisle. Behind one wall, a slow leak had quietly fed a thin line of mold. The "never-stain" carpet was treated with stain-guard chemicals that don't just stay in the fibers — they slowly shed into dust and indoor air, hitchhiking on the very dust she breathed in every day. The plastic plant off-gassed more VOCs every afternoon when the sun hit it. The plug-in atomized synthetic fragrance — including phthalates and other compounds — into the air her brain needed to think.

At home, she microwaved leftovers in plastic containers because it was fast. She drank hot coffee from a scratched non-stick travel mug she'd had for years. Her water pitcher looked fancy but barely removed the contaminants in her area. She loved scented candles and fabric softener because they made the house "feel clean."

Claire wasn't broken.

Her body was simply processing far more than its fair share.

She had been working hard on the levers she could see — sleep, food, movement, schedule — while another set of levers, the invisible ones, stayed untouched. Her biology was like a worker trying to repair a house while someone quietly kept punching new holes in the roof.

This chapter is about those holes.

Not to scare you. To help you see what your body has been seeing all along — and to show you how a few simple changes can unlock energy, clarity, and sleep you may have given up on.

Water: Clear Isn't Always Clean

Most people assume clear water is safe water. It often isn't that simple.

Your tap may carry things you cannot see or taste:

- PFAS ("forever chemicals")
- Lead and other metals from old pipes
- Industrial by-products from upstream
- Agricultural residues

None of these make the water cloudy. None of them give it a smell.

All of them tell your liver: "You'll be busy today."

Moving from no filtration to a good, independently tested carbon filter or reverse-osmosis system is already a meaningful step. Over time, cleaner water means a lighter backpack and a quieter workload for your body.

Air and Dust: The Invisible Highway

We think of air as "fine" or "polluted." In reality, indoor air lives on a spectrum — and you have far more power over it than you think.

Dust is like a taxi for chemicals:

- Flame retardants from couches and mattresses
- Stain guards from carpets and upholstery
- Pesticides tracked in on the soles of shoes

- VOCs from fresh paint, glues, and plastics
- Mold spores from tiny leaks and damp corners

You don't need an engineering degree to make things better. Small habits help a lot:

- Shoes off at the door so the outside doesn't ride in on your floors
- Damp-dust once a week instead of just pushing dust around
- Vacuum with a HEPA filter, especially in bedrooms and carpets
- Fix leaks early; don't let "a little damp" become "a quiet mold problem"
- Run kitchen and bathroom fans; crack windows when outdoor air is decent
- Consider a small HEPA + carbon air purifier in the bedroom so your brain and lungs get eight hours of cleaner air while you sleep

These are not boutique wellness hacks.
They are boring, beautiful ways to stop loading your system while you rest.

The Kitchen: Heat, Plastic, and Old Non-Stick

The kitchen should be where healing begins. Often it's where another layer of exposure sneaks in.

Three simple principles carry most of the benefit:

1. **Don't heat food in plastic.**
   Microwaving in plastic containers or covering hot dishes with plastic wrap nudges tiny amounts of chemicals into your food, especially with oily or acidic sauces.

2. **Retire flaking non-stick.**
   Deep scratches or peeling coatings belong in the trash, not on your stove. Favor stainless steel, cast iron, or enamel for most cooking. If you keep any non-stick, use it at lower heat and replace it if it nicks.

3. **Watch the hot water path.**
   Super-hot water forced through plastic pods and plastic tubing can leach microplastics and other compounds into your morning coffee. Where possible, let hot water meet glass or stainless steel instead.

These are not dramatic moves.
They're quiet acts of protection your future self will thank you for.

Fragrances: When "Clean" Smells Dirty to the Body

Most people's homes smell like something: fresh linen, ocean breeze, seasonal spice, floral mist.

To the body, that often translates to one word: load.

Plug-in air fresheners, heavily scented candles, room sprays, fabric softeners, strongly perfumed detergents and cleaners — all of them send volatile organic compounds into your air. For some people, they are the single biggest trigger for:

- Headaches
- Brain fog
- Sinus congestion
- Irritability
- Sleep disruption

You don't have to live in a scent-free monastery. Just choose:

- Unplug plug-ins.
- Reserve intense scents for special occasions, not 24/7 background.
- Make the bedroom fragrance-free so your nervous system has one room where it doesn't have to negotiate with chemicals all night.

Clean doesn't need a smell.
It can simply feel like calm air.

Mold: The Quiet Saboteur

Mold is everywhere in nature. Your body can handle traces.

Trouble starts when water stays where it doesn't belong — behind walls, under carpets, in basements, around windows — and feeds a colony.

Not everyone is mold-sensitive. But for those who are, even small exposures can mean:

- Fatigue that makes no sense on paper
- Brain fog and word-finding glitches
- Sinus trouble, cough, asthma flares
- Sleep that feels "shallow" and unrefreshing

If you've had leaks, dampness, visible growth, or a musty smell that never quite goes away, take it seriously. You don't need fear; you need a plan: fix the moisture, assess the space, remediate properly if needed.

Heavy Metals: Mercury and Friends

Two under-appreciated sources you already know:

- Big predatory fish (tuna, swordfish, king mackerel, shark)
- Old "silver" dental fillings (which are about half mercury)

Over time, low-level mercury exposure can show up as:

- Brain fog
- Headaches
- Low mood
- Stubborn fatigue

You don't have to fear the ocean. You just need to eat lower on the food chain most of the time: wild salmon, sardines, anchovies, trout.

If your fillings are cracked or failing, don't rush to a random drill. Mercury-containing fillings should be removed only by a dentist trained in safe protocols (SMART/IAOMT), with proper suction, barriers, and ventilation.

Your body's clearance systems love:

- Cruciferous vegetables (broccoli, cabbage, arugula, sprouts)
- Enough fiber to keep stools regular
- Hydration
- Nutrients like vitamin C and selenium

More advanced supports like NAC or glutathione sometimes help — but only after the basics are in place, and ideally with professional guidance.

The point isn't panic.

It's smarter sources, safer dentistry, and better exits.

A Quiet Question in the Grocery Aisle

Picture a normal day:

- Oat cereal in the morning
- A granola bar mid-morning
- Crackers with lunch
- Pasta at night
- A cookie after dinner
- A salad "for balance"

Nothing wild. Just grocery-store life.

When independent labs tested these kinds of foods, they found that some oat-based cereals and snack bars carried glyphosate residues in the low thousands of parts per billion. Still within current legal limits — but higher than most people realize.

If someone eats several of these foods in a single day, their intake can add up to measurable doses of pesticide — again, not an acute poison, not illegal, but also not something most people know they're eating.

This chapter isn't here to settle the debate about any one chemical.

It's here to ask a simple question:

If a chemical is traveling in your food, shouldn't you at least know it's there?

We already label sugar.

We label fats, allergens, colors, and preservatives.

Adding a simple note about pesticide residues wouldn't restrict anyone's freedom. It would simply give people one more moment to pause and ask:

"Is this what I want to eat today?"

And once you ask that question about glyphosate, you begin to see the broader picture: phthalates drifting from perfumes into your lungs. PFAS baked into nonstick surfaces and food packaging. Dyes, emulsifiers, and preservatives slipping into meals. None of them on a bold front label. None of them announcing themselves to the tired parent in the aisle trying to do their best.

The real issue is not one chemical.

It's the principle: Do people have the right to see what they're bringing into their bodies before they decide?

You do, now.

The First Line of Detox Is Not a Pill

You will see many products promising to "detox," "cleanse," "reset," or "pull toxins" from your system. Some have their place.

But for most people, the first line of detox is not a supplement. It is your life. It is:

- Cleaner water
- Cleaner air
- Less heated plastic
- Less unnecessary fragrance
- Less dust and mold
- More fiber

- More sweat from walks, chores, warm baths, or sauna when appropriate
- More bowel regularity
- More sleep

Only after you reduce what comes in and support what goes out does it make sense to consider targeted binders, antioxidants, or more advanced protocols — and even then, carefully, with guidance, and never in a body that is already constipated, underslept, and under-fed.

Detox that makes you dramatically sicker is not a badge of honor.

It is usually a sign that your bucket was already overflowing.

Claire's Second Chapter

Claire didn't move to the countryside.

She didn't turn her life into a lab.

She filtered her drinking and cooking water.

She unplugged the plug-ins and put heavy scents away.

She stopped microwaving in plastic and bought a few glass containers.

She retired her oldest nonstick pan and scratched mug.

She took her shoes off at the door, damp-dusted once a week, and added a small purifier to her bedroom.

No dramatic "detox."

No extreme protocol.

Just fewer stones in the backpack.

Two weeks passed. Not much changed.

By week four, she noticed she hadn't had a midday headache in a while. Her brain felt a little clearer in afternoon meetings. Her sleep felt deeper. She woke up feeling just slightly less burdened.

It wasn't a miracle.

It was her biology finally able to do its job.

Your body is not trying to betray you.

It is trying to protect you in a world that keeps quietly loading your pack.

Lighten the load, and the systems you thought were "broken" often start working again.

What You Need to Remember

You cannot — and do not need to — eliminate every toxin.
You can:

- Stop heating food in plastic
- Store and reheat in glass
- Cook most meals on stainless, cast iron, or enamel
- Filter your water
- Run a HEPA purifier where you sleep
- Unplug unnecessary fragrances
- Fix leaks
- Choose lower-mercury fish
- And ask, gently but firmly, "What's in this?" before you bring it home

Small, boring changes done every day will protect you more than any three-day cleanse ever will.

Your body wants to heal.

If you give it cleaner inputs and lighter surroundings, it often will — quietly, steadily, faithfully.

You don't need to fear the invisible.

You just need to know it's there.

Then, step by step, you can choose differently.

PART IV

LIVING WITH THE COMPASS

If you're reading this page, you already did what most people never do:
you stopped long enough to tell the truth.
You looked at health from every angle — sleep, food, movement, stress, environment, connection, and meaning. And here's what matters most:

You already know enough.
Not enough to master every molecule.
Enough to know what changes a real life.
Sleep is repair.
Real food, in rhythm, steadies the whole system.
Walking is medicine.
Your nervous system was never meant to live at redline.
Light, water, air, toxins, and screens quietly steer your biology.
Relationships and meaning aren't extras — they're the center.
And love, alignment, and a deeper order can steady the heart.
So here is what you don't need:
a perfect plan, more rules, or permission from any expert — including me.

What you need now is trust.
Trust that small, honest changes count.
Trust that the same intelligence keeping your heart beating can guide your next step.
The bridge from knowing to living is not more information.
It's the quiet turn inside that says: *This time, I'm not just reading. I'm walking.*
Not yesterday's choices. Not old regrets.
Today's choices:
One earlier bedtime.
One walk after dinner.
One real-food meal.
One glass of water before coffee.
One "no" to what drains you.
One minute of prayer, gratitude, or stillness.
They look small. But they are votes — cast in the direction of life.
If you've finished the 101 days and you've made progress, celebrate it.
And if you want more, don't hunt for a new plan. Walk the journey again.
The first lap rebuilds rhythm and trust. The second builds resilience and staying power.

From this moment forward, see yourself as someone already on the path.
Not starting Monday. Not after the next crisis. Now.
You don't need to walk perfectly.
You only need to keep walking.
And as you close this book, here is my wish for you:
May you remember your body is not random parts,
but a living instrument designed for rhythm, joy, and service.
May you remember you already know enough to begin—
and that beginning is worth more than a lifetime of waiting.
May you be protected from perfectionism.
May small steps feel meaningful.
May setbacks become teachers, not verdicts.
May wisdom, grace, and love guide your hand
as you choose how to eat, move, rest, connect, and live.
The path is under your feet.
Walk it — one loving choice at a time—
and let the next chapter of your life begin.

One last Invitation…
If this book was gifted to you and it helped in any way,
    please consider gifting it forward to someone you care about.
    It will do more good in their hands than sitting quietly on a shelf.

A permission to share
If one of these daily entries really helped you, you're welcome to share a small part of it with someone you love — a line, a short paragraph, or a quick photo.
    Little pieces, passed from hand to hand, are how this book will quietly find the people who need it most.
    And if you have a moment, please consider leaving a short review on Amazon.com. Your words help others who are tired and discouraged
    to find something that might finally help them too.
    Thank you for reading.
    Thank you for choosing to care for your health.
    I'm grateful you walked this journey with me.

BONUS: "THE COMPASS"

A closing poem to return to when you drift.

"THE COMPASS"

In the quiet pulse of dawn
I choose rhythm over rush.
Enduring principles — true balance —
the key to life's riddle.
I greet the morning light like an old friend,
long before the glow of screens.
At day's end, the sunset sings me into stillness;
with every shiver of the soul I know:
nothing ends but lives forever in light beyond sight.
Feasts and fasts honor the body's ancient clocks.
My home is a sanctuary, free of hidden harms.
I am a river finding the sea,
growing stronger as I follow nature's mandates.
I have walked the valley by night,
stumbled where you stumble —
so I know the way through.
With this compass
and the tools of healing in hand,
I turn toward true health —
my true north and the purpose of life.
— A. Smyrlis, MD

NOTES & SOURCES

How to use these notes: In the 101-Day Guided Journey, each Quick Science section includes a single superscript number (for example, [7]). That number matches the Day number.

To find the sources for a Day, go to the Quick Science Index by Day below and look up that Day. The index will point you to one or more endnote clusters (EN01–EN39). Then go to those cluster entries for the full citations.

Example: If you see [7] in the text, look up Day 7 in the index. It will point you to EN17.

Quick Science by-Day Mapping

Day	EN cluster(s)	Quick topic cue (first bullet)
1	EN01	Biological age is an estimate of how much "wear and tear" your body has accumulated, and scientists can approximate it using tests like DNA methylation ("epigenetic clocks") and other biomarkers.
2	EN02	Smartphones and blue-light screens at night suppress melatonin and disturb circadian rhythms, leading to poorer sleep quality and higher long-term health risks.
3	EN07, EN06	Brief walking bouts (5–10 minutes) can improve alertness and mood within minutes and help stabilize blood sugar when done after meals.
4	EN03, EN04	Sleep loss impairs emotional regulation and decision-making, making you more impulsive, more irritable, and more likely to choose unhealthy foods and behaviors.
5	EN02, EN09	A consistent morning routine is linked with better mood and lower perceived stress.
6	EN09	Returning quickly ("never miss twice") keeps small slips from turning into full drop-offs.
7	EN17	Genuine laughter reduces stress hormones like cortisol and adrenaline while increasing endorphins, your body's natural pain-relieving and feel-good chemicals.
8	EN11	Constant multitasking and task-switching increase mental fatigue and reduce efficiency; you lose time and quality every time you jump between tasks instead of focusing on one.

9	EN12	Even mild dehydration (1–2% loss of body weight in water) can impair attention, memory, and mood — you feel more tired, scattered, and irritable.
10	EN13	Reducing mental and digital clutter lowers stress hormones like cortisol and can improve focus and decision-making.
11	EN09, EN30	Visible tracking increases follow-through because progress is motivating.
12	EN18	Strong social connection and community involvement are linked with lower risk of death from many causes and better heart health.
13	EN36, EN33	Many essential substances — including water, vitamins, and minerals — have a therapeutic window: too little causes deficiency, too much causes toxicity.
14	EN01, EN22	Epigenetic mechanisms (like DNA methylation and histone modification) respond to lifestyle inputs — sleep, food, stress, and movement can literally change how certain genes are expressed.
15	EN22	Protein and healthy fats slow stomach emptying, which smooths the rise and fall of blood sugar and provides amino acids for neurotransmitters (brain chemicals) that regulate mood and focus.
16	EN14	Longer exhales increase vagal tone and help downshift the fight-or-flight response.
17	EN15, EN09	Psychological flexibility is linked to lower distress, better health behaviors, and higher persistence.
18	EN13, EN30	Chronic sympathetic overdrive raises blood pressure, tightens blood vessels, and blunts immune function.
19	EN13, EN15	Low motivation and heavier fatigue can reflect overload and stress physiology — not personal weakness.
20	EN17	Play and creative activities can reduce perceived stress and improve mood by engaging brain circuits tied to reward, curiosity, and exploration.
21	EN11	Quiet, reflective time can help your nervous system downshift and settle.
22	EN20	Telling people what they "must" do often triggers psychological reactance — a defensive pushback that makes them less likely to change.
23	EN06	Higher daily step counts are consistently associated with lower all-cause and cardiovascular mortality.
24	EN30, EN07, EN22	Lifestyle changes (nutrition, movement, weight loss, alcohol reduction, and stress management) can meaningfully improve blood pressure, blood sugar, and cholesterol — and for some people can be comparable to first-line medications, especially when combined.

25	EN03	Chronic sleep debt (regularly <6–7 hours per night) raises insulin resistance, blood pressure, and inflammation, all of which damage the endothelium and increase cardiovascular risk.
26	EN20	A strong sense of purpose is linked with lower all-cause mortality and better cardiovascular outcomes.
27	EN22, EN26	Soluble fiber (like the pectin in apples and the fiber in berries) slows glucose absorption and feeds healthy gut bacteria.
28	EN02, EN23	Morning outdoor light helps entrain the brain's master clock (the suprachiasmatic nucleus, SCN), synchronizing circadian rhythm and supporting energy, mood, and hormone timing.
29	EN14	Paced breathing — especially with longer exhales (for example, in for 4 seconds, out for 6) — can increase parasympathetic activity (vagal tone) and help the body downshift; over time it may support lower resting heart rate and blood pressure.
30	EN11	Task switching carries measurable "switch costs" — it slows thinking, increases errors, and raises subjective fatigue.
31	EN33	Chemicals like PFAS, phthalates, and certain VOCs can act as endocrine disruptors and immune irritants, subtly influencing hormones, inflammation, and metabolism over time.
32	EN09, EN35	Repeating a small behavior in the same context (same time, same cue) strengthens neural pathways in the basal ganglia, turning effortful actions into easier, automatic habits.
33	EN04	Slow-wave sleep (SWS) — the deepest, most physically restorative stage — peaks in the first half of the night and is crucial for metabolic repair, immune function, and hormone balance.
34	EN08	Regular stair climbing in short bouts improves cardiovascular fitness and VO2 max, even when total exercise time is modest.
35	EN22, EN24	Real food changes signals. Meals higher in fiber, protein, and unsaturated fats tend to flatten glucose spikes, improve satiety, and reduce inflammatory stress on blood vessels (endothelial function).
36	EN18	Social connection is reliably associated with better longevity and cardiovascular outcomes.
37	EN21, EN13	After basic financial security is met, additional income tends to bring smaller gains in day-to-day well-being.
38	EN32, EN15	Matching pace to current capacity lowers injury risk and burnout, and helps you keep going long enough to improve.
39	EN23, EN22	Eating to comfortable satisfaction (often described as ~70–80% full) can improve post-meal glucose control and may reduce markers of oxidative stress.
40	EN09	Writing down a clear goal and seeing it often (on a card, screen, or wall) "primes" the brain — making choices that match that goal easier and more automatic.

41	EN13, EN32	Bodies adapt best to cycles of stress and recovery. Constant high stress without rest drives allostatic load — the wear-and-tear of never turning off — which is linked to fatigue, depression, and chronic disease.
42	EN15	Self-compassion practices (kind self-talk, hand-over-heart) are associated with lower shame and anxiety, and greater emotional resilience.
43	EN13	High gear (sympathetic activation) is essential for focus and performance, but chronic overactivation without enough parasympathetic time is linked to hypertension, impaired immunity, and burnout.
44	EN29	Living in greener environments and spending time in parks and forests are associated with lower mortality, better mental health, and improved cardiovascular outcomes.
45	EN31	Preventive health behaviors — such as not smoking, regular movement, mostly whole-food eating, and adequate sleep — substantially reduce the risk of chronic diseases that are costly in both money and quality of life.
46	EN31	Small, steady lifestyle changes — more walking, fiber-rich whole foods, earlier sleep — can start improving blood pressure, blood sugar, and triglycerides within a few months, even before the scale moves much.
47	EN11, EN17	High exposure to distressing media is associated with higher perceived stress and anxiety, and a more pessimistic view of the world.
48	EN21	Financial stress is associated with anxiety, depression, poor sleep, high blood pressure, and increased risk of cardiovascular disease.
49	EN13	Chronic over-giving without recovery can keep the stress response elevated, which can weaken sleep, mood, and immune resilience over time.
50	EN02	Morning outdoor light activates specialized cells in the retina that signal the suprachiasmatic nucleus (SCN), the brain's master clock, anchoring circadian rhythm.
51	EN05	Alcohol may shorten the time it takes to fall asleep, but it fragments the night, suppresses REM, and worsens sleep quality — especially in the second half of the night.
52	EN31, EN02, EN30	Lifestyle interventions — nutrition, movement, sleep, and stress reduction — are associated with lower risk and better outcomes across many chronic conditions.
53	EN19	The quality of a close relationship is associated with health outcomes: supportive, low-conflict relationships are linked with better longevity and cardiovascular markers, while chronic high-conflict relationships are linked with higher stress and worse health over time.

54	EN13	Chronic fear and worry keep the body's stress response activated, which can contribute to high blood pressure, blood sugar problems, digestive issues, and immune changes.
55	EN27	Naming emotions (I feel angry, I feel hurt) reduces reactivity in the brain's alarm centers and increases activity in regions involved in control and decision-making.
56	EN28	Motor imagery (mentally rehearsing a movement) activates many of the same brain regions as physical practice and can improve learning and performance.
57	EN09	Habits automate behavior by shifting control from effortful decision-making to more automatic brain circuits; this reduces reliance on willpower and makes healthy actions easier to repeat.
58	EN02, EN10, EN09	Boundary-setting around light, noise, and digital input is associated with better sleep and lower perceived stress and anxiety.
59	EN06	Walking improves circulation, oxygenation, and lymph flow, lowering clot risk and supporting recovery. Movement increases cerebral blood flow and boosts brain growth factors tied to mood, memory, and learning.
60	EN25, EN24	Grass-fed and pasture-raised beef and dairy generally contain more beneficial fats (like omega-3s and CLA) and antioxidants, while grain-fed and confinement products tend to lean toward more omega-6 and fewer of some protective nutrients.
61	EN37	Repeated micro-arousals fragment deep sleep even when total hours look "normal."
62	EN17, EN30	Randomized gratitude interventions (like writing down blessings) are associated with improved sleep quality, optimism, and overall well-being, and in some studies reduced diastolic blood pressure.
63	EN16	Meditation and contemplative prayer can reduce reactivity to daily stressors and support steadier emotional regulation.
64	EN09, EN17	Action creates internal feedback and a small sense of reward that reinforces new behaviors.
65	EN31	Midlife patterns — sleep, movement, diet, smoking, stress — are linked to later risk for heart disease, stroke, cognitive decline, and disability.
66	EN10	Designing your environment ("choice architecture") can shape behavior more consistently than motivation alone.
67	EN09, EN11	Self-chosen structure reduces decision fatigue and preserves willpower for meaningful choices.
68	EN31, EN13	Body systems (hormones, gut, nerves, immune signals, and the heart) constantly talk to each other; a shift in one area can show up somewhere else.
69	EN13, EN32	Healthy systems rely on oscillation — stress followed by true recovery.

70	EN30	A strong therapeutic alliance (good relationship between clinician and patient) is associated with better adherence, satisfaction, and in some cases better health outcomes.
71	EN18, EN38	Higher perceived social support is linked with lower stress markers and better health outcomes.
72	EN11, EN16	Focusing fully on a single task (present-moment attention) can reduce mental noise and stress, freeing up cognitive resources for accuracy, learning, and recall.
73	EN27, EN09	Reframing can change how stress feels in the body. Interpreting stress as a challenge rather than a threat can shift nervous-system response and influence recovery over time.
74	EN20	Focusing on process rather than outcome reduces performance anxiety and improves consistency.
75	EN06, EN29, EN18	Gardening can increase daily physical activity (walking, bending, lifting) in an enjoyable, low-pressure way.
76	EN32	After a stressor (exercise or deep learning), the body can rebound above baseline — often described as super-compensation — especially when recovery is real.
77	EN16, EN17	Compassion and loving-kindness practices can reduce sympathetic arousal and may support steadier blood pressure over time.
78	EN21, EN11	Chasing constant "more" — more alerts, more purchases, more stimulation — can keep the reward system revved up, which may leave you feeling restless and empty instead of satisfied.
79	EN17	Generous acts can activate reward circuits in the brain and may increase chemicals linked with bonding and meaning (like dopamine and oxytocin).
80	EN39	Living in alignment with your core values is associated with lower stress, better psychological wellbeing, and greater life satisfaction.
81	EN11	Chronic noise exposure is associated with higher stress hormones and higher cardiovascular strain over time.
82	EN32, EN22, EN04	Tissue repair follows phases (inflammation → repair → remodeling); loading too hard or too early can disrupt healing and cause re-injury.
83	EN09	Habits tend to become more automatic after repetition: practicing the same small action in the same context (same time, same cue) makes it easier to repeat.
84	EN09	Tiny, consistent behaviors are often easier for the brain to accept, which can help habits form with less internal resistance.
85	EN11	Short rest breaks can improve decision-making and reduce errors.
86	EN20	A strong sense of purpose is associated with lower risk of heart disease, depression, and earlier death in observational studies.

87	EN27, EN32	Reframing stress as a challenge (instead of a threat) can improve performance and reduce physiological stress reactivity.
88	EN30	Patients who prepare questions and express their priorities tend to have better understanding of their conditions and are more likely to follow through with agreed plans.
89	EN21, EN18	The "high" from new possessions often fades quickly as your brain adapts, while stable relationships, meaningful work, and simple pleasures contribute more to long-term wellbeing.
90	EN17, EN06	Positive emotion is associated with better adherence to health behaviors and can support resilience over time.
91	EN19, EN27, EN03	Hostility carried over months and years is associated with higher rates of cardiovascular disease and shorter lifespan.
92	EN20	Gentle awareness of mortality (processed in a healthy way) can nudge people toward more value-driven, prosocial choices in some studies.
93	EN13, EN31	Your body responds to what you repeat. Small daily stressors (short sleep, sitting, ultra-processed food, chronic stress) add up into cumulative "wear and tear" — higher blood pressure, worse insulin sensitivity, and more inflammation over time.
94	EN11, EN13	Chronic overload keeps the stress response activated, raising stress signaling (including cortisol and adrenaline), which over time can impair memory and increase cardiometabolic strain.
95	EN21, EN20	Chasing only external rewards (money, status) is associated with higher stress and lower wellbeing than pursuing values-aligned goals.
96	EN34	Loss of structure and roles in retirement is associated with worsening sleep, lower activity, and higher risk of low mood and cognitive decline in some studies.
97	EN31	Many chronic diseases (like heart disease and type 2 diabetes) are influenced by lifestyle factors such as smoking, inactivity, diet quality, sleep, and chronic stress.
98	EN35, EN11	Repeated thought patterns strengthen related neural circuits ("neurons that fire together, wire together"), making those patterns easier to return to over time.
99	EN19, EN13	Chronic conflict or coldness at home can raise stress signaling, disrupt sleep, and worsen physical symptoms, even if work stress stays the same.
100	EN20	Health behaviors driven by intrinsic motives (love, values, purpose) are more likely to stick than those driven only by fear or shame.
101	EN16, EN20	Regular spiritual practices (prayer, meditation, reflective worship) are associated with better coping, lower perceived stress, and greater resilience in many studies, especially during illness or loss.

Chapter Mapping (Ch. 8–19)

Chapter 8 — Why You're So Tired: EN13, EN03, EN18, EN31
Chapter 9 — It's Not You — It's Your Clock: EN02, EN23, EN03
Chapter 10 — How Your Life Fell Out of Rhythm: EN09, EN35, EN11
Chapter 11 — Your Roots: EN13, EN11, EN20
Chapter 12 — Your Energy Grid: EN13, EN14, EN15, EN16
Chapter 13 — The Domino Game: EN09, EN10, EN20
Chapter 14 — Sleep: EN02, EN03, EN04, EN05
Chapter 15 — Movement: EN06, EN07, EN08, EN32
Chapter 16 — Food: EN22, EN23, EN24, EN25
Chapter 17 — Gut Health: EN26, EN22
Chapter 18 — From Redline to Rhythm: EN13, EN14, EN15, EN16, EN17, EN18
Chapter 19 — Hidden Saboteurs: EN33, EN36

Endnote clusters (EN01–EN39)

EN01 — Biological age & epigenetic clocks
Supports claims about "biological age" (distinct from chronological age) and how epigenetic biomarkers can estimate aging processes and healthspan risk.

Horvath S. DNA methylation age of human tissues and cell types. Genome Biology. 2013.

Levine ME, Lu AT, Quach A, et al. An epigenetic biomarker of aging for lifespan and healthspan. Aging (Albany NY). 2018.
Jylhävä J, Pedersen NL, Hägg S. Biological age predictors. EBioMedicine. 2017.

EN02 — Light/screens & circadian rhythm
Supports claims that evening light/screen exposure can delay circadian timing and melatonin onset, and that morning light helps entrain the circadian clock.

Chang AM, Aeschbach D, Duffy JF, Czeisler CA. Evening use of light-emitting eReaders negatively affects sleep, circadian timing, and next-morning alertness. PNAS. 2015.

Hattar S, Liao HW, Takao M, Berson DM, Yau KW. Melanopsin-containing retinal ganglion cells: architecture, projections, and intrinsic photosensitivity. Science. 2002.
American Academy of Sleep Medicine (AASM). Clinical/consumer guidance on light exposure and sleep (screen use and evening light).

EN03 — Sleep loss & sleep duration (health outcomes)
Supports claims that insufficient sleep is linked with worse mood/cognition and higher cardiometabolic risk over time.

Watson NF, Badr MS, Belenky G, et al. Recommended amount of sleep for a healthy adult: a joint consensus statement of the AASM and SRS. Sleep. 2015.

Spiegel K, Leproult R, Van Cauter E. Impact of sleep debt on metabolic and endocrine function. The Lancet. 1999.
Cappuccio FP, D'Elia L, Strazzullo P, Miller MA. Quantity and quality of sleep and incidence of type 2 diabetes: systematic review and meta-analysis. Diabetes Care. 2010.

EN04 — Sleep architecture, glymphatic system, memory & immune function
Supports claims that deep sleep contributes to restoration, brain waste clearance, immune regulation, and memory consolidation.

Xie L, Kang H, Xu Q, et al. Sleep drives metabolite clearance from the adult brain. Science. 2013.

Diekelmann S, Born J. The memory function of sleep. Nature Reviews Neuroscience. 2010.
Besedovsky L, Lange T, Born J. Sleep and immune function. Pflügers Archiv. 2012.

EN05 — Alcohol/sedatives & restorative sleep
Supports claims that alcohol (and some sedatives) can alter sleep architecture and reduce restorative sleep quality.

Ebrahim IO, Shapiro CM, Williams AJ, Fenwick PB. Alcohol and sleep: a systematic review. Sleep Medicine Reviews. 2013.

Sateia MJ, Buysse DJ, Krystal AD, Neubauer DN, Heald JL. Clinical practice guideline for the pharmacologic treatment of chronic insomnia in adults. Journal of Clinical Sleep Medicine. 2017.
Roehrs T, Roth T. Sleep, sleepiness, and alcohol use. Alcohol Research & Health. Review article (various editions).

EN06 — Physical activity, step counts, sedentary time & mortality
Supports claims linking regular movement/steps to lower mortality risk and the harms of prolonged sitting.

World Health Organization. WHO guidelines on physical activity and sedentary behaviour. 2020.

Saint-Maurice PF, Troiano RP, Bassett DR Jr, et al. Association of daily step count and step intensity with mortality among US adults. JAMA. 2020.
Ekelund U, Steene-Johannessen J, Brown WJ, et al. Does physical activity attenuate the association of sitting time with mortality? The Lancet. 2016.

EN07 — Short bouts of movement & post-meal walking (glucose and cardiometabolic markers)
Supports claims that brief activity breaks — especially after meals — can improve post-meal glucose handling and related markers.

DiPietro L, Gribok A, Stevens MS, Hamm LF, Rumpler W. Three 15-minute bouts of postmeal walking improves 24-hour glycemic control in older people at risk for impaired glucose tolerance. Diabetes Care. 2013.

Benatti FB, Ried-Larsen M. Effects of breaking up prolonged sitting on postprandial glucose and insulin: systematic review and meta-analysis. Sports Medicine. 2015.
American Diabetes Association. Standards of Medical Care in Diabetes (physical activity guidance for glycemic management; current edition).

EN08 — Stair climbing and "exercise snacks" (fitness gains from brief intensity)
Supports claims that brief stair climbing/interval-style activity can improve cardiorespiratory fitness over time.

Boreham CA, Wallace WF, Nevill A. Training effects of accumulated daily stair-climbing exercise in previously sedentary young women. Preventive Medicine. 2000.

Gibala MJ, Little JP, Macdonald MJ, Hawley JA. Physiological adaptations to low-volume, high-intensity interval training. The Journal of Physiology. 2012.
Stamatakis E, et al. Studies on vigorous intermittent lifestyle physical activity (VILPA) and cardiometabolic outcomes. (Representative 2020s cohort literature.)

EN09 — Habit formation, implementation intentions, self-monitoring & behavior change
Supports claims that small repeated actions can become more automatic, and that planning and monitoring improve follow-through.

Lally P, van Jaarsveld CHM, Potts HWW, Wardle J. How are habits formed: modelling habit formation in the real world. European Journal of Social Psychology. 2010.

Gollwitzer PM. Implementation intentions: strong effects of simple plans. American Psychologist. 1999.

Gollwitzer PM, Sheeran P. Implementation intentions and goal achievement: a meta-analysis. Advances in Experimental Social Psychology. 2006.
Harkin B, Webb TL, Chang BP, et al. Does monitoring goal progress promote goal attainment? A meta-analysis. Psychological Bulletin. 2016.

EN10 — Choice architecture & environment design ("nudges")
Supports claims that adjusting defaults, friction, and visibility can shape behavior without relying on willpower alone.

Hollands GJ, Shemilt I, Marteau TM, et al. Altering micro-environments to change health-related behaviour: a systematic review and meta-analysis. (2013–2015 literature.)

Cadario R, Chandon P. Which healthy eating nudges work best? A meta-analysis of field experiments. Marketing Science. 2020.
Thaler RH, Sunstein CR. Nudge: Improving Decisions About Health, Wealth, and Happiness. 2008.

EN11 — Multitasking, task switching, cognitive load & restorative breaks
Supports claims about task-switch "switch costs," mental fatigue, and the benefits of closing loops and taking short breaks (especially near bedtime).

Rubinstein JS, Meyer DE, Evans JE. Executive control of cognitive processes in task switching. Journal of Experimental Psychology: Human Perception and Performance. 2001.

Raichle ME, MacLeod AM, Snyder AZ, Powers WJ, Gusnard DA, Shulman GL. A default mode of brain function. PNAS. 2001.
Scullin MK, Krueger MA, Ballard HK, Pruett N, Bliwise DL. The effects of bedtime writing on sleep difficulty and duration. Journal of Experimental Psychology: Applied. 2018.

EN12 — Hydration, blood volume & cognitive performance
Supports claims that mild dehydration can worsen mood, perceived effort, and some aspects of cognition.

Lieberman HR. Hydration and cognition: a critical review and recommendations for future research. Journal of the American College of Nutrition. 2012.

Armstrong LE, Ganio MS, Casa DJ, et al. Mild dehydration affects mood in healthy young women. Journal of Nutrition. 2012.
Masento NA, Golightly M, Field DT, Butler LT, van Reekum CM. Effects of hydration status on cognitive performance and mood. British Journal of Nutrition. 2014.

EN13 — Stress physiology, allostatic load & chronic sympathetic activation
Supports claims that chronic stress drives "wear and tear" (allostatic load) via stress mediators and downstream cardiometabolic and immune effects.

McEwen BS. Protective and damaging effects of stress mediators: central role of the brain. New England Journal of Medicine. 1998.

McEwen BS, Stellar E. Stress and the individual: mechanisms leading to disease. Archives of Internal Medicine. 1993.
Cohen S, Janicki-Deverts D, Miller GE. Psychological stress and disease. JAMA. 2007.

EN14 — Breathing techniques, HRV & autonomic regulation
Supports claims that paced breathing (often with longer exhales) can reduce physiological arousal and shift autonomic balance.

Balban MY, Neri E, Kogon MM, et al. Brief structured respiration practices enhance mood and reduce physiological arousal. Cell Reports Medicine. 2023.

Zaccaro A, Piarulli A, Laurino M, et al. How breath-control can change your life: a systematic review. Frontiers in Human Neuroscience. 2018.
Lehrer PM, Gevirtz R. Heart rate variability biofeedback: how and why does it work? Frontiers in Psychology. 2014.

EN15 — Psychological flexibility (ACT) & self-compassion
Supports claims that psychological flexibility and self-compassion can improve resilience, reduce distress, and support sustained behavior change.

A-Tjak JGL, Davis ML, Morina N, Powers MB, Smits JAJ, Emmelkamp PMG. Efficacy of acceptance and commitment therapy: meta-analysis. Psychotherapy and Psychosomatics. 2015.

Kirby JN, Tellegen CL, Steindl SR. A meta-analysis of compassion-based interventions. Behavior Therapy. 2017.
Sirois FM, Kitner R, Hirsch JK. Self-compassion, affect, and health-promoting behaviors. Health Psychology. 2015.

EN16 — Mindfulness/meditation/compassion practices (and contemplative prayer)
Supports claims that contemplative practices can reduce stress and anxiety and support well-being (and sometimes sleep or blood pressure outcomes).

Goyal M, Singh S, Sibinga EMS, et al. Meditation programs for psychological stress and well-being: systematic review and meta-analysis. JAMA Internal Medicine. 2014.

Zeng X, Chiu CPK, Wang R, Oei TPS, Leung FYK. Loving-kindness meditation and positive emotions: meta-analysis. Frontiers in Psychology. 2015.
Koenig HG. Religion, spirituality, and health: research and clinical implications. ISRN Psychiatry. 2012.

EN17 — Positive emotion: laughter, gratitude, kindness & prosocial behavior
Supports claims that brief positive emotion practices can reduce perceived stress and are associated with improved well-being (and sometimes sleep/stress markers).

Emmons RA, McCullough ME. Counting blessings versus burdens: gratitude and subjective well-being. Journal of Personality and Social Psychology. 2003.

Dickens LR. Gratitude interventions: meta-analyses on effectiveness. Basic and Applied Social Psychology. 2017.

Dunn EW, Aknin LB, Norton MI. Spending money on others promotes happiness. Science. 2008.
Berk LS, Tan SA, Fry WF, et al. Neuroendocrine and stress hormone changes during mirthful laughter. American Journal of the Medical Sciences. 1989.

EN18 — Social connection, loneliness & health/longevity
Supports claims that social integration and support are linked to lower mortality risk, while loneliness and isolation confer meaningful risk.

Holt-Lunstad J, Smith TB, Layton JB. Social relationships and mortality risk: meta-analytic review. PLoS Medicine. 2010.

Holt-Lunstad J, Smith TB, Baker M, Harris T, Stephenson D. Loneliness/social isolation as mortality risk factors: meta-analysis. Perspectives on Psychological Science. 2015.
Office of the U.S. Surgeon General. Our Epidemic of Loneliness and Isolation: Advisory on Social Connection. 2023.

EN19 — Relationship quality, conflict, hostility & cardiometabolic health
Supports claims that relationship strain/conflict and hostility are linked with worse stress physiology and cardiometabolic outcomes over time.

Robles TF, Slatcher RB, Trombello JM, McGinn MM. Marital quality and health: meta-analytic review. Psychological Bulletin. 2014.

Chida Y, Steptoe A. Anger/hostility and future coronary heart disease: meta-analysis. Journal of the American College of Cardiology. 2009.
Kiecolt-Glaser JK, Gouin JP, Hantsoo L. Close relationships, inflammation, and health. Neuroscience & Biobehavioral Reviews. 2010.

EN20 — Purpose/values, intrinsic motivation, autonomy & psychological reactance
Supports claims that purpose and autonomous motivation are linked with better outcomes, and that controlling messaging can trigger pushback (reactance).

Alimujiang A, Wiensch A, Boss J, et al. Life purpose and mortality among U.S. adults older than 50 years. JAMA Network Open. 2019.

Deci EL, Ryan RM. The "what" and "why" of goal pursuits: self-determination theory. Psychological Inquiry. 2000.

Teixeira PJ, Carraça EV, Markland D, Silva MN, Ryan RM. Self-determination theory and exercise: systematic review. International Journal of Behavioral Nutrition and Physical Activity. 2012.
Rains SA. Psychological reactance revisited: meta-analytic review. Human Communication Research. 2013.

EN21 — Income, time affluence, financial stress & hedonic adaptation
Supports claims about diminishing returns of income on daily well-being, the value of "buying time," and adaptation to possessions.

Kahneman D, Deaton A. High income improves evaluation of life but not emotional well-being. PNAS. 2010.

Killingsworth MA. Experienced well-being rises with income, even above $75,000 per year. PNAS. 2021.

Whillans AV, Dunn EW, Smeets P, Bekkers R, Norton MI. Buying time promotes happiness. PNAS. 2017.

Diener E, Lucas RE, Scollon CN. Beyond the hedonic treadmill: revising adaptation theory. American Psychologist. 2006.
Brickman P, Coates D, Janoff-Bulman R. Lottery winners and accident victims: is happiness relative? Journal of Personality and Social Psychology. 1978.

EN22 — Nutrition: glycemic response, fiber/protein/fat, vinegar, added sugar/fructose
Supports claims about meal composition and glucose spikes, benefits of fiber, and metabolic effects of added sugars (including fructose).

Reynolds A, Mann J, Cummings J, Winter N, Mete E, Te Morenga L. Carbohydrate quality and human health: systematic reviews and meta-analyses. The Lancet. 2019.

Johnston CS, Kim CM, Buller AJ. Vinegar improves insulin sensitivity to a high-carbohydrate meal in insulin-resistant subjects. Diabetes Care. 2004.

Stanhope KL, Schwarz JM, Keim NL, et al. Fructose-sweetened beverages increase visceral adiposity and worsen insulin sensitivity. Journal of Clinical Investigation. 2009.
American Heart Association scientific statements on added sugars and cardiometabolic risk.

EN23 — Meal timing, time-restricted eating & chrono-nutrition
Supports claims that late eating and circadian misalignment influence metabolic outcomes, and that earlier eating windows can improve markers even without weight loss.

Sutton EF, Beyl R, Early KS, Cefalu WT, Ravussin E, Peterson CM. Early time-restricted feeding improves insulin sensitivity, blood pressure, and oxidative stress without weight loss. Cell Metabolism. 2018.
Scheer FAJL, Hilton MF, Mantzoros CS, Shea SA. Adverse metabolic and cardiovascular consequences of circadian misalignment. PNAS. 2009.

EN24 — Ultra-processed foods & health outcomes
Supports claims linking ultra-processed diets to higher calorie intake and weight gain under controlled conditions, and to poorer health outcomes in population research.

Monteiro CA, Moubarac JC, Cannon G, Ng SW, Popkin B. Ultra-processed products are becoming dominant in the global food system. Obesity Reviews. 2013.
Hall KD, Ayuketah A, Brychta R, et al. Ultra-processed diets cause excess calorie intake and weight gain: randomized controlled trial. Cell Metabolism. 2019.

EN25 — Food quality: omega-3 (grass-fed/pasture) and pesticides/organic exposure
Supports claims about fatty acid profile differences in grass-fed vs grain-fed animal products and evidence that organic interventions can reduce pesticide metabolite burden.

Daley CA, Abbott A, Doyle PS, Nader GA, Larson S. Review of fatty acid profiles and antioxidant content in grass-fed vs grain-fed beef. Nutrition Journal. 2010.

Oates L, Cohen M, Braun L, Schembri A, Taskova R. Reduction in urinary organophosphate pesticide metabolites after a week-long organic diet intervention. Environmental Research. 2014.
USDA Pesticide Data Program (PDP). Annual reports on pesticide residues in foods.

EN26 — Gut microbiome, dietary fiber, SCFAs & gut–brain axis
Supports claims that dietary fiber shapes the microbiome and that microbiome-derived metabolites influence immune and brain signaling.

Cryan JF, Dinan TG. Mind-altering microorganisms: gut microbiota and brain/behaviour. Nature Reviews Neuroscience. 2012.

Makki K, Deehan EC, Walter J, Bäckhed F. Dietary fiber and gut microbiota in health and disease. Cell Host & Microbe. 2018.
Sonnenburg JL, Bäckhed F. Diet–microbiota interactions as moderators of metabolism. Nature. 2016.

EN27 — Emotion labeling, cognitive reappraisal & stress reappraisal
Supports claims that naming emotions and reframing stress can reduce reactivity and improve coping/performance.

Lieberman MD, Eisenberger NI, Crockett MJ, Tom SM, Pfeifer JH, Way BM. Putting feelings into words: affect labeling disrupts amygdala activity. Psychological Science. 2007.

Webb TL, Miles E, Sheeran P. Emotion regulation strategies: meta-analysis. Psychological Bulletin. 2012.
Jamieson JP, Mendes WB, Blackstock E, Schmader T. Reappraising arousal improves performance and physiological responses. Journal of Experimental Social Psychology. 2010/2012.

EN28 — Motor imagery & neural activation
Supports claims that mentally rehearsing movement activates overlapping neural circuits and can support learning and rehabilitation.

Jeannerod M. Mental imagery in the motor context. Neuropsychologia. 1995.
Decety J. The neurophysiological basis of motor imagery. Behavioural Brain Research. 1996.

EN29 — Nature/green space/forest bathing & health
Supports claims that green space and nature exposure are linked with improved mental health and some physiological markers.

Twohig-Bennett C, Jones A. Health benefits of greenspace exposure: systematic review and meta-analysis. Environmental Research. 2018.

Bratman GN, Hamilton JP, Hahn KS, Daily GC, Gross JJ. Nature experience reduces rumination and subgenual PFC activation. PNAS. 2015.

Li Q. Effect of forest bathing trips on human health: a review. International Journal of Environmental Research and Public Health. 2010.

EN30 — Blood pressure: lifestyle, DASH, home monitoring & shared decision-making
Supports claims that lifestyle changes can lower blood pressure, that home BP monitoring improves diagnosis/management, and that shared decision-making supports adherence.

Whelton PK, Carey RM, Aronow WS, et al. 2017 ACC/AHA guideline for high blood pressure in adults. Hypertension. 2018.

Siu AL; U.S. Preventive Services Task Force. Screening for high blood pressure in adults: recommendation statement. Annals of Internal Medicine. 2015.

Appel LJ, Moore TJ, Obarzanek E, et al. DASH trial: dietary patterns and blood pressure. New England Journal of Medicine. 1997.

Uhlig K, Patel K, Ip S, Kitsios GD, Balk EM. Self-measured BP monitoring in hypertension: systematic review and meta-analysis. Annals of Internal Medicine. 2013.

EN31 — Lifestyle patterns & long-term chronic disease/cognitive decline risk
Supports claims that combined lifestyle factors shape long-term cardiometabolic and cognitive outcomes.

Livingston G, Huntley J, Sommerlad A, et al. Dementia prevention, intervention, and care: Lancet Commission report. The Lancet. 2020 (and subsequent updates).

Li Y, Schoufour J, Wang DD, et al. Healthy lifestyle and life expectancy free of major chronic disease. BMJ. 2020.

Ngandu T, Lehtisalo J, Solomon A, et al. FINGER trial: multidomain intervention to prevent cognitive decline. The Lancet. 2015.

EN32 — Recovery, tissue repair phases, deconditioning & return-to-activity
Supports claims that tissues heal in phases and that graded loading and recovery reduce reinjury risk and support adaptation.

Järvinen TAH, Järvinen TLN, Kääriäinen M, Kalimo H, Järvinen M. Muscle injuries: biology and treatment. American Journal of Sports Medicine. 2005.

Sports medicine consensus statements on graded return-to-play and progressive loading principles (representative guidelines).

EN33 — Environmental exposures: PFAS/phthalates/VOCs/mold/heavy metals/microplastics
Supports claims that common environmental exposures can affect endocrine, respiratory, neurologic, or immune health and that exposure reduction can lower burden.

National Academies of Sciences, Engineering, and Medicine. Guidance on PFAS exposure, testing, and clinical follow-up. 2022.

Steinemann A. Volatile emissions from common consumer products. Air Quality, Atmosphere & Health. 2015.

Allen JG, MacNaughton P, Satish U, Santanam S, Vallarino J, Spengler JD. Cognitive function scores and CO_2/ventilation/VOC exposures in office workers: controlled exposure study. Environmental Health Perspectives. 2016.

Institute of Medicine. Damp Indoor Spaces and Health. 2004.

World Health Organization. Indoor air quality guidelines: dampness and mould. 2009.

Centers for Disease Control and Prevention (CDC). Lead exposure and health effects (clinical guidance; updated periodically).

FDA/EPA consumer guidance on mercury in seafood (updated periodically).
Hernandez LM, Xu EG, Larsson HCE, Tahara R, Maisuria VB, Tufenkji N. Plastic teabags release microparticles and nanoparticles into tea. Environmental Science & Technology. 2019.

EN34 — Retirement transitions & health/cognition
Supports claims that retirement can change health and cognition through shifts in structure, routine, purpose, and social engagement (effects vary by context).

Rohwedder S, Willis RJ. Mental retirement. Journal of Economic Perspectives. 2010.
Bonsang E, Adam S, Perelman S. Does retirement affect cognitive functioning? Journal of Health Economics. 2012.

EN35 — Neuroplasticity, attention, and repeated thought patterns
Supports claims that repeated thoughts and behaviors strengthen neural pathways over time (a foundation for habit loops and attention training).

Hebb DO. The Organization of Behavior: A Neuropsychological Theory. 1949.
Research reviews on Hebbian learning and neuroplasticity (representative modern review literature).

EN36 — Dose–response, hormesis, and U/J-shaped curves
Supports claims that many inputs have a therapeutic window (too little/too much can be harmful) and that some relationships are U- or J-shaped.

Calabrese EJ, Baldwin LA. Hormesis: the dose-response revolution. Annual Review of Pharmacology and Toxicology. 2003.

Arem H, Moore SC, Patel A, et al. Leisure time physical activity and mortality: pooled analysis of dose–response. JAMA Internal Medicine. 2015.
Modern toxicology references on dose–response and chronic low-dose exposure (therapeutic window principle).

EN37 — Sleep-disordered breathing / obstructive sleep apnea (OSA) Supports claims that airway obstruction causes repeated micro-arousals, intermittent hypoxemia, sympathetic activation/ overnight BP strain, and that diagnosis/treatment improves sleep quality and daytime symptoms.

Peppard PE, Young T, Palta M, Skatrud J. Prospective study of the association between sleep-disordered breathing and hypertension. *N Engl J Med.* 2000;342(19):1378-1384. doi:10.1056/NEJM200005113421901.

Yeghiazarians Y, et al. Obstructive Sleep Apnea and Cardiovascular Disease: A Scientific Statement From the American Heart Association. *Circulation.* 2021;144(3):e56-e67. doi:10.1161/CIR.0000000000000988.

Kapur VK, et al. Clinical practice guideline for diagnostic testing for adult obstructive sleep apnea. *J Clin Sleep Med.* 2017;13(3):479-504.

Prabhakar NR, Kumar GK. Mechanisms of sympathetic activation and blood pressure elevation by intermittent hypoxia. *Respir Physiol Neurobiol.* 2010;174(1-2):156-161. doi:10.1016/j.resp.2010.08.021.
Montesi SB, Edwards BA, Malhotra A, Bakker JP. Effect of continuous positive airway pressure treatment on blood pressure: systematic review and meta-analysis of randomized controlled trials. *J Clin Sleep Med.* 2012;8(5):587-596.

EN38 — Perfectionism, role overload & burnout

Supports claims that maladaptive perfectionism (especially perfectionistic concerns/self-criticism) relates to burnout and psychological distress, and that reducing overload/supporting flexibility can improve wellbeing over time.

Hill AP, Curran T. Multidimensional perfectionism and burnout: a meta-analysis. *Pers Soc Psychol Rev.* 2016;20(3):269–288.
Limburg K, Watson HJ, Hagger MS, Egan SJ. The relationship between perfectionism and psychopathology: a meta-analysis. *J Clin Psychol.* 2017;73(10):1301–1326.

EN39 — Environmental noise, sleep disturbance & cardiovascular strain

Supports claims that chronic environmental noise can disturb sleep (even without full awakening), increase stress physiology, and is associated with hypertension and cardiovascular risk.

Basner M, Babisch W, Davis A, et al. Auditory and non-auditory effects of noise on health. *Lancet.* 2014;383(9925):1325–1332. doi:10.1016/S0140-6736(13)61613-X.

Münzel T, Gori T, Babisch W, Basner M. Cardiovascular effects of environmental noise exposure. *Eur Heart J.* 2014;35(13):829–836. doi:10.1093/eurheartj/ehu030.

World Health Organization, Regional Office for Europe. *Environmental noise guidelines for the European Region.* 2019. ISBN: 9789289053563.
van Kempen E, Babisch W. The quantitative relationship between road traffic noise and hypertension: a meta-analysis. *J Hypertens.* 2012;30(6):1075–1086. doi:10.1097/HJH.0b013e328352ac54.

ACKNOWLEDGMENT

I'd like to thank Chisom Ezeh of The Publishing Pad for her steady support with formatting, cover-design input, and thoughtful feedback that helped me clarify several ideas. I'm grateful for her patience, skill, and reliability throughout the process.

MEET THE AUTHOR

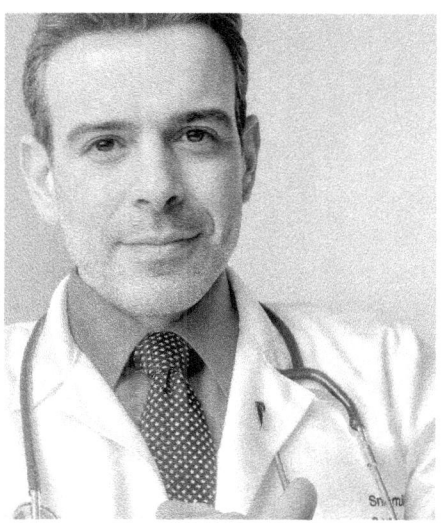

Athan Smyrlis, MD, FACC

Dr. Smyrlis is an interventional cardiologist who treats the heart in high-stakes moments. Over time, a quieter pattern kept showing up in his office: people who weren't "sick enough" for a diagnosis, yet didn't feel well enough to live fully — fatigue, brain fog, poor sleep, and a persistent sense of being run down, even when routine testing looked normal. That gap is what led him to write.

After more than two decades in medicine, he has seen both its miracles and its blind spots. He values medications and procedures and uses them when needed — but his approach is evidence-informed and integrative: he focuses on the daily foundations — sleep, food, movement, stress, and environment — so medication becomes a bridge, not a destination.

In his practice and writing, he translates complex physiology into plain language and helps people make lasting change through a practical, trust-based partnership. He lives on Long Island, New York, with his wife and two daughters.

www.ingramcontent.com/pod-product-compliance
Lightning Source LLC
Chambersburg PA
CBHW020529030426
42337CB00013B/789